Counseling Asian Indian Immigrant Families

Varughese Jacob

Counseling Asian Indian Immigrant Families

A Pastoral Psychotherapeutic Model

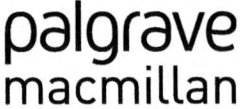

Varughese Jacob
Ben Taub General Hospital
Houston, Texas
USA

ISBN 978-3-319-64306-9   ISBN 978-3-319-64307-6   (eBook)
DOI 10.1007/978-3-319-64307-6

Library of Congress Control Number: 2017952607

Cover design by Ran Shauli
Cover photo (©) Varughese Jacob

Printed on acid-free paper

This Palgrave Macmillan imprint is published by Springer Nature
The registered company is Springer International Publishing AG
The registered company address is: Gewerbestrasse 11, 6330 Cham, Switzerland

This work is dedicated to my brother, Thomas Thekkecharuvil Jacob who sacrificed his education, privileges and prospects for the sake of his family in the absence of our father and encouraged me to continue my theological journey with all his support. His life has been a model of compassion and service which, taught me that caring for others is a calling and not a profession

FOREWORD

Dr. Varughese Jacob's book, *Counseling Asian-Indian Immigrant Families: A Pastoral Psychotherapeutic Model* breaks new ground in the area of pastoral care and counseling. There is a surfeit of literature in the area of counseling today, on such topics as clinical, historical, descriptive, biblical and theological interpretations of the importance and need for pastoral counseling, dealing with: materials on various approaches; theories, therapies and models of counseling; methodological tools proposed to be used in research in pastoral counseling; paradigm shifts in understanding and practicing of counseling; shifting the focus from dealing with individual personal problems to dealing with the larger problems such as the socioeconomic, cultural, and religious problems in counseling; materials on experiences of individuals and group intervention/ prevention; as well as advocacy done in counseling. I can go on.... but even in the midst of such riches any Asian counselors do eagerly await new approaches for counseling. Dr. Jacob's book is an answer to this quest. This book comes as another dish from the banquet – important, well desired, and long awaited.

A salient feature of this book is its authenticity, as it has been written from Dr. Jacob's experience of living in two cultures: born and brought up in India, and then crossing the seas to the USA. He writes from the experience of a decade of living in the USA, observing his people—Indians, their struggles of adjustment, conflict with their children, youth living in a twilight zone of not knowing who they are and their conflicts with parents, coupled with problems of their own developmental stages.

Furthermore, the author breaks new ground in three ways: first, he brings a new corrective into the counseling approach as he challenges the need to understand Indian culture in counseling. He does this by not judging or defending Indian culture, but explaining the culture, belief system and religion, as well as their children's plight, living in two cultures as they do. Meanwhile, he gently dismantles an established theory of DSM classifying certain personality traits as pathological. Unfortunately, some of those traits are seen among immigrant Indians, which is a hindrance in counseling. As such, traits are immediately dismissed and classified as mental illness. The problems of immigrant Indians are viewed as mental illness rather than normal problems needing management. His concern needs to be appreciated as he reiterates the concern of Asian and African counselors trained in the West— that theories in DSM are rooted in Western culture – known culture – and any personality theory contrary to this standard is considered as pathological. Dr. Jacob does not approve of such a universal approach and swings the pendulum to the "Other's Culture" as distinctive, unique, rooted in a rich ancient culture, but he is willing to expose the weakness of the absoluteness of the culture as well as people's narrow, defensive, naïve understanding of their culture, and of parenting resisting change.

Second, this book describes graphically the conflict between the second and first generations of Indians settled in the USA and the effects on their families. Such conflicts resulting in dysfunctional families are a serious concern of many immigrant families in the USA, and it spills over into India as most of the immigrant population families live in India. This book will also help immigrant Indians to understand their own problems and seek ways to deal with their problems themselves, in addition to preparing those who are or will be parents for the difficulties that could potentially lie in store for second-generation children.

Third, Jacob prescribes the model of an integrated approach, borrowing from various theories, integrating spirituality into his approach. He doesn't stop at describing the problems, but rather goes another step and attempts to test his model with two case studies.

Dr. Jacob's book is timely for clinicians and practitioners in Western cultures, where Indians or Asians with similar cultures have settled. Not only can it provide insight and cultural sensitivity in the practice, training, and professional development of therapists as they encounter these families in their own practice, it can serve as a tool to bring awareness to those same clinicians and practitioners as they seek to provide support to community organizations, cultural and religious centers, and other institutions looking for guidance in how to better serve their newest members.

The book does justice both to psychological and theological perspectives of the understanding of a person, of self-object, and of relationship among family members. I am glad that he has pursued this topic, and I am extremely proud of not only Jacob, but also Dr. Immanuel Lartey, my friend, for his valuable contributions, insights, feedback and patience, as he walked Varughese through the process. Dr. Jacob's persistence, motivation and hard work have been rewarded. This book is the outcome of all his struggles, and will certainly add to the existing pool of knowledge. I recommend this gem to be read and interacted with widely. Many Blessings to Dr. Jacob as he undertakes his faith journey–I find a compassionate and sharp counselor budding in the area of Pastoral Care and Counseling.

Dr. Nalini Arles
Professor and Chairperson of the Dept. of Christian Ministry,
UTC Bangalore (Rtd.)
Former President, ICPCC
Former President, APC on PCC
Founder & President of Association of Theologically
Trained Women in India
Visiting Professor of Graduate Theological Union, Berkeley, CA, USA
Lutheran Theological seminary, Saint Paul, MN, USA
St. Thomas University, Miami, FL, USA

PREFACE

This book explores the factors contributing to intergenerational family conflict among Asian-Indian immigrant families living in the Western cultural world, particularly in the United States. The findings indicate that this conflict is largely a product of difference in cultural values and identity, acculturation stress, and the experience of marginality. Because these immigrants' family issues are stressful and significantly influenced by cultural factors, clinical students and therapists caring for these families must be aware of the cultural and emotional dynamics at play within and between their clients. Cultural sensitivity is required to work with these clients to improve individual and family functioning. Components of the allocentric Asian-Indian culture may be seen as pathological when viewed through the lens of Western psychological diagnostic frameworks such as DSM-IV/V. Since many of their problems are culturally formed and connected with culture, therapists should be able to meet counselees at their culturally shaped needs.

After setting a stage for the readers to see the Asian-Indians from a cultural perspective, this book analyzes and interprets empirical data collected from questionnaires measuring sources of family conflict distributed among two hundred families. The data show that the one-way interaction from parents, cultural value conflicts, and intergenerational conflict lead to individual and family dysfunctionality. The data from the questionnaire are interpreted through two different theoretical approaches, first from a psychological perspective and then from a theological perspective. Based on the self psychology of Heinz Kohut, Sudhir Kakar's psychoanalytic understanding of communal identity or self, and Young Lee's theology of marginality, a five-step counseling model named "Praxis–Reflection–Action" (PRA) model is developed to address the immigrant family issues and intergenerational conflicts in the Asian-Indian immigrant families. "Praxis–Reflection–Action" (PRA) model is the very first pastoral psycho-therapeutic counseling model developed to deal with immigrant family issues from the Asian-Indian Cultural perspective.

The Praxis–Reflection–Action (PRA) model is developed to provide culturally sensitive pastoral psychotherapy/counseling for immigrants' issues and sees their issues through a cultural lens rather than a psychopath-ological lens. The five-stage PRA model of pastoral counseling presented here is intended to help meet the pastoral care needs of Asian-Indian immigrants through a culturally sensitive model. The premise of this model is changing the individuals within the context of the system.

Ben Taub General Hospital   Varughese Jacob
Houston, TX
USA

ACKNOWLEDGEMENTS

I am deeply indebted to many people who have played crucial roles in this project. My sincere appreciation and thanks go to my dissertation committee who helped me with their scholarship, experience, and dedication to complete this book. It is their close attention and constant guidance that helped me to materialize initially this as a satisfactory dissertation and now in the form of a book. My particular thanks go to Dr. Scheib for the immense support, committed help and words of wisdom that I could always count on. I am grateful to Dr. Emmanuel Lartey and Dr. Bill Harkins, extraordinary teachers, pastoral counselors, pastoral theologians, authors and mentors to me for their enthusiastic support and many rich inputs.

I gratefully acknowledge the encouragement and support I received from my former professors Drs. Nalini and the Late Siga Arles, friends Mathews Valliaveetil and family, Cherian K. Varughese and family, Hepsiba James, Pastor Jeff and Cyndi Padgett, and all other Asian-Indians who supported me with their experiences and stories throughout these years. In addition, I am grateful to Dr. Iris Devadason, Rev. Kim LeVert and Stephanie Schmidt for reading and editing this book. I am also indebted to Mr. Baiju A. Thomas and Mr. Shijomom Joy for designing and developing the cover of this book.

I thank my family for their constant prayers and support in helping me to reach this important milestone in life. In the midst of several challenges, the ongoing prayer support of my mother and sister Sherly and her family with other family members who sustained me to reach this point.

Finally, with a grateful heart and tearful eyes I acknowledge the grace and mercy of God, which I have received during my journey to complete this book and thank Him for the same. He is worthy of all my praises.

CONTENTS

About the Author

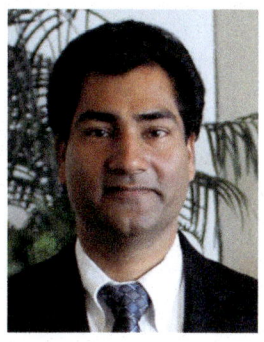

Varughese Jacob PhD, is a professional chaplain for hospital and hospice patients. As an ordained Christian minister, Jacob has served Indian and international communities in various capacities such as Pastor, Pastoral Counselor, and Associate Professor of Pastoral Care and Counseling. Currently Dr. Jacob is working for Harris County Health System and Buckner Hospice, both in Houston, TX.

LIST OF ABBREVIATIONS

ABCD Complex	American Born Confused Desi
ABCD Complex	American Born Confident Desi
ADDRESSING	Age and Generational Influences, Developmental and Acquired Disabilities, Religion and Spiritual Orientation, Ethnicity, Socioeconomic Status, Sexual Orientation, Indigenous Heritage, National Origin and Gender.
DSM IV and V	*Diagnostic and Statistical Manual of Mental Disorders*
GPA	Grade Point Average
PRA	Praxis-Reflection-Action Model
WASP	White Anglo-Saxon Protestant

LIST OF FIGURES

CHAPTER 1

Introduction and Overview

Asian-Indian individuals and families who immigrate to the United States often find themselves caught between differing values and cultural patterns of their home country and their adopted country. While this experience itself is painful at various levels of life, it becomes all the more painful when a family experiences this difference between two or more generations living under the same roof. Therefore, the purpose of this book is to offer a pastoral psychotherapeutic model for intervention with Asian-Indian individuals and families caught between two conflicting cultures, namely the Indian and American/Western cultures. It is an undertaking that calls for a liberative pastoral care praxis.

In order to develop this model, I have drawn on Heinz Kohut's self-psychological understanding of human development, and Indian psychoanalyst Sudhir Kakar's psychosocial understanding of shared psychological experiences, which pervade and govern Indian childhood. I also use the pastoral theological work of Jung Young Lee, a Korean-American theologian who analyzes immigrant family issues from the perspective of marginality.[1]

Kakar says human development in the Indian culture is an interplay between the universal process of human development and the Indian cultural milieu, which includes religious ideals, historical traditions, and some social institutions that are specific, if not exclusive to Indian society.[2] According to Kakar, what constitutes a common Indian identity is the predominance of family and community in everyday life. Kohut's understanding of the importance of empathy (care/grace) in the development

© The Author(s) 2017
V. Jacob, *Counseling Asian Indian Immigrant Families*,
DOI 10.1007/978-3-319-64307-6_1

and healing of persons is applicable and relevant to the lives of Indian immigrants. He believes that the child's relationships with the mother and father during the formative period are important for normal healthy development of the self. Though his major focus of attention is the "human self" (i.e., a self-centered approach), his emphasis on relationality and empathy is relevant and consistent with the Asian-Indian emphasis on the importance of relationships and caring. In Indian culture, relationship and caring are considered as norms for familial and communal vitality, gifts given to individuals from the Creator through their peers.

Lee, as a marginal immigrant, explains how the experiences of being an immigrant, an ethnic minority person on the margins of society, affects one's way of doing theology. According to Lee, ethnicity is the most important, the primary, determinant that creates marginality and minority status in all areas—political, social, educational, economic and many more—for Asian immigrants in the United States. Everyone's ethnicity includes their racial origin and cultural preferences. "As an Asian American, all other determinants are relative to but of lesser significance than the racial origin and cultural differences."[3] Along with identity issues and cultural value conflicts, the frustration that results from the marginal status of immigrants in the United States exacerbates intergenerational conflicts.

The following narrative illustrates some of the intergenerational tensions experienced by Indian immigrant families:

Mr. and Mrs. Thomas, respectively a software engineer and a registered nurse, and their son Tom (age 17) were referred to me for family therapy by their pastor, John, 15 years after they immigrated to the United States. A younger son, Tim (age 12) and a daughter Toni (age five), completed the family. At the interview the parents, in particular the mother, presented a long and detailed list of Tom's problems, which included partying on the weekends and staying out later than his parents approved, staying overnight at an American friend's home without parental permission, drinking beer (the family was Pentecostal), dressing and having his hair cut in ways unacceptable to his parents, and most damaging, wishing to major in fine arts rather than in medicine, which his parents expected of him. According to Mrs. Thomas, Tom had been a model child until approximately one year prior to entering therapy. She said, "He listened to his parents and did not give us trouble." All that changed in his sophomore year in high school when he joined the varsity soccer team and began to associate more closely with his American peers on the teams. Mrs. Thomas attributed Tom's behavioral and attitudinal changes to the negative influences of three specific teammates whom she accused of corrupting Tom such that he had become "more like an American child than the Indian child they believed they were raising."

Mrs. Thomas' perception of American children and parents, in particular adolescents and their parents, was very negative. She believed herself to be a much better parent than her American counterparts. As a result of parental displeasures, Tom was withdrawn from the soccer team and much of the freedom he previously enjoyed was severely curtailed. Mrs. Thomas' displeasure with the American culture intensified when the soccer coach visited the parents in an effort to persuade them to allow Tom to rejoin the team. Mrs. Thomas concluded that the coach was more interested in Tom "becoming a football player than being a good boy who listens to his parents." Tom did not rejoin the team.

Tom was very critical of his mother. He accused her of "liking to be in America for the money but not liking Americans" and "thinking that she is better than everybody and wanting me to be Indian in America." From his perspective, the behavior his mother found objectionable was necessary for him to "fit in" with his peers. Tom pointed out that he still maintained a very high grade point average (GPA) in high school, and was a member of the chess and mathematics clubs. Furthermore, he did not complain much when his parents, primarily his mother, refused to buy him a car, "even though my parents can afford it."

Mr. Thomas did not say much, but what he said was less intense than what his wife offered. He acknowledged the difficulty of raising children in the United States given "the night and day" differences concerning expectations for children's behavior in the United States and India. He also acknowledged "Tom is a good boy and everything is different for all of us." He solicited my assistance to find the family "a workable middle ground." Accordingly, therapy focused on helping Tom and his parents explore compromises and alternatives to being polarized, within a workable middle ground. Among the many similar cases I have encountered, the Thomas' situation represents in a stark manner the intergenerational issues among immigrant families.

Having been a parish minister for 18 years and a theological teacher for 16 years in India prior to entering a doctoral program in the United States, I am familiar with the traditional Indian way of helping and caring for people. However, due to the influences of globalization, various kinds of new issues and problems have risen. Thus, at times, I sensed that the traditional methods were inadequate to help people who were going through complex issues.

During my doctoral studies, I had encountered several more immigrant families in which parents and children are in distress due to cultural issues. I have witnessed sharp disputes between parents and children based on the widely disparate cultural values the children and parents hold. I have also been invited into several homes to talk to the children. As a first-generation immigrant, at times I felt ignored, at least by some second-generation immigrants, due to the judgmental attitude that they experienced from first-generation immigrants. In such situations, I tried to listen and apply the theoretical skills I have learned from my Western education. However, I found myself pushed to the point of having to question the applicability of the supposed hegemonic methods of care currently reported in the literature.

Methods of care and counseling that claim cultural sensitivity in the attentiveness of the therapist on the one hand whilst highlighting/privileging Euro-Western lenses of judging other cultures on the other are counterproductive to the healing of the intended recipients. Therefore, I realized that the diagnostic tools and self-centered concepts in both my course work and practicum required a great deal of transformation to fit people of different cultural backgrounds who are grounded in a communal personhood. This book is the result of that conviction.

THE CONTEXT OF THIS BOOK

The English education brought by the British to India in the eighteenth century greatly facilitated the improvement of human life and the development of the nation. Those who received an English education began to communicate with the English-speaking nations and to migrate to those countries seeking jobs. Though people initially migrated for work purposes, in the course of time they began to settle in their host countries because of the improved living conditions, job security, and economic gains. Such people used to come back to India to get married and then return to their host countries with their spouses. Those people—hereinafter referred to as first-generation immigrants—were born, raised, and spent a considerable amount of their life in the typical traditional Indian culture and carried that culture (values, attitudes, perspectives, and biases) into their everyday immigrant lives. Even though they made some changes in their lifestyles and dress code, the basic tenets of their beliefs, values, behavior, and thought patterns remained very close to the cultural tenets they inherited from their home country. Though I am aware that culture is not stagnant but is under constant transition and change, here the clue is that this first generation of immigrants, distanced from their homeland, have internalized what it unconsciously understood as stagnant and normative.

However, their children—hereinafter referred to as second-generation immigrants—born in an alien country or their parents' host country, are raised in that specific culture, which is entirely different from their parents' cultural inheritance. While this second generation was being raised in alien countries, the culture of those countries naturally became the culture of the second-generation immigrants. Therefore, they adopted that particular cultural lifestyle as part of their everyday life.

These second-generation immigrants, like any other children, grow under the disciplinary system of their parents during their childhood. However, when they enter school and enter the teenage years, they move into the realm of Western, individualistic society that emphasizes individuation, differentiation, and autonomy of individuals over family and community. These opposite norms and values create an inevitable clash with the cultural values, outlooks, and practices of their parents.

For instance, dating, clubbing, pregnancy out of wedlock, divorce, and single parenthood are taboo and stigmatized in traditional Indian culture. If the member of a traditional Indian family gets involved in such issues and this is made public, that whole family is looked down upon in the community and ostracized. In most cases, people would avoid initiating a marriage relationship with such families. However, most of the second-generation immigrants who grow up in mainstream American culture often consider many of these traditional attitudes unimportant.

One of the major concerns here is the family and community values which are inherent in Indian culture, in contrast to the mainstream American culture that tends to promote individualism and consumerism. K. Ahmed observes that "the United States is typically considered an individualistic culture and European-American parents generally raise their children to be autonomous, assertive, and self-reliant."[4] When second-generation immigrants fail to follow the culture of their parent's home country, the community of first-generation immigrants starts questioning, gossiping, and isolating such families in the community. Moreover, such news will be relayed to others in the home country of the first-generation immigrants.

In the Indian culture, the name and fame brought by one member of the family is the name and fame of the whole family. In the same way, shame and guilt brought by one member of the family is considered as the shame and guilt of the entire family. Second-generation immigrants who are born and raised in an individualistic, consumer culture do not grasp or subscribe this fact and are indifferent to it. For instance, Dave, a second-generation Indian American, told me in an interview that "we work hard, we pay our bills and we live. We don't care what people think about us; maybe my parents do, but not I." In this context, often what is normal to the second-generation immigrants is very abnormal to the first-generation immigrants. Consequently, family members may experience isolation, a sense of shame and guilt, and may be ostracized by their community.

Intergenerational conflicts within families can create stress, emotional rifts, and, often, fights between the first and second generations. Family dysfunctions resulting from intergenerational conflicts may appear as lack of communication, refusal to participate in family-ascribed roles, and open disobedience to parental rules. In order to understand intergenerational conflict, we need to consider three factors. The first factor is stress due to emotional rifts and family dysfunctions that may be initiated by the first-generation immigrants as a result of their sense of shame, guilt, and isolation in the community. The second factor is second-generation immigrants' lack of full awareness of the meaning of their "parental culture" and its original values, though they do have some knowledge of Indian cultural and community values and the emotional difficulties of their parents related to it. And the third factor includes the marginality status of the immigrants, peer pressure from the school, work and society, and the lack of safe space to vent their feelings. In many families, it is observed that face-to-face communication or quality communication between the first- and second-generation immigrants is rare since the parents are busy with their jobs and children are involved in their activities. Contributing to the lack of face-to-face quality communication is the often unconscious assumption of first-generation immigrants that the second generation knows and understands the parental culture they have observed in their parents' lives.

Through working with families as a pastor and counselor, I have observed that while most first-generation immigrants are not fully aware of and concerned about the peer pressure on their children, neither are the second-generation immigrants fully aware of their parents' emotional pain, stress, and (often justified) fear of social stigma. This lack of awareness on the part of both groups often leads to further quarrels, fights, and temporary moving-out, which is another sensitive issue in the Indian cultural context. I believe that a significant factor contributing to generational conflict is an understanding of self. While the first generation holds to and values "communal identity" and "communal self," the second generation seeks more of an "individual identity" and an "individual self." Existing literatures also show that generational conflicts between parents and children are becoming the norm as the children get older and have to deal first-hand with a set of conflicting expectations.[5]

These two groups of people living in two cultural worlds, often under the same roof, bring challenges to personal and family functioning. These challenges may manifest themselves in different forms such as anger, isolation, fear, confusion, and a kind of paranoia. Pastoral care and counseling may not be meaningful to this community unless caregivers and therapists are aware of the cultural nuances and worldviews with which these peoples' identities are shaped. If these challenges to personal and family functioning, made manifest in different forms, are viewed through the American cultural lens, they may be considered as psychopathology.

It is in the light of such prevailing conditions and experiences that this book has become necessary. I decided to explore the formation of individuals' cultural identity and the need for a culturally sensitive therapy for this group of people. Consequently, my major concerns were focused on four areas: (1) the first-generation Indian immigrants who follow a particular cultural life style with changes here and there for the sake of survival and their cultural identity issues; (2) the second-generation immigrants who struggle to live in between two cultures and their cultural identity issues; (3) the marginality status and acculturation stress, which influence and shape the identity of both generatons; and (4) the consequent impact of conflict between first and second generations on the functioning of personal and family life.

Western therapists may assume that second-generation Indian immigrants are fully assimilated into the American culture since they seem to hold American cultural values. This assumption, however, can impede effective healing since many second-generation immigrants are struggling to survive between two cultural worlds and to find meaning and identity in their lives. On the other hand, the first generation is often labeled as "less assimilated" into the mainstream American culture and seen as struggling with the fear of "family dissolution." Realistically, it is the "existence of family," which gives worth and meaning to the lives of first-generation immigrants. What is family for them is defined by the cultural values they retain and pass on to the next generation as the members of a household harmoniously living within a specific cultural frame. Second-generation family members, who are generally more Westernized in their life style, make their parental community sensitive, suspicious, angry, and fearful, as they cannot keep their Westernized children within their own cultural world.

As a pastoral psychotherapist working with Asian-Indian immigrant families, one of the major issues I observed was a lack of culturally appropriate therapy that would address the cultural conflicts within these families. Their care needs were deeply rooted in the struggle to deal with the dictates of a Western culture that emphasizes individualism, unlike Indian culture, which is communally oriented. Asian-Indians are culturally formed in their understanding of what it means to be human. This presents challenges when they seek help and are presented with foreign resolutions to their problems.

My therapy experience with Asian-Indian families has revealed to me that though there are several books that discuss the cultural and psychological needs of the Asian-Indian immigrant families, there is almost nothing in terms of a psychotherapeutic model that accommodates the particular needs of the Asian-Indian immigrant families in the Western World.

Frequently, the therapy available to Asian-Indian immigrants in the United States and Western world is based on developmental and diagnostic theories and counseling practices developed by and for those living in a Eurocentric or Western culture. Too often, these theories and practices have been applied to immigrants without regard to the cultural background that informs their way of life in times of joy and pain. Even when their culture is manifest, it tends to either be ignored or evaluated by the standards of another culture either due to ignorance or disregard.

I have seen families torn apart and persons subjected to alienation or loneliness due to therapists pushing them to be independent. Oftentimes this push comes from a culturally insensitive therapist or the perpetuation of the dominant, so-called "First-World" culture over so-called "Third-World" culture. Approaches that focus on development of an autonomous self are limited because they fail to meet the Asian-Indian's communal-centered concept of personhood.

It is important to address the cultural background of those immigrating so that we are able to understand the depth of their problems and, thereby, engage their culture in therapy. Addressing their cultural background will help the therapist to truly connect with clients and understand the experience of their inner world. This understanding is important for pastoral care because therapists must meet their clients at their point of need in order to provide effective healing. Different cultures shape the development of their members in different ways. Thus, even in a condition of extreme stress, the individuals take from their culture its conventions of traditions in implementing and giving form to an idiosyncratic disorder, with the culture providing, as it were, the patterns of altered conduct.

Using exclusively Western psychological theories to assess the needs of immigrant families will do more harm than good, for there is a great danger of overlooking the values and norms present in the other cultures. It can also create additional problems for the intended recipients of care. One of the common limitations of this approach is that it may cause the family to disintegrate or to stop coming for therapy, as the therapy is incompatible with their family-oriented and communal-centric identity.

Since the lifestyle, English accent, and cultural practices of the parental generation are different from the second-generation immigrants, the latter develop a negative attitude to their parental culture. The American education they receive is also partly responsible for this attitude. Therapists trained in Western psychological theory, too, may hold a negative attitude towards Indian cultural values. This negativity that the dominant culture has propagated against Indian cultures—for example with regard to arranged marriage, the caste system, dating, and much more—has impacted the way people see individuals who come from India, and thus has created negative stereotypes of their culture, labeling it inferior to mainstream American or Western culture.

Siby, one of the second-generation respondents in this study, who sought therapy following the divorce of his parents, was sarcastically asked by his American therapist, "Are you going to follow in the footsteps of your parents?" Siby asked for clarification, "What do you mean?" The counselor said, "I mean an arranged marriage." This teenager quit counseling because of the counselor's stereotyped understanding and flippant attitude regarding the arranged marriage and divorce of Siby's parents.

Therefore, the pastoral care and psychotherapeutic model that I propose here in this book is one that considers the culture of persons as a primary source of their healing. It is to be treated with the same respect as other sources, such as personality developmental and psychological theories. In other words, the model I propose considers all resources, including psychological, diagnostic, and personality theories, within the framework of a person's cultural background. I maintain that Western-based theories cannot be considered as a normative frame in the healing process of a person from the non-Western world. Even if there is a contradiction between the Western-based resources and a person's cultural background, an effort must be made to reconsider and reinterpret those resources within the cultural framework of that particular person.

Any attempt to counsel Asian-Indian immigrants should be considered as an inquiry or a kind of research. In other words, the counselor must be open to the dictates of the counselee, the field text, the "living human document."[6] Any action or behavior on the part of the counselee/client that might be considered deviant based on a therapeutic assumption of the dominant culture should be approached with an objective curiosity and cultural sensitivity rather than considering it as a symptom of disease. For example, while direct eye contact is seen as sign of attention to and engagement with the speaker in Western culture, it is seen as a sign of disrespect in Indian culture, especially when it occurs with persons of the opposite gender. Indian women will generally avoid eye contact as a result of gender expectations. If this behavior is not understood in terms of its cultural meaning, female counselees may be seen as avoidant or excessively passive. Ignoring culturally shaped gender expectations, especially for women and children from Asian India, can have a negative effect on the course of therapy. Similarly, a therapist who demands to see family members individually, without the whole family (especially a wife without husband in a family conflict) can create divisions and differences of opinion within families. This can also create suspicion that will reduce the level of cooperation among family members necessary to the healing process.

The community for whom this psychotherapeutic counseling model is advocated has a strong history of traditional methods of healing. It has much to offer in the process of healing and so members of this immigrant community must be considered co-therapists and conversation partners with valuable information that will help in the caring process. Cultural identity issues and the influences of globalization demand new ways of healing that will not negate counselees' cultural norms and values.

Previous studies have shown that immigration demands considerable adjustment and generates cultural problems for people migrating into new cultures.[7] Another layer of challenge is added in cases when families migrate at different times and have different levels of acculturation.[8] This problem is further increased when different generations—those who immigrated from one culture to another and the generation born and raised in the host culture—now live under the same roof.

It is common for frustrations to run high among immigrants. An earlier immigrant may be pushing new arrivals to change so fast that they may feel they are being forced to assimilate[9] rather than being given the grace of time to learn how to survive in the new culture as they interact with members of the family who have achieved better levels of acculturation. This is a period of enculturation[10] for the new arrivals, and the push by earlier immigrants can increase the intensity of stress for them if family members/friends do not give them ample space for the acculturation process to happen at its own pace. This issue is significant for first-generation parents and second-generation children as the level of enculturation differs greatly between the generations. Feeling forced to assimilate creates a problem for immigrants that entails feelings of subjugation and oppression. Hence, a sense of inferiority, low self-esteem, and feelings of lost identity may develop. This experience is the opposite of what the immigrants expected of life in America or in any Western country, a place where they had understood that people were accepted for who they were. It is my contention that when therapy fails to respect the cultural norms and values held so dearly and dutifully by Asian-Indian families, it will not lead to healing. Further, I believe that people seeking care are not taken sufficiently seriously when we do not anchor our psychotherapy and counseling in the solid foundation of their cultural milieu. By ignoring the importance of culture, a valuable source of holistic care is being denied. When it ignores the cultural values of first-generation Asian-Indian parents in therapy and assumes that second-generation immigrants are assimilated into the host-country culture, Eurocentric American therapy disrespects clients as fully human and is limited in the ability to heal.

Most first-generation Asian-Indian immigrant parents already fear the "death of family or home"[11] because they are unable to pass on their cultural values to their children born and raised in American/Western culture. While they seek help addressing that fear and confusion of the "dying family or home" experience, therapy, if it disregards their cultural values, inflicts more pain on them, exacerbating their fear. At the same time, second-generation immigrants born and raised in American culture also face rejection from both American society and their parental cultures. They are trying hard to survive, even in the face of rejection by both the dominant and immigrant cultures/communities. In these situations, when therapists assume that the second-generation immigrants are already assimilated into the American cultures, therapy fails to externalize their issues, gain their trust, and build up a strong therapeutic relationship.

DESCRIPTION OF THE SOURCES OF THIS BOOK

To develop a pastoral care and psychotherapeutic method that provides an informed pastoral intervention for Asian-Indian immigrant families living in two different cultural spaces (Indian and American/Western), I explored a number of factors contributing to intergenerational conflict. An informing conviction was a serious consideration of the life stories and experiences of Asian Indians and their children. A guiding assumption of this book is that for effective and appropriate pastoral practice to be meaningful and helpful to counselees, it must meet them at their level and point of need. This calls for an integrative approach that understands and privileges the cultural embeddedness of the Asian-Indian immigrants.

Based on my experience as a pastor, teacher, and counselor, I have observed a number of factors that can contribute to intergenerational conflict in Indian immigrant families. The research and questionnaire designed for this book sought to determine the prevalence of these factors. The eight apparent factors explored through this study are:

1. In-depth and quality communication between first- and second-generation Indian immigrants rarely takes place in those families.
2. Intra-family relationships between the first and second generation are often conflictual, resulting from family dysfunctions of Indian immigrants in the United States.
3. The power struggle in the family due to American laws concerning child rearing, corporal punishment, individual culture, and children's access to information systematically discourages in-depth interactions between the first- and second-generation family members regarding any ongoing conflict.
4. Mutual acceptance of culture is lacking among first- and second-generation Indian immigrants, leading to intergenerational conflicts in the family.
5. Religious institutions and social organizations fail to address the need for cultural integration and quality improvement of family functionality among Indian immigrant families in the United States.
6. An overemphasis on the superiority of one culture conveniently ignores the peer pressure and social stigma experienced by both the first- and second-generation Indian immigrants in the United States.

7. Hiding family stress between first and second generations due to the
   social stigma attached to disclosing family issues to someone outside
   the family (the therapist) creates dysfunction.
8. Lack of integration of both United States and Indian cultural values
   leads to family dysfunctions among Indian immigrants in the United
   States.

Based on the findings of a structured questionnaire which explored these
eight factors affecting intergenerational conflict and family functioning,
I propose a culturally sensitive and culturally competent psychotherapeutic
model that examines the practice of doing appropriate and effective pastoral
psychotherapy and counseling with Asian-Indian immigrant families dealing
with alienation resulting from immigration. Certain theoretical concepts of
Kohut, Kakar, and Lee have been incorporated into my model. All pastoral
care praxis has the components of a valid research method because every
counseling and therapeutic encounter in which I have engaged included
information gathering, engagement of social and behavioral sciences, theological engagement, critical correlation, and application phases. I experienced this type of research-in-practice as one in which the counselees
become co-researchers with the therapist or counselor as they helped in
the validation of the insights of this endeavor.

The research was conducted among Asian-Indian immigrants who had
migrated from different states of India to states in the southeastern region of
the United States. Only respondents from four states (Texas, Florida,
Alabama, and Georgia) were selected for this study. One hundred first-
generation and 100 second-generation Asian-Indian immigrants were
selected as study samples from these states, with an equal representation
of males and females. The second-generation immigrants selected for this
study were over 17 years of age, born and raised in the cultural context of
the United States. The first-generation immigrant respondents were born
and raised in India and migrated to the United States in their late twenties,
thirties, or early forties. Their current ages ranged from 45 to 65 years. In
this study, the stratified random sampling method was applied for the
selection of the subjects.

OPERATIONAL DEFINITIONS

A number of key terms are used throughout the book. Their definitions
follow:

First-Generation Indian Immigrants: People who migrated from India to the United States with different visa status seeking jobs and financial benefit. Born and raised in India, their identity is shaped by the Indian cultural context. Their lifestyle and perceptions still cling to traditional Indian cultural values that formed them before immigration even in the midst of ongoing cultural changes in India.

Second-Generation Indian Immigrants: Children of first-generation Indian immigrants, born and raised in the United States, or brought to the United States with their parents as infants. It includes youngsters who are not clear about the culture of their parents and unable to read and write their parents' language fluently, though speaking a few words here and there. Simply stated, "the 'second-generation' consists of children of immigrants."[12]

Culture: Often, the term 'culture' is used in a broad sense to refer to all the learned and shared ideas and products of a society. It is "a shared way of life that includes values, beliefs, and norms transmitted within a particular society from generation to generation. It consists of symbols, language, values, beliefs, worldviews, myths, ideologies, and norms."[13] The interaction between two cultural communities always involves borrowing from each other's culture, and over a period of time this import and export process results in the evolution of entirely new cultural forms.

Cultural Identity: Cultural identity refers to an individual's orientation that arises when people live interculturally. Cultural identity also refers to thoughts and feelings about belonging to one's ethnocultural group (ethnic identity) and to the larger society (national identity). It is a sense of belonging to, or attachment with either or both these cultural groupings.[14] Language issues (including language proficiency and use) also arise during intercultural living: which languages are learned, and which are used and in which kind of interactions, are all decisions that are made daily and are part of cultural identity. The pattern of social contacts and interactions with members of one's own group and with others is also a crucial part of cultural identity.

Cultural Integration: The fundamental aspect of unity that connects different groups of communities of a society is called integration. According to Gaikward, integration means, "operationally, the observable enduring dispositions of the individuals in any given group to co-ordinate their actions closely towards each other or in respect of each other. It is meaningless to speak of integration unless it is understood to exist in degrees which must be measurable and definable in quantitative terms."[15] Integration can be measured by the study of frequency, regularity, scatteredness, and nature of diverse action patterns. In this sense, it is qualitative as well. A favorable attitude and emotional attachment to different overt and covert symbols of identification indicates the presence of integration. However, in this book integration does not mean an identification or assimilation of a minority culture to the dominant one; rather it is internal integration of acceptance.

Ethnic Identity. A construct which refers to one's sense of belonging to an ethnic group and the part of one's thinking, perceptions, feelings, and behavior that is due to ethnic group membership. Psychologist Jean Phinney states "ethnic identity is a dynamic, multidimensional construct that refers to one's identity or sense of self, as a member of an ethnic group the attitudes and behaviors associated with that sense."[16] The involvement in the social and cultural practices of one's ethnic group is the most widely used indicator of ethnic identity.[17] The ethnic group is usually one in which the individual claims heritage. Ethnic identification, therefore, may also refer to identification or feeling of membership with others regarding the character, the spirit of a culture, or the cultural ethos based on a sense of commonality of origin, beliefs, values, customs, or practices of a specific group of people.

However, ethnic identity is not a fixed categorization, but rather a fluid and dynamic understanding of self and ethnic background. Ethnic identity is constructed and modified as individuals become aware of their ethnicity, within the large (sociocultural) setting.[18] Similarly, Joanne Nagel suggests ethnicity is a socially constructed process, and ethnic boundaries, identities and culture are negotiated, defined and produced through social interaction inside and outside ethnic communities.[19]

Asian-Indian Culture. Asian-Indians are a heterogeneous group in themselves. In this book, the terms 'Indian' and 'Asian-Indian' are used interchangeably. As Saran states, "each regional subgroup of India has its own unique history, practices, languages, values, and customs."[20] Yet there are a lot of cultural beliefs, values and practices, related to family, marriage, child-rearing, and community in common, and such common cultural values, beliefs, and practices are discussed in this book. Hence, the term "Indian culture" in this book only refers to those common cultural values. Asian-Indian cultural values referred to in this book focus only on communal nature of Indian culture (interdependence), pressure from parents to maintain traditional cultural values, family bonds, parental control, specifically in education, careers, dating and marriage, child-rearing, and parental expectations based on gender roles.

American Culture: America is a nation of many cultures. Predominant white, middle-class European-American culture, African-American culture, and many other cultures are found in the United States. Though I am aware that there is no "American culture," often the mainstream, predominant white, middle-class European-American culture that emphasizes individual autonomy, gender egalitarianism, concept of family, child-rearing with the focus of individuation and freedom of choice are considered as the major elements of American/Western culture.

Intergenerational Conflict: An intergenerational conflict is either a conflict situation between teenagers and adults or any conflict between two generations. It will often involve all-inclusive prejudices against another generation. Furthermore, intergenerational conflict describes cultural, social or economic discrepancies between generations. These can be caused by value shift or conflict of interest between younger and older generations. Intergenerational conflict is also a term associated with the "generation gap." Intergenerational conflict refers to the collective tension, strain, and antagonism between older and younger generations. Indian families have a deep sense of obligation to take care of one another; and the individual is viewed as a part of a larger family and community, and members of an extended family will go to great lengths to support any individual in the family. The conflict arises when this closeness and caring leads to attempts to stifle an individual's desire to hold some values that are contrary to the family or cultural values.[21]

Family Function/Dysfunction: A dysfunctional family in this study is one in which conflict, misbehavior, and abuse on the part of individual members of the family occur continually, leading other members to accommodate such actions. Family dysfunction is examined based on family functionality in traditional Indian cultural understanding. As in any culture, the presence of a direct verbal communication with warmth, love, and care, is one of the major criteria that decides whether the family functions or is dysfunctional. In this study, mutual

respect and care, maintaining family structure, fulfilling family responsibilities, maintaining family ties (depending on cultural understanding), and so on are factors that measure family functionality or
dysfunction. If the harmony of the family is broken in relation to its
cultural practices, such a family is considered as dysfunctional. For
instance, if there is verbal, physical and emotional abuse, no open
communication or reciprocal relationship following the moving-out
of a daughter or dating of a son, such a family is considered as
relatively dysfunctional. In other words, when fathers and sons do
not bond, mothers and daughters do not communicate, parents,
grandparents and elders are disrespected, heritage is not transferred,
and family bond weakens there is probably growing dysfunctionality.

The research described in this book is exclusively limited to Asian Indian
immigrants in the southeast region of the United States. Hence, it does not
focus on similar experiences outside the region. Further, it is strictly limited
to the experience of intergenerational immigrant families. Thus, first-generation or second-generation Indian immigrants who live without their
parents and children are not included in this book. Thirdly, only five specific
areas and related topics are selected for discussion: (1) in-depth intrafamily
relationships between first- and second-generation immigrants; (2) communication, mutual acceptance; (3) respect for cultural values and practices,
(over)emphasis on the superiority or inferiority of one culture over the other
(level of acculturation) and related issues of marginality status;
(4) intergenerational conflict and individual/family functionality; and
(5) the role of religious and social institutions in educating the immigrants
on cultural integration. There are clearly other dimensions, but they are not
the focus of this work.

The model I propose in this project is culturally sensitive to the Asian
Indians in that it is communally and culturally centered. The model primarily focuses on group dynamics rather than the one-on-one model that is self-
centric in nature. The model also calls for a reorientation of the therapeutic
context to include cultural communal nuances.

Finally, this model is developed in the context of Asian-Indian families
living in multiple cultural spaces in the United States of America. Therefore,
it may not be entirely relevant to other immigrants living in the United
States or Asian-Indian families who have immigrated to other Western
countries. I do not claim that this model is *the* model for Asian Indians at
all times. Rather, it provides a starting point for counseling Asian-Indian

immigrants and, hopefully, other immigrant groups, as well. The model of pastoral counseling being proposed in this book is intended to contribute to the literature of pastoral counseling theory, calling for diversity of approaches when engaging persons from different cultures other than the dominant culture in the United States.

NOTES

1. One of the major sources used in this research is Jung Yung Lee's *Marginality: The Key to Multicultural Theology* (Minneapolis, MN: Fortress Press, 1995).
2. Sudhir Kakar, *The Inner World: A Psychoanalytic Study of Childhood and Society in India*. (Delhi: Oxford University Press, 1978), 1.
3. Lee, *Marginality*, 33.
4. K. Ahmed, "Adolescent Development for South Asian American Girls," in *Emerging Voices: South Asian American Women Redefine Self, Family and Community*, ed. S. R. Gupta (Walnut Creek, CA: AltaMira Press, 1999), 37–49. See also S. Jambunathan, "Comparison of Parenting Attitudes among Five Ethnic Groups in the United States," *Journal of Comparative Family Studies* Vol. 31, no. 4, (Autumn, 2000): 395–406.
5. M. K. Aravamudan, "Conflict Continuity and Change: Indian Americans Negotiate Ethnic Identity and Gender through Decisions about Dating and Marriage" (PhD diss., Northwestern University 2003).
6. Henry J. Nouwen, "Anton T. Boison and Theology through Living Human Documents," *Pastoral Psychology* 19, no. 7 (September, 1968): 49.
7. Ram Gidoomal, "Displacement: Effect of Immigration on Families," in *Caring for the South Asian Souls*, eds. Thomas Kulanjiyil and T. V. Thomas (Bangalore: Primalogue Publishing & Media, 2010).
8. The term "acculturation" is used in this book to refer to the process by which persons learn aspects of a culture that is not theirs whereby they learn to incorporate some of its aspects that will enable them to survive in their new environment. See also the definition by George K. Hong and Mary Anna Domokos-Cheng Ham in *Psychotherapy and Counseling with Asian American Clients: A Practical Guide* (Thousand Oaks, CA: Sage Publications, Inc., 2001), 37.
9. The term "assimilation" in this book refers to persons giving up their original culture and accepting the dominant culture. See also Hong and Ham, 36–37.
10. Enculturation refers to the process of learning aspects of a culture from one's own peers that allows the immigrant learning to feel that they are doing it in community and as a way of enhancing their identity.

11. The phrase "death of family or home" is used to indicate the end of transmitting or passing on to their children the cultural values, beliefs, and practices that the first-generation parents hold so dearly and dutifully. For them, home means their life with their family members as that is who they are, culturally.

12. M. Zhou, "Growing Up American: The Challenges Confronting Immigrant Children and Children of Immigrants," *Annual Review of Sociology* 23, no. 1 (August, 1997): 6395; J. Bacon, "Constructing Collective Ethnic Identities: The Case of Second Generation Asian Indians," *Qualitative Sociology* 22, no. 2 (Spring, 1999): 141–160.

13. Raymond Scupin, *Ethnicity in Race and Ethnicity* (Englewood Cliffs: NJ: Prentice Hall, 2003), 69.

14. John W. Berry, Jean S. Phinney, David L. Sam, and Paul Vedder, eds., *Immigrant Youth in Cultural Transition: Acculturation, Identity and Adaptation Across National Contexts* (Hillsdale, NJ: Lawrence Erlbaum Associates, 2006).

15. V.R. Gaikward, *The Anglo Indians: A study in the Problems and Process Involved in Emotional and Cultural Integration* (Bombay: Asia Publishing House, 1965), 5.

16. Jean Phinney, "Ethnic Identity and Acculturation," in *Acculturation: Advances in Theory, Measurement and Applied Research*, eds. K. Chun and G. Marin (Washington, DC: American Psychological Association, 2003), 63. Also see Phinney, J. and Alipuria, L. "Ethnic Identity in Older Adolescents from Four Ethnic Groups." Paper presented at the Biennial Meeting of the Society for Research in Child Development, Baltimore (1987), 36.

17. Jean Phinney, "Ethnic Identity in Adolescents and Adults: Review of Research," *Psychological Bulletin* 108, no. 3 (November, 1990): 499–514.

18. Phinney, "Ethnic Identity and Acculturation," 63.

19. Joanne Nagel, "Constructing Ethnicity: Creating and Recreating Ethnic Identity and Culture," *Social Problems* 41, no. 1 (February, 1994): 153.

20. Parmatma Saran, *The Asian Indian Experience in the United States* (Cambridge, MA: Schenkman Publishing, 1985).

21. V. Rao, S. Channabassavanna, and R. Parthasarathy, "Transitory Status Image of Working Women in Modern India," *Indian Journal of Social Work* 45, no. 2 (1984): 198–202.

CHAPTER 2

Historical and Cultural Factors in Ethnic Identity Formation of Asian-Indian Immigrants: Understanding the Context of Care

INTRODUCTION

This chapter sets the stage for the development of a model of pastoral psychotherapeutic care that fits the needs of Asian-Indian immigrants in the United States of America, based on an understanding of a fuller picture of who they are and how they have come to be who they are. I explore the complex cultural identity of Asian-Indians based on their cultural values, belief systems, and lifestyle, while trying to delineate some of their fears, including a sense of isolation, they may experience while they are living in the United States. I also explore how Indian immigrants respond to the unique stress of immigration and try to reshape their lives in the United States in the midst of various post-immigration challenges and struggles. Asian-Indians warrant separate research and exploration since their culture is distinct from other Asian groups. Asian-Indians are, however, a heterogeneous group in themselves. Parmatma Saran[1] states that each regional subgroup of India has its own unique history, practices, languages, values, and customs. Yet, there are many cultural beliefs, values, and practices related to family, marriage, child-rearing, and community in common among Indians. This chapter discusses those common cultural values, beliefs, and practices. Hence, the term "Indian culture" in this book only refers to those common cultural values. Highlighting the importance of Asian-Indian traditional culture or the cultural context of Asian-Indians neither negates the reality of the good and positive elements that come from other cultures nor does it claim that the best is only found in the

© The Author(s) 2017
V. Jacob, *Counseling Asian Indian Immigrant Families*,
DOI 10.1007/978-3-319-64307-6_2

traditional context. Attending to cultural assumptions of Asian-Indians allows us to understand the important role these play in formulating and providing informed care.

ASIAN-INDIANS IN THE UNITED STATES OF AMERICA

The earliest record of the presence of an Asian-Indian in North America is to be found in a colonial diary. In 1790, an Indian from Madras (Chennai) visited Salem, Massachusetts. He is believed to have accompanied a British sea captain who was plying a trading vessel between New England ports and such coastal towns as Bombay (Mumbai), Madras (Chennai), and Calcutta (Kolkotha). According to the diary of Rev. William Bentley, a clergyman in Salem, Massachusetts, dated December 29, 1790,

> The Indian had the pleasure of seeing for the first time a native of the Indies from Madras. He is of dark complexion, long straight black hair, soft countenance, tall and well proportioned. He is said to be darker than Indians in general of his own caste, being much darker than any native Indians of America. I had no opportunity to judge his ability, but his countenance was not expressive. He came to Salem with Capt. Gibaut and has been in Europe.[2]

Bentley does not say anything further about the Indian from Madras, whether he remained in Salem or just passed through. However, 61 years later, in 1851, there is a report stating that in Salem, half-a-dozen Asian-Indians participated in the fourth of July parade of the East India Marine Society.[3]

Asian-Indian Migration to the United States: The First Wave

By the late nineteenth century, there were many recruitment drives for laborers to work in the lumber towns of Washington, laying railroads in Oregon, and working in the agricultural fields of California. By 1920, some 6400 Indians had entered the United States.[4] This is often referred to as the first wave of Indian immigration. Most of these first-wave immigrants were single men, and the men to women ratio was almost 75 : 1, and many ended up marrying other ethnic immigrants.[5]

Asian-Indian Migration to the United States: The Second Wave

Though Asian history of migration to the United State begins centuries ago, the Indian part of it commences from the turn of the first quarter of the twentieth century. The last major immigration act, The United States Immigration Act of 1965, put an end to the period of the discriminatory, selective immigration. Following the passing of that act, people were permitted to come from every part of the world with an established limitation of 20,000 as the quota to be filled by citizens of any one nation, irrespective of color, creed, ethnic, or national origin.[6] The objectives of that legislation were plainly stated in President John Kennedy's message to congress on July 23, 1963. According to Kennedy,

> The most urgent and fundamental reform I am recommending relates to the national origins quota system of selecting immigrants. Although the legislation I am transmitting deals with many problems, which require remedial actions, it concentrates attention primarily upon revision of our quota system. The use of a national origins system is without basis in either logic or reason. It neither satisfies a national need nor accomplishes an international purpose. In an age of interdependence among nations, such a system is an anachronism for it discriminates among applicants for admission into the United States on the basis of the accident of birth. But the legislation I am submitting will insure that progress will continue to be made toward our ideals and toward the realization of humanitarian objectives.[7]

This liberal immigration act opened the way for Asian-Indians, along with several other ethnic groups, to migrate to the United States, and accounts for the steep rise in the Indian immigrant population from 10,000 in 1965 to 525,000 twenty years later, crossing the million mark in 1997.[8]

The second wave of newcomers was strikingly different from the earlier immigrants. According to Fong, "the post-1965 Asian immigrants are more geographically dispersed, better educated, and better off economically than the pre-1965 Asian immigrants."[9] Unlike the railroad workers and farm laborers of the first-wave immigrants, the second-wave immigrants were better educated, highly skilled, and came with job-related experience.[10] They were urban professionals while the earlier wave was largely rural farmers. The second-wave immigrants came with their families or brought them soon afterwards, while in the earlier wave it was mostly single men that immigrated. While their predecessors were native Indian language speakers, the latter immigrants were fluent in English and performed well in cross-cultural work settings. The bright, educated, and ambitious men and women were more likely to explore opportunities overseas. From the early 1970s through the mid1980s more than 15,000 engineers and more than 15,000 physicians came to America from India.[11]

According to United States Census Bureau 2000, the educational achievement of Asian-Indians was the highest of any ethnic group in America. Almost 65 percent of the entire Indian American population has at least a bachelor's degree, 21 percent a master's, and almost 5 percent a doctorate. The earning of Asian-Indians is the highest among immigrant groups in the United States, exceeding even the Japanese who were the top earners for many decades.[12] *India-West*, a widely published weekly Indian newspapers in the United States, cited a Pew Research Center study that recently reported that more than 80 percent of Indian Americans hold college or advanced degrees.[13] According to that research, Indian Americans also have the highest income levels, earning $65,000 per year, with a median household income of $88,000, far higher than the United States household average of $49,000.[14]

Despite such remarkable socio-economic advancements, the Indian community has its share of problems. Racism is one, with perhaps the worst example being the New Jersey "dot busters"—a group of thugs who sought out ethnic Indians and mugged them or attacked their properties in the late 1980s and 1990s.[15] The dot was reference to the *bindi* worn by Hindu women on their forehead. In post-9/11 America, men in the Sikh community came under suspicion for their long beards and turbans. The shooting at a Wisconsin Sikh Temple, killing seven and leaving several injured on August 5, 2012, is a recent example of this racist discrimination. It is also a fact that many Indian immigrants are living in poverty, contrary to the popular notion that Indians in America are all affluent. Nationwide, 10.13 percent of Indian-American children under 17years old and 23.04 percent of Indian Americans aged 18–24 old live in poverty.[16] Along with this, their cultural identity issues reflected in various walks of their life precipitate the need for pastoral care and counseling for this community.

Based on the United States Bureau of the Census 2010, Asian-Indians in the United States are currently 3.2 million in number, make up the third-largest Asian population, and representing one of the fastest-growing immigrant populations in the United States.[17] This number includes all those who identify themselves as Indian-American or Asian-Indian, irrespective of the immigration classification to which they belong. As per the details released by United States Census Bureau 2010, the total United States population grew by 9.7 percent, from 281.4 million in 2000 to 308.7 million in 2010. However, the Asian population increased more than four times faster than the total United States population, growing 43 percent from 10.2 million to 14.7 million. According to the United States Census Bureau, of all the detailed Asian alone-or-in any combination groups that had a population of a million or more, the Indian-American population grew the fastest (by 68 percent), followed by the Filipino (44 percent), Vietnamese (42 percent), Chinese (40 percent), and Korean (39 percent) populations.[18] *South Asian Chronicle* reports that people of Indian origin are close to making up 1 percent of America's population of 308.7 million, with their numbers shooting up by a whopping 69.37 percent over the last decade.[19] Indians are now the largest of 25 Asian subgroups in the United States, mainly in the South and Midwest. This makes India the main driver in the population growth of Asian Americans, according to an analysis of the United States 2010 census data by the California-based *India-West* newspaper.[20] In 2002, it was predicted that the Indian population living in United States would increase to 2 million by the year 2050.[21] However, this prediction came to fruition 40 years early and superseded all expectations.

Asian-Indian Cultural and Ethnic Identity

Identity-formation is the process by which an individual develops a distinct personality or a set of characteristics by which he/she becomes recognizable or known. According to Jean Phinney and Linda Alpuria, ethnic identity is "an individual's sense of self as a member of an ethnic group and the attitudes and behaviors associated with that sense."[22] Further, they note that it is the "process of development from an unexamined ethnic identity through a period of exploration, to arrive at an achieved ethnic identity."[23] According to Mao Sotomayor, "ethnic identification may also refer to identification or feeling of membership with others regarding the character, the spirit of a culture, or the cultural ethos based on a sense of commonality of origin, beliefs, values, customs, or practices of a specific group of people."[24] Additionally, identity refers to a person's sense of belonging in a society based on his/her social experience.[25] Donald R. Atkinson and Ruth H. Gim propose that the development of ethnic identity follows five distinct stages:

- Conformity—preferences of values of the dominant culture instead of one's own cultural group;
- Dissonance—confusion and conflict regarding the dominant culture's system and one's own group's cultural system;
- Resistance and immersion—active rejection of the dominant system and acceptance of one's own cultural group's traditions and customs;
- Introspection—questioning the values of both the majority and minority cultures;
- Synergistic articulation and awareness—resolution of conflicts in previous stages and developing a cultural identity that selects elements from both the dominant and minority cultural groups' values.[26]

Though Atkinson's and Gim's theory provides a basis for investigating identity development among Asian-Indians, the theory is created neither on the basis of the Asian-Indian experience nor with the collectivistic emphasis and the layers of influence contained across an Asian ethnic population.

In order to fully understand Asian-Indian identity development, we must have some knowledge of the cultural context in which this identity is formed. Indian psychologist Sudhir Kakar provides a culturally informed understanding of identity development in Indian society. He states that

> Many of the salient aspects of the Indian society like family-centeredness, religion, regional affiliation, language, caste/class and many more play a crucial role in the development of the self-concept. An individual self is seen within a communal self, individual accomplishments are valued only if it improves the wellbeing and/or status of one's family and community. In conflictual situations, everyone always regards their collective self over their personal self.[27]

In the Indian culture, identity is more ascribed by birth, family, community, caste, status, and religion than by achievement. The ascribed identity tends to restrict choices open to the individual and, to a large extent, tends to be the reflection of the familial and social norms of expectations. Personal interests, goals, welfare, and glory are secondary to those of the family. In order to attain harmony within the family, it is essential for an individual to surrender or merge into his/her family, which, in turn, results in less differentiation of his/her individual self.[28] The achieved notion of identity according to the Western understanding and the ascribed notion of identity according to the Eastern understanding converge in second-generation Asian-Indians, creating a pull in opposite directions, tearing the "self" of this generation. The tension seems more acute within members of the second-generation Asian-Indians than in any other of the ethnic communities.[29]

The identity of the first generation is developed and shaped around the family. Speaking about family in the Indian culture is a part of one's self-identity. Every individual has a certain role in his/her family and in society. Therefore, individual identity is formed in relation to family identity. As a result, every individual is understood as a part of the greater social system and no one behaves in an individuated way. Since one's identity and roles are already established within the family and community, the concept of "finding one's self" may be difficult to comprehend in traditional Asian-Indian families. This, again, is rather different from the typical Western concept of individuation and differentiation, perceived as a normal part of personal development.[30]

During the process of identity development, Indian Americans, unlike those stemming from individualistic cultures, select and integrate their private, public, and collective selves. Increasing individuation and disengagement from the family is not understood as a normal way of growth from an Indian perspective.[31] There is fear of shame and stigmatism not only for oneself, but of one's family members within the community. Lavina Melwani, quoting Sunaina Maira of the Harvard Graduate School of Education, notes that

> Classic conceptions of adolescence in American psychology has stressed increasing individuation and disengagement from the family as central to this rite of passage, which are not necessarily emphasized in traditional notions of this stage in Indian families. What is considered normal in American society suddenly gets a bad or rebellious connotation in the Indian value system. And the kids are made to feel un-Indian and parents lose face.[32]

The Indian expression, "lose face," conveys that one has damaged their good family name and reputation in the eyes of others. "Saving face" plays a fundamental role in the process of Asian-Indian identity development. Saving face is the avoidance of humiliation and embarrassment, as well as the preservation or redemption of one's own and one's family's dignity. Tony O'Sullivan highlights the practice of saving face, noting that while "the Asian community has a process called saving face . . . in America it is called 'putting on a good face."[33] O'Sullivan offers a short list, in no particular order, of things people put on a good face about or "forget" to tell relatives about: divorce, remarriage, children out of wedlock, mental illness, sexual abuse, living together rather than marrying, dropping out of college or high school, quitting or losing a job, criminal record, incarceration, and drug/alcohol addiction—just to name a few.[34] The common denominator between these cultural features is that people would rather lie than come clean and face the possible embarrassment they might suffer in front of friends or relatives. O'Sullivan notes that "in Asian cultures, dirty laundry is something that is kept under tight wraps. They don't want anyone knowing about that bit too much. Come to think of it, most cultures keep their family secrets quiet."[35]

THE QUESTION OF WORLDVIEW

Worldview is a sense of how the social world is organized, how persons are related to one another, and to the entire complex of social relations that constitute a society. It is the product of a person's experience in his/her culture of origin. This is because "world view represents one's beliefs, values, and assumptions about people, relationships, nature, and activity in the world. It includes group and individual identity, values and belief systems."[36] As Clifford Geertz points out, a worldview provides a model or map of reality by structuring one's perceptions of reality.[37] George Alexander explains the term worldview as follows:

> Worldviews "includes the cognitive aspect of belief, ideas and attitudes that are learned early in life and seldom verbalized. Its function is to explain, validate, reinforce, integrate and adopt in order to bridge the gap between the subjective world in one's mind and the objective world outside. Taking together cognitive, affective, and evaluative assumptions provide people with a way of looking at the world that makes sense of it and gives them a feeling of being at home and that reassures them they are right. The worldview serves as the foundation on which they construct their explicit belief and value systems, and the social institutions within which they live their daily lives."[38]

Certainly, a great variety exists in the ways individuals within a common culture think about their social world. I believe that people from a common cultural background generally share an understanding of the way their culture thinks about social relationships. Even a person who holds views different from most people or different from his/her own parents has a shared understanding, if not acceptance, of the dominant worldview. To the extent that people share a cultural milieu that surrounds and delimits their particular experiences of language, religion, caste, gender, family, education, work, and politics, they share the worldview constitutive of their common cultural background. This is not to say that worldviews entail complete and coherent sets of articulated ideas passed down from generation to generation. Rather, each individual, in the process of growing up or living in a particular cultural milieu, gradually constructs a set of ideas about the social world based on his/her experience of everyday life.

I am aware that the existence of a common culture that serves as the basis for a shared worldview has been widely debated. Both cultural boundaries (who is to be included in the culture) and cultural consensus (is there really a single culture that is shared by all) are problems that challenge the notion of a common culture. Here, my stand is an emic approach, an approach that accepts as a cultural unit any group that talks about itself as belonging to a particular cultural tradition, such as being Indian or being American. The fact that "Indian culture" may mean different things to different people does not undermine the importance of the concept of those who use it.[39]

Briefly, the term "worldview" is a set of assumptions, ideas, and beliefs that are in some sense constructed on the fly over the course of time by each individual as a way of making sense of the social world in which he/she lives. Some of these notions, however, will become articulated as people discuss their ideas about the nature of social life, particularly when they perceive a difference in the way "we" believe versus the way "they" behave. In this sense, worldview is both public and private.

When Asian-Indians immigrate to America, they carry with them a worldview grounded in their culture of origin, which is primarily communal and collectivistic. Likewise, people born and raised as Americans share an understanding of an American worldview that emphasizes individuality, human rights, personal freedom, and equality. Though the term "American culture" is complicated in its ideal sense, yet despite individual, regional, and social group variation, there is a commonly recognized American worldview, no matter if the American belongs to the white middle class, is African American, or rural American. Research indicates that worldview is an integral component of the adjustment process of individual immigrants, their families, and immigrant communities.[40] To the extent that the immigrant's worldview differs from the worldview dominant in America, a type of adjustment must occur that differs from the more observable adjustment of language, dress, food, demeanor, work roles, or family relations. Immigrants must come to terms with the types of persons they see themselves as and the types of persons they are raising their children to be, while immersed in a society founded upon a worldview that may be radically different from their own.

WORLDVIEWS: AN EXAMPLE

The following story offers an illustration of the worldview of two different generations. Leela is a 40-year-old Indian female who migrated to Los Angeles, California, in her late twenties with her husband and two children—her 5-year-old son, Ashish, and 3-year-old daughter, Anisha—and later became a United States citizen. One day when Leela went to a United States post office with her children, they saw the American flag in front of the post office and Leela asked her children, "What flag is that?" "American flag," said Anisha, while Ashish said, "It is our flag." Then Ashish looked at his mother for the confirmation and again asked, "Right, mama?"

It took a moment for Leela to answer. All of a sudden, she remembered a different tricolor Indian flag of orange, white, and green, the way it flew in breeze in front of her school, to indicate the Indian independence, Indian Republic Day, and so much more. Though she loves America and is proud of being an American citizen, all of a sudden, at her son's answer, her thoughts went to the past. However, Leela said to her son, "Of course, it is sweetheart, it is our flag." But she states that it was not what she wanted to really tell her son. Leela further narrates that she could not sleep that night. She began to think what it meant for her to be Indian and what it meant for her children to be American. Though both she and her children speak English, they do so with an entirely different form of English, in terms of accent.

America is synonymous with immigration. Migration to any country in general and to United States in particular brings unique categories of cultural and emotional stress and struggles to the immigrants. Though America is a land of great opportunities, immigration to a new land is generally both a boon and bane. Immigration is a boon in terms of education, career opportunities, freedom of movement, speech, and thought, while a bane in terms of the loss of extended family—grandparents, uncles and aunts, even cousins of cousins—and the comfortable sense that your parents' house is only one of the many homes in which you belong.[41]

Leela's case indicates the unfathomable psychological pain experienced by a mother due to acculturation, a process that is infested with threats to ethnic identity, sense of betrayal and guilt, nostalgia, sense of loss, perceived sense of prejudice and discrimination, and culture shock. Cognitively, one feels an allegiance to the new country and new culture, but constant dissonance is caused by the awareness and intensity of bonding to the native country and cultural ties that are hard to break. For first-generation immigrants, it is hard to find psychological solace and serenity in the new culture because too many acculturative vultures[42] gnaw at their heart.

The tricolor Indian flag was an insignia of national pride and childhood memories for Leela. The thought of separation from that flag made her feel a surprising twinge in her heart and made her think about patriotism, ancestry, and complexities of cultures. A deep sense of tragic loss is caused by the great gap created upon migration into a new culture when generations of a family are deeply divided and become strangers, as was the case for Leela. Like many other Indian immigrants, for Leela the psychological and emotional pain of losing one's culture may be intensified when it is involuntary. For many Indian men, migration is voluntary, whereas women's migration is generally involuntary. Though they are interested in living with their husbands or parents, often the decision to immigrate is primarily made by their parents or husbands.

CULTURAL VALUES AND BELIEFS AMONG ASIAN-INDIANS

As has already been mentioned, Asian-Indians warrant separate research and exploration since their culture is distinct from other Asian groups and because they are a heterogeneous group in themselves. Each regional subgroup of India has its own, unique history, practice, languages, values, and customs.[43] For instance, an Asian-Indian may feel they have little in common with another Asian-Indian immigrant who has come from a different Indian state.[44] Therefore, it is also extremely difficult to explain the cultural values, practices, and belief system of Indians in general. However, there are certain cultural values that are held in common by every Indian. And whenever those values are affected, the homeostasis of the family is disturbed. Even with globalization, those common cultural values are consciously or unconsciously practiced by most Indians, both in India and overseas. Therefore, what I emphasize in this chapter is limited to such common cultural values practiced and reinforced by the Indian immigrants in the United States, and the impact of observing those practices on family functioning as they live in the individualistic culture of the United States.

Asian-Indians enter the United States with a set of cultural beliefs, values, mores, and traditions for family members. This is especially true for children in the areas of family norms, child-rearing practices, and parent–child and spousal relationships that are entirely different from the Western/Euro-American understanding of marriage, family, and hospitality (briefly explained later in this chapter). As a result, Asian-Indian immigrants are considered "different" and are treated "differently." This creates for those immigrants a sense of rejection and alienation in the emotional world of the community simply because they have a racially and culturally diverse understanding that does not fit into the mainstream, normative American cultural framework. This situation urgently demands pastoral care, psychotherapy, and counseling for Asian-Indian families in the United States.

Researchers have considered the culture of the United States to be primarily individualistic and the culture of India to be collectivistic.[45] Collectivistic societies place greater importance on the group (or the family) than on that of the individual. For instance, in collectivistic societies, an individual is typically expected to make sacrifices for the good of the family. In the Asian-Indian culture, a strong attachment and sense of responsibility to the family form the very core of the Asian-Indian culture.[46] The Indian family structure has typically been patriarchal, extended, and interdependent,[47] with gender roles and expectations clearly defined. Men are the primary wage earners, decision-makers, and disciplinarians of the household. Along with career responsibilities, women act as primary caretakers and nurturers of the family. Children are expected to respect their elders, obey authority implicitly, and bring honor to the family.[48]

Family harmony and interdependence are also highly encouraged among Asian-Indian families.[49] The common patterns found in the Indian family generally contrast with those of the typical European-American family, where family structure is often nuclear, egalitarian, and individualistic.[50] Though these socially accepted cultural values and characteristics are under transition primarily due to globalization and modernization, the roles and responsibilities characteristic of a collectivist or communal culture are still practiced among the majority of Asian-Indians.

Decisions made in Asian-Indian families are often highly influenced by parents, primarily because it is generally believed that parents are more experienced and that their children do not have enough life experience to make certain decisions.[51] Additionally, a greater level of aversive control is imposed upon Asian-Indian children in order to instill a sense of obligation to the family and to encourage interdependence. In Asian-Indian culture, parents usually have a strong influence on the career choices of their children and, more importantly, on the choice of a marriage partner. Though these cultural practices are in transition, they are still practiced among the majority of the Indian population. Therefore, when Asian-Indian immigrants enter the United States, they are surrounded by a culture that holds very different views of the family as compared to their own.

Goals related to child-rearing may be the other most significant difference between European-American families and Asian-Indian families. European-American parents generally raise their children to be autonomous, assertive, and self-reliant.[52] European-American parents generally use inductive reasoning with their children, allow choices for their children, and encourage children to be active explorers of their own environment,[53] encouraging their children to think for themselves or become their own person.[54] Therefore, it may be natural for persons born, raised, and socialized within the cultural context of the United States to experiment individually with choices such as vocational aspirations or dating relationships that are suitable for them. Unlike their European-American peers, Asian-Indian children—both female and male—are socialized not to be autonomous, but rather to be interdependent on family. Women in particular are socialized to be dependent at every stage of life—first, on parents, next on a husband, and finally on sons.[55] Ramani S. Durvasula and Gaithri A. Mylvaganam state that for Asian-Indians, "the goal of parenting is not to provide the children with sufficient skills to leave the family but to instill a sense of obligation and duty"[56] to the family. Beginning at a young age and continuing throughout adulthood, Asian-Indian parents encourage children's interdependency on the parents and family.[57] Since one's identity and roles are already established within the family and community, the concept of finding one's self is difficult for the traditional Asian-Indian families to grasp.[58]

The concept and value of marriage in the Indian culture differ from those of Western culture. Marriage is seen as a permanent alliance, not only between two individuals, but also between two families.[59] In traditional Indian culture, arranged marriage—where parents, relatives, and/or significant elders find a suitable marriage partner for an individual—is the most common form of marriage. Arranged marriages continue to be common, even among Asian-Indian immigrants who have been in the United States for a long period of time.[60] Since divorce is highly stigmatized in their culture, the divorce rate among Asian-Indians, both in India and among those who live in America, is typically low.[61] Casual dating is strongly discouraged, in general, and sexual purity—more so in girls—is enforced. One of the major reasons for this restriction is the social stigma placed on the family by the community if an unwed woman in a family becomes pregnant through dating. It is then very difficult for men from reputed families to come forward to marry either the pregnant woman or the other daughters in that particular family.

Some researchers, such as Uma A. Segal,[62] reveal that Asian-Indian parents often fear dating will lead to sexual involvement or sexual assault on girls. Other scholars, such as Dasgupta, Durvasula, and Mylvaganam,[63] theorize that Asian-Indian parents fear dating may lead to their children marrying interracially or even outside of their subgroup, thereby losing their culture. Furthermore, since the divorce rate is higher in the United States than in India, Asian-Indian parents in the United States may also worry that interracial marriage may end in divorce.[64] Therefore, selection of a marriage partner is rarely done autonomously. Instead, a marriage is arranged through familial and community involvement. However, unlike previous generations where a potential bride or groom had little say in the final marriage decision, "modern" arranged marriages allow the prospective bride and/or groom to have considerable influence on the final decision.[65]

As in the case of spousal choice, Indian parents also have a strong influence on the career choice of their children. Asian-Indians are often achievement-oriented and set high aspirations for their children's success.[66] Even at the preschool age, parents value academic training for their children and facilitate the development of their cognitive skills.[67] Asian-Indian children are typically encouraged to attend college and pursue professional degrees in medicine, law, or business, while degrees in liberal arts and social sciences are often discouraged.[68] Current statistics show Asian-Indians make up the highest proportion of the total United States population with a bachelor's degree or higher.[69] High educational achievement is also a part of bringing honor to the family name.

An additional characteristic of the allocentric (group oriented) Asian-Indian culture is the role the community plays in the life of an individual. It is clearly evident that there is a sense of obligation to both family and to the group as a whole.[70] Ethnic group approval plays a significant role in Asian-Indian families in preserving cultural identity.[71] The Asian-Indian community is a close-knit group, and an individual's social network can be quite extensive. The strong sense of support and unity within the community can be highly adaptive and invaluable for an individual. However, the tight-knit nature of the culture forces parents to pressure the next generations to maintain a good reputation since others in the community are "always watching."[72]

Beginning in early childhood, children are aware of and taught to protect the honor of the family and to preserve a good family name.[73] Conformity and behaviors promoting group harmony are highly encouraged. Therefore, parents may restrict their children from engaging in behaviors that could possibly dishonor the family. For instance, restrictions may be placed on time spent outside the home with friends, with members of different ethnic groups, and with members of the opposite gender. The cultural value of preserving the family name may also be one explanation for the high level of parental control in Asian-Indian families.

To summarize, Asian-Indian culture has been identified as an allocentric culture, where great importance is placed on the family/group rather than on the individual. A deep obligation and commitment to the family forms the foundation of Asian-Indian culture. Often, parents and elders play a significant role in decision-making for the major life-events of their children. Children, in turn, are expected to bring honor to the family name by obeying their parents and elders, and by maintaining a good reputation within the Asian-Indian community.

Religion generally plays a significant role in the lives of most Asian-Indians, and its function in the culture cannot be underestimated. In the lives of Indian immigrants, religious institutions have often been identified as means to create a community and transmit cultural values. Such values often contrast starkly with those of the dominant cultural norms of the United States. Therefore, when Asian-Indians immigrate to the United States, they are surrounded by a culture that holds different views of the family compared to that of their own, and they are faced with the challenging experience of adapting in a new, unfamiliar cultural context.

SECOND-GENERATION ASIAN-INDIANS AND THEIR CULTURAL VALUES

The term second-generation Asian-Indian refers to the children of the first-generation Indian immigrants who are both born and raised in the United States or those who are brought to the United States with their parents during their infancy. These youngsters are often not well informed about the culture of their parents. Neither do they read and write their parents' language fluently, though they may be able to speak a few words.

Sociologist Phillip Abrams has a two-tiered definition of generation. In his view, the sociological significance of generation depends on the specific historical experiences, which connect individual identities with momentous social changes.[74] The history of most traditional societies is representative of only one sociological generation. By contrast, a sociological generation can theoretically include many biological generations, and occurs only under specific conditions. As Abrams further notes, "if a new sociological generation is to emerge, a new configuration of social action, the attempts of individuals to construct identity, must coincide with major and palpable historical experiences in relation to which new meanings can be assembled."[75]

Second-generation Indian immigrants occupy a position between two cultural spaces, suggesting marginal competency and sensitivity in both cultures while often living in a bicultural environment.[76] It is a complex experience of loneliness and struggle to belong to two separate cultures and generations. This struggle is not only based on a generational gap within a culture, but also on the conflicting values between cultures.[77] Although Asian-Indians constitute a large segment of the North American population, little research focusing on second generations is available.[78] Much of the current research on second-generation Asian Americans deals with the experience of other ethnic groups such as Chinese, Korean, Vietnamese, and Filipino youth.[79]

Children of Asian-Indian immigrant parents may experience confusion in identity development.[80] Generally, second-generation Asian-Indians are exposed to two very different cultural patterns as they attempt to establish their own identity through personal struggle and contemplation and/or parental influence and social guidance.[81] As they seek to develop their identity, they are faced with an opposing and conflicting set of forces; one, a Western force, which is based on autonomy and individual choice, the other, an Indian force, which is based on collective and predetermined choices.[82] As Min Zhou notes, the contrasting values of Asian-Indian families in terms of individualism and collectivism lead to clashes between parents and children over the degree of autonomy in making important life-decisions.[83]

Second-generation Indian immigrants live in two diverse worlds: the immigrant world of their parents' culture and community and the American world of their peers shaped by their education and media that influences their resident culture. Being shuttled between American schools and Indian homes, Indian children grow up in a double bind. On the one hand, their parents tend to teach collectivism, religious commitment, and gender role differentiation. On the other hand, American schools and the wider society promote individualism, secularism, and gender equality. The tension this double bind creates in children can lead to great psychological stress.[84] The ongoing negotiation necessary to transit between cultures requires that one constantly define and redefine one's ethnic identity between the self and the external world.[85]

Studies show that most second-generation youths feel torn between being Indian and being American, a predicament shaped by their Indian upbringing and American socialization. This leads to their confusion in terms of developing their own identity.[86] Generally, second-generation Asian-Indians are exposed to two very different cultural patterns in terms of determining their identity as they attempt to establish their own identity through personal struggle and contemplation and/or parental influence and social guidance. They are faced with opposing sets of forces that attempt to shape their ethnic identity.[87] These consist of a Western force, which is based on their individual choices. The other is an Indian force, which is based on collective and predetermined choices. Therefore, their lives seem to be bifurcated between the land of their parents and the land of birth or adoption. It seems that they are pulled in one direction at home and another direction at school. They speak their ancestral language at home and English elsewhere.

Ronald Takaki highlights the experience of Japanese Americans, which is similar to that of Indian immigrants:

> Their lives and identities were bifurcated between the land of their parents and the land of their birth, folk stories about boy Momotaro and children's tales about the Jack and Beanstalk, the Japanese love song their mothers sang in the kitchen and the popular songs they heard on the radio, the summer *obon* dances and the weekend jitterbug dances, Japanese New Year's day and Christmas, the annual *kenjinkai* picnics and high school outings, *banzai* to the Emperor's health and the pledge of allegiance to the flag of the United States.[88]

Likewise, Sam George describes the very similar experience of the bicultural life of second-generation Asian-Indians in the United States:

Because of their sense of religiosity, traditions and family culture, the younger generation is caught between ethnicities and assimilation tendencies. . . . In spite of the pervasive presence of the American socializing agents such as public schools, churches, social organizations and popular media, the progenies of the immigrant generation starts out the mainstream society. They are neither here nor there, caught up in the complex web of influences and struggle without much help.[89]

Living in this in-between space and traveling between cultures requires, as Radha Hedge notes, constant definition and redefinition of one's own ethnic identity and the ability to "negotiate between the self and the external world."[90] Similarly, Chen states that "although many ethnic children are used to integrating their own ethnic culture and the host culture, they often complain that the situation of being caught between two cultures makes them feel marginal."[91] The development of an Americanized identity is countered by the concomitant pull of the ethnic identity. The issues of skin color, languages, and stereotypes, as well as other issues related to identity, make things difficult for second-generations. Compared to their parents, they often become much more assimilated into the dominant society and, thus, have less ethnic identification. However, the consciousness, adoption, and application of the ethnic identity will ebb and flow, depending on one's life experience. Ethnic identity is shaped by the harsh reality of racism, which may lead one to reject or enhance his or her ethnic identity.

Having grown up in a homogenized culture in India, I observe that first generations are often unaware and are insensitive to the struggle of second generations in discovering their identities in a new land.[92] The disconnect between parents and children is illustrated by one respondent in my study who said, "My parents in the church sing old Malayalam devotional songs, read Malayalam Bible, and pray in Malayalam, but I prefer contemporary worship songs in English. Since I don't know those songs they sing, I am often reluctant to attend the church."[93] Here, difference is experienced not just in the language, but also in the genre of music. However, in Indian culture, any personal choice inconsistent with family wishes is perceived by family as a threat to parental status and the parental right to control children's behavior.[94] Obligation to family and community is central in Asian-Indian culture and is required in relationships of ascribed roles and status, such as parents/child and employer/employee. The socialization process usually employs shame and loss of face to reinforce prescribed sets of obligations. The strongest obligation is to one's parents. Because an individual always seeks to maintain harmonious interpersonal relationships, family obligations are communicated indirectly and without confrontation.[95]

Although many Indian-American children are used to integrating their own ethnic culture and the host culture, they often complain that the situation of being caught between two cultures makes them feel marginal.[96] They feel they are neither fully Indian (as are their parents), nor are they fully American. They are the "halfway" generation, stuck between two cultures and required to participate in the social worlds of their foreign-born parents and their native-born peers.[97] As marginal persons, they may feel rejected and alienated by one or both parents, by home, or by school.[98]

The struggles that the second generation experience are mostly due to the intermingling of Asian-Indian and Western values.[99] The identity conflict that results from balancing Indian culture and American culture leads to various labels for the halfway generation, including the American Born Confused *Desi* (ABCD complex—*Desi* means locals); the coconut generation (externally brown and internally white), *Chai* (Indian tea—a blend of brown extract from tea leaves and white milk), and Banana—externally yellow and internally white. The heart of the problem is that, although they were born and raised in America, the American majority culture still views them as foreigners and although they were not raised in India, they are expected to identify with and to be proficient in Indian culture.[100] Though these labels are simply descriptive and are used pejoratively, in my personal conversations with several ABCDs, many state with a sense of humor mixed with a sense of shame and anger that "we are not American-born *confused desies,* but we are American-born *confident desies.*"[101]

However, the situation in many families worsens as time passes and children learn local principles, which leads to mutual misunderstanding between generations. As Ravindra S. Johal notes, "it is commonly believed that the "culture clash" is prevalent in Asian-Indian youth in Canada too, with its originating source being home, school, and media. Such a divergence in beliefs, norms, and values is negatively impacting identity development among second-generation Asian-Indians."[102] The trend of the second-generation immigrants to fit more with their adopted Western culture increases the risk of intergenerational conflict within families. Unfortunately, such situations often lead to conflicts, as well as alcohol and drug use among Asian-Indian teenagers.[103] This particular group is unique as its members experience United States society at birth and they are never displaced from their country of birth.

Many second-generation Indian women attempt to understand and redefine themselves and their gender-roles in their families and their communities as they search for a bicultural identity.[104] These women who are born in America and grow up in that cultural context are also living amidst the values and practices of an Indian cultural background and history in their homes, which can lead to an ambiguous personal and cultural identity. Reaching bicultural adulthood can be difficult for anyone. It is even more difficult for children of immigrants who must reconcile conflicting gender influences.

Perhaps the most important area in which Indian-American young women struggle is the area of gender biases and stereotypes, such as the expectation that women will be dependent on their parents in childhood, on their husbands in adulthood, and on their children in old age. Women face a variety of difficulties, such as trying to gain equal status, removing language barriers, trying to find an identity, and battling with various stereotyped gender roles and unrealistic marital expectations.[105] Economic independence, along with an emphasis on individualism and unique social conditions in the United States, forces Indian women to re-examine their traditional gender roles in the context of a newly adopted mainstream American culture. When Indian women start changing from their passive and docile roles as wives at home and begin to be more active and independent, marital conflict looms large. When Indian women work, Indian men consider their new household responsibilities demeaning and an insult to their masculine identity and masculine roles. When changed gender roles generate marital conflicts, psychological stress increases due to the task of maintaining marital bonds.[106] Asian-Indian women living in the United States are particularly likely to experience cultural value conflicts between the more egalitarian gender role expectations in terms of decision-making in contrast to the traditional collectivistic Indian culture that requires strict adherence to hierarchical gender expectations. Women more often seek interracial marriage, which may be a result of the desire of second-generation women to avoid men who hold to traditional Indian female roles.

The effect of ambiguous personal and cultural identity is exacerbated for young Indian-American women when they are pressurized to be a dutiful and very "Indian" daughter at home. Researchers such as K. Ahmed and Gupta have argued that as a result of these dynamics, young women feel torn between individualism and the obligations they have towards their families. It has also been discovered that young South Asian-Indian women often feel as though they are living two very different lives as they resort to lying and hiding important aspects of their lives from their parents in order to actually have a life. This may lead to a sense of not feeling whole in either of their two worlds.[107]

The media's role in the socialization of Indian Americans also contributes to the backlash of Indian culture. The desire for whiteness is demonstrated in depth by a second-generation Asian-Indian activist and theatre artist, Sheila James. In her personal narrative, she chronicles how she unnaturally became a blond. As Poonam Arora quotes James, she says:

> Most of the actresses on TV, film and magazines were blond-haired and blue eyed. I figured I could adjust the color in my hair to fit the role. Underlying the desire for 'whiteness' is a racist ideology, which interprets the world associated with the dark skin of Indian and African people with danger, savagery, primitiveness, intellectual inferiority, and the inability to progress beyond a childlike mentality. Meanwhile whiteness is equated with purity, virginity, beauty, and civility.[108]

I also believe it is a part of the socially stereotyped understanding that white, is fair, superior, beautiful, and is the best; while black or dark is evil, not good, and inferior.

CONFLICTS OF CULTURAL VALUES

Cultural value conflict, according to Arpana Inman, Madonna Constantine, and Nicholas Ladany, is "an experience of negative affect (e.g., guilt or anxiety) and cognitive contradictions that result from contending simultaneously with the values and behavioral expectations that are internalized from the culture of origin (Asian-Indian culture) and the values and behavioral expectations imposed on the person from the new culture (white, American culture)."[109] The second-generation immigrants who are socialized or exposed to the double binds previously mentioned are often caught in cultural value conflicts as they bring the internalized American values, which are nuclear, egalitarian, and individualistic, into the Indian families where family harmony and interdependence are highly encouraged.

First-generation immigrants have experienced much of their socialization in India and, therefore, may feel less pressure to conform to Western values since Indian values have been internalized by them. They may find it easier to reconcile values from the host culture and culture of origin. Conversely, second-generation Asian-Indians who are born and raised in the United States may have more difficulty finding a balance between the two cultures. For them, the sensation of being the in-betweens is particularly accentuated. Like their parents, when the second-generation Asian-Indians compartmentalize their life, conflicts become inevitable from the cultural clash of American individualism versus Indian communitarianism as the two positions become polarized.[110] For instance, a second-generation Indian-American's desire to pursue an undergraduate degree in the fine arts will not be supported by the family. Career decisions are based on the impact upon the family's financial well-being, not the individual's interests. The conflict in practicing values and unfulfilled role expectations eventually leads to intergenerational conflicts at home. In this process, both first and second generations are left with feelings of betrayal, anger, and resentment. Efforts of second-generation children to question or clarify their parents' unfair demand or their own position are considered as acts of defiance or disloyalty and seen as destructive behavior resulting from the influence of "American culture."

Though shame and guilt exist in all cultures, and the emphasis on shame and guilt varies from culture to culture, most Asian cultures are predominantly shame-bound cultures, while most of the Western cultures are predominantly guilt-based cultures.[111] In Eastern cultures, the social consequence of "getting caught" is seen as more important than the individual's feeling. The experience of defilement or contamination is a bigger issue than depravity itself. In Western cultures, guilt seems to be more of an issue than shame. Guilt basically implies "I made a mistake," while shame implies "I *am* a mistake." If my behavior is wrong, I can correct and change it. However, if my very being is flawed, I am without hope for change. Guilt is a feeling that arises while we violate our conscience. Guilt cultures emphasize punishment and forgiveness as ways of restoring the moral order, while shame cultures stress self-denial and humility as ways of restoring the social order.[112]

A shame-based culture primarily emphasizes communal identity and values while a guilt-based culture primarily emphasizes individualistic identity and personal values. In shame-based cultures, one maintains self-respect not by choosing what is good over what is evil but by choosing what is expected of one. Shame is removed and honor restored only when a person does what society expects of him/her in the situation.[113] For second-generation immigrants, where both cultures converge, both guilt and shame are experienced. As they simultaneously and repeatedly live in between guilt- and shame-based cultures, their woes are multiplied. Their unique experience of being the emerging generation in a multicultural and postmodern world toughens their exteriors, but like all young adults, their inner cores are looking for meaningful relationships in order to discover themselves and their mission in this world. My research is a response to that "inner core of softness."

In conclusion, first generations (parents) strive to hold onto the culture and traditions that they brought to the West from India, while second generations' identification with modern, North American culture threatens the continuation of those traditions. Many families feel threatened by the thought that their culture may eventually diminish at the hands of their relatively more "Americanized" children. This, in essence, causes conflicts between parents and their children.[114] Researchers such as Gauri Bhattacharya,[115] and Romola Dugsin[116] have acknowledged that intergenerational conflict is the main issue in the experience of growing up South Asian in America. As Bhattacharya notes, "Studies indicate that the magnitude of intergenerational conflict is highest for first-generation immigrants from a "distant" culture and their second-generation children, who were born and socialized in the host culture."[117] In terms of dealing with this conflict, Portes and Rumbaut argue that the best and most successful strategy for the second generation is to follow what is referred to as a process of "selective acculturation" where they incorporate themselves into mainstream society while at the same time retaining portions of their parents' culture and remain connected to the family and the community.[118]

FAMILY FUNCTIONING

Traditionally, Indian families have been greatly influenced by a patriarchal, extended family system, with parents, grandparents, and other elders playing significant roles in socializing young children into culturally expected behaviors. Characteristically, a majority of Asian-Indian immigrant parents' relationship with their children is formal. That is, with regard to age and gender, communication and authority flow downward consistent with a hierarchical order of position and status. Asian-Indian parents accept their duty to care for their children, the children's reciprocated duty is to unquestionably respect and honor their parents. In this context, parents expect children to defer to parental wishes and to behave in ways that reflect well upon the family, including the extended family. A majority of Asian-Indian immigrant parents rely on the inculcation of guilt and shame to keep the children, regardless of age, focused on the importance of family obligation and to behave in ways that do not "bring shame" to the family. Accordingly, obligation to the family, based on "we" rather than "I" values, is the dominant philosophy that undergirds the life and values of the first-generation Asian-Indian immigrants.

Asian-Indian parenting practices typically include an authoritarian parenting style and emphasize academic achievement, familial bond, and solidarity (e.g., importance of family and respect for elders).[119] Because of the history of the caste system in the Asian-Indian culture, marriage within the same community and religion is encouraged. Dating is socially and culturally discouraged and premarital sexual relations are generally condemned. Since religion is considered as a means of transmitting cultural values, religious beliefs and activities play an important role in parenting practices. These beliefs and practices are often required implicitly, rather than explicitly, through a culturally determined learning process.[120] Like many other immigrant parents, Asian-Indian immigrants continue to emphasize specific values and goals for their second-generation children—values that were instilled during their own upbringing (e.g., pride in cultural heritage and familial interdependence). However, through the process of immigration, Asian-Indians experience a sense of displacement when the prescriptive parameters of their original environment no longer function within the new environment.

Living in a culturally incongruent community, first-generation parents perceive themselves as having the sole responsibility of imparting cultural values to their children, which results in restrictive behaviors by the parents.[121] Within this context, actively reproducing the traditional culture and establishing a cultural identity in their children become important parenting goals for these immigrants.[122] Indian immigrants raising a family in the United States face challenges of acculturation, assimilation, and socialization. It is observed that tensions are caused when homeland-oriented and tradition-bound first-generation immigrants attempt to impose their ideas and values on their increasingly Americanized children. Additionally, double standards for male and female offspring occur in most Asian-Indian households. Females are expected to assume gender-specific chores and duties (including cleaning and cooking), whereas males are not obliged to participate in household responsibilities. Das rightly points out that at no other time do the trials of the Asian-Indian immigrant family reach such severity as when it is involved in the socialization of its children, especially adolescents.[123] Culture conflict is experienced in a most turbulent way as the immigrant family tries to navigate its course through the usual tumult of raising adolescent children.[124] Hence, intergenerational, cultural conflicts are a chief source of strain among immigrating Asian-Indian parents and their children.

David A. Baptiste contends that the primary concerns that Indian immigrant parents experience in the United States are fear of losing children to the United States culture, loss of parental authority over children (including the ability to choose a spouse), and loss of face within the Asian-Indian community due to children's out-of-culture behaviors.[125] Segal, in her study, observes that parents perceived adolescents to be "rebellious" and "contaminated" by American culture when arguments arise about dating and gaining independence.[126] Conflict between parents and adolescents may be fairly normal and expected in American society. However, this concept is distressing for Asian-Indian immigrant parents who value interdependence, family harmony, and implicit obedience to authority.[127]

Studies of second-generation adolescents and adult immigrants, such as Segal's[128] and Dugsin's,[129] reveal experiences of family conflicts due to disagreements in areas such as parental control, poor communication, dating and marriage, educational excellence, and career choices. For instance, adolescents in Segal's study describe two issues that cause tension in the family: communication with parents is experienced as generally being one-sided, and Asian-Indian parents place pressure on their adolescents to excel and pursue only favorable careers.[130] In that study, several adolescents and young adults who were average achievers experienced low self-esteem or felt like failures for not being above-average achievers. Additionally, given the contrasting perspectives on love between American and Indian cultures, family conflicts in the area of marriage and dating are particularly salient within Asian-Indian families.[131]

Among Asian-Indian parents, complicated and almost contradictory strategies are used to reconcile cultural differences in parenting.[132] As mentioned earlier, compared to their counterparts in the dominant, white, middle-class American culture, Asian-Indian parents often exert stronger levels of parental control with their female children than with their male children. Stronger parental control may be a means by which parents attempt to reconcile intergenerational conflicts by not allowing their children to be exposed to American culture and friends. Females, however, may be exposed to stronger degrees of aversive (parental) control since they are traditionally seen as the preservers and transmitters of culture.[133]

Asian-Indian parents like to maintain authority over their children for the sake of emphasizing a strong emotional commitment to their families and to being Indian. To reproduce the dense matrix of relationships of their national cultures, Indian parents bind themselves to their children in sentimental systems of rights and duties. They expect their children to respect and obey their judgments about the host society and about India.[134] In doing this, Indian parents are conveying and reinforcing ideas of pride and respect. However, their second-generation children have an entirely different orientation and perspective on life, which clashes with the value expectation of their parents, resulting in family disharmony and conflict.

Though the idea of bicultural socialization is embraced to a certain extent by the first-generation immigrants, when traditional values are challenged, the second-generation immigrants are advised to steer clear of American culture. Usually, up until dating and mate selection become issues, most Indian parents, in an effort to ensure their children's success, encourage and aid their children in the utilization, internalization, and manifestation of American modes of behavior. This support is then directly contradicted when the children try to choose a mate, which is considered anti-Indian.

Thus, it is clear that the Asian-Indian population in the United States has split into generations. First-generation immigrants, of course, preserve more of their homeland flavor and traditions, while their children born in United States share only a certain part of their parents' cultures and are more assimilated into American culture. This obviously is a source of conflicts within families. Therefore, these second-generation experiences cannot be understood in isolation. Dynamics surrounding immigration and family experiences can significantly influence how parents socialize their children. Thus, understanding Asian-Indian parents' immigration experiences becomes imperative in contextualizing second-generation experiences. In Chap. 3, I discuss some of my personal observations on those issues that precipitate intergenerational conflicts within Asian-Indian immigrant families. Some of those points are also identified and supported by different authors, such as David Baptiste.[135]

NOTES

1. Parmatma Saran, *The Asian-Indian Experience in the United States* (Cambridge, MA: Schenkman Press, 1985), 26.

2. William Bentley, *The Diary of William Bentley* (Salem, MA: The Essex Institute, 1962), 228.

3. George P. Alexander, *New Americans: The Progress of Asian-Indians in America* (Cypress, CA: P & P Enterprises, 1997), 16.

4. Karen I. Leonard, *The South Asian Americans* (Westport, CT: Greenwood Press, 1997), 69.

5. Karen I. Leonard, *Making Ethnic Choices: California's Punjabi Mexican Americans* (Philadelphia, PA: Temple University Press, 1992), 113; Leonard, *The South Asian Americans,* 58.

6. S. Chandrasekar, ed., *From India to America: A Brief History of Immigration: Problems of Discrimination, Adaptation, and Assimilation* (La Jolla, CA: Population Review Publication, 1984), 63.

7. John F. Kennedy, message to Congress on July 23, 1963, quoted in M. N. Srinivas, *Social Change in Modern India* (Berkley, CA: University of California Press, 1966), 139.

8. Sam George, *Coconut Generation: Ministry to the Americanized Asian-Indians* (Niles, IL: Mall Publishing Co., 2006), 22.

9. Timothy Fong, *The Contemporary Asian American Experience: Beyond the Model Minority* (Englewood Cliffs, NJ: Prentice Hall, 2002), 73.

10. Meena Sharma, *Walking a Cultural Divide: The Lived Experiences of Second Generation Asian-Indian Females in Canada and the United States* (Detroit, MI: Wayne State University, 2008), 24; Leonard, *The South Asian Americans.*

11. Paul M. Ong, Lucie Cheng, and Leslie Evans, "Migration of Highly Educated Asians and Global Dynamics," *Asian and Pacific Migration Journal* 1, nos. 3–4 (1992): 545.

12. Census Bureau of United States, 2000, Figures 9 and 12, http://www.census.gov/prod/2002pubs/c2kbr01-16.pdf (accessed March 10, 2012).

13. Sunita Sohrabji, "Indian Americans Most Educated, Richest, Says Pew Report," *India West,* June 29, 2012.

14. Ibid.

15. Elizabeth Gutierrez, "The Dotbuster Attacks: Hate Crime against Asian-Indians in Jersey City, New Jersey," *Middle States Geographer 1996,* 30–38 http://geographyplanning.buffalostate.edu/MSG%201,996/5_Gutierrez.pdf (accessed August 29, 2012).

16. George, *Coconut Generation.* 26.

17. "Indian Americans Third Largest Asian Community in US," *South Asian Chronicle,* March 30, 2012.

18. Ibid.
19. "Indian Origin People Close to Being in 100 Americans," *South Asian Chronicle*, April 6, 2012.
20. Ibid.
21. Gordon C. Nagayama Hall and Sumie Okazaki, eds., *Asian American Psychology: The Science of Lives in Context* (Washington, DC: American Psychological Association, 2002), 5.
22. Jean S. Phinney and Linda Line Alpuria, "Ethnic Identity in Older Adolescents from Four Ethnic Groups," (paper presented at the biennial meeting of the Society for Research in Child Development, Baltimore, MD, April 30, 1987), 36.
23. Ibid.
24. Mao Sotomayor, "Language, Culture, Ethnicity in Developing Self-Concept," *Social Case Work* 111, no. 4 (1997): 195.
25. Fong. 27.
26. Donald R. Atkinson and Ruth H. Gim, "Asian American Cultural Identity and Attitudes towards Mental Health Services." *Journal of Counseling Psychology* 36, no. 2 (1989): 210.
27. Sudhir Kakar, *The Inner World: A Psychoanalytic Study of Childhood and Society in India* (Delhi: Oxford University Press, 1978), 120–122.
28. V. Dhruvarajan, "Ethnic Cultural Retention and Transmission among First Generation Hindu Asian-Indians in Canadian Prairie City," *Journal of Comparative Family Studies* 24, no. 1 (Spring 1993): 67; V. M. Ranganath and V. K. Ranganath, "Asian-Indian Children" in *Transcultural Child Development: Psychological Assessment and Treatment*, eds. William Arroyo, Gloria Johnson-Powell, Joe Yamamoto, and Gail Wyatt (New York, NY: John Wiley & Sons, 1997), 36–50.
29. Parmatma Saran and E. Eames, *The New Ethnics: Asian-Indians in the United States* (New York, NY: Praeger, 1991), 31; U. Segal, "Cultural variables in Asian-Indian Families," *Families in Society* 72, no. 4 (1991): 233–241.
30. Sudhir Kakar, *Identity and Adulthood* (Delhi: Oxford University Press, 1992). x–xi
31. Sudhir Kakar, *Culture and Psyche: Selected Essays*, 2nd ed. (Delhi: Oxford University Press, 2007), 22.
32. Sunaina Maira, *Desis in the House: Indian American Youth Culture in NYC* (Philadelphia, PA: Temple University Press 1969), quoted in Lavina Melwani, "Forging an Indian American Identity: How Authentic an Indian Are You?" *Little India*, October 31, 1995.
33. Tony, O'Sullivan, *Asian-American Affairs: A Face Saved is a Face Earned* (New York, NY: Russell Sage, 1999), 7.
34. Ibid.

35. Ibid.
36. T.A. Kulanjiyil, "Landscape: Mental Health Needs of South Asian-Indians," in *Caring for the South Asian Soul*, ed. T.A. Kulanjiyil and D.V. Thomas (Bangalore: Primalogue), 22.
37. Clifford Geertz, "Myth, Symbol and Culture," *Journal of the American Academy of Arts and Sciences* 101, no.1 (Winter, 1972):169.
38. George P. Alexander, *New Americans: The Progress of Asian-Indians in America* (Cypress, CA: P&P Enterprises, 1997), 33.
39. Alexander, *New Americans: The Progress of Asian-Indians in America*, 34.
40. Kulanjiyil, "Landscape: Mental Health Needs of South Asian-Indians," 22.
41. George. *Coconut Generation*, 36.
42. See footnote 5, Chap. 1 for clarification.
43. Saran P. *The Asian-Indian Experience in the United States*, 43. Also see footnote 2 in this chapter.
44. R. S. Durvasalu and G. A. Mylvaganam, "Mental Health of Asian-Indians: Relevant Issues and Community Implications," *Journal of Community Psychology* 22, no. 2 (April, 1994): 97–108.
45. Segal, "Cultural Variables in Asian-Indian Families," 234.
46. E. Prathikanti, "East Indian Families," in *Working with Asian Americans: A Guide for Clinicians*, ed. Evelyn Lee (New York, NY: Guilford Press, 1997), 113–125; U. Segal, "Asian-Indian Families," in *Ethnic Families in America: Patterns and Variations*, eds. C. Mindel, R. Habenstein, and R. Wright, Jr. (Upper Saddle River, NJ: Prentice Hall, 1998), 331–360.
47. Segal, "Asian-Indian Families," 335.
48. Ranganath and Ranganath, "Asian-Indian Children," 107.
49. Dhruvarajan, "Ethnic Cultural Retention and Transmission among First Generation Hindu Asian-Indians in Canadian Prairie City," 65.
50. Ranganath and Ranganath, "Asian-Indian Children," 105.
51. Segal, "Asian-Indian Families," 336.
52. K. Ahmed, "Adolescent Development for South Asian American Girls," in *Emerging Voices: South Asian American Women Redefine Self, Family and Community*, ed. S.R. Gupta (Walnut Creek, CA: Alta Mira Press, 1999), 37–49; Saigeetha Jambunathan, Diane C. Burts, and Sarah Pierce, "Comparison of Parenting Attitudes Among Five Ethnic Groups in the United States," *Journal of Comparative Family Studies* 31 no. 4 (Autumn, 2000): 395–406.
53. Jambunathan, Burts, and Pierce. "Comparison of Perception of Self-Competence among Five Ethnic Groups of Preschoolers in the United States," 562.
54. Ahmed, "Adolescent Development for South Asian American Girls," 37.
55. Segal, "Asian-Indian Families," 337.

56. Durvas Ramani, Suryakantham Durvasula, and Gaithri A. Mylvaganam, "Mental Health of Asian-Indians: Relevant Issues and Community Implications," 98.
57. Jambunathan, Burts, and Pierce, "Comparison of Perception of Self-Competence among Five Ethnic Groups of Preschoolers in the United States," 651–660.
58. Ahmed, "Adolescent Development for South Asian American Girls," 38.
59. A. K. Das and S. F. Kemp, "Between Two Worlds: Counseling South Asian Immigrants," *Journal of Multicultural Counseling and Development* 25, no. 1 (January, 1997): 23–34.
60. D. Baptiste, "Family Therapy with East Indian Immigrant Parents Rearing Children in the United States: Parental Concerns, Therapeutic Issues, and Recommendations," *Contemporary Family Therapy, An International Journal* 27, no. 3 (September, 2005): 345–366.
61. Saran, Eames and Prathikanti, *The New Ethnics: Asian-Indians in the United States*, 235.
62. Uma A. Segal, "Cultural Variables in Asian-Indian Families," 236.
63. S. Dasgupta, "Gender Roles and Cultural Continuity in the Asian-Indian Immigrant Community in the United States," 955.
64. Segal, "Asian-Indian Families," 338.
65. S. Gupta, "Forged by Fire: Indian-Americans Reflect on Their Marriages, Divorces, and on Rebuilding Lives, in *Emerging Voices: South Asian American Women Redefine Self, Family, and Community*, ed. S. R. Gupta (Walnut Creek, CA: AltaMira Press, 1999). 193–221.
66. Saran and Eames, *New Ethnics Asian-Indian in the United States*. 236.
67. Jambunathan, Burts, and Pierce, "Comparison of Perception of Self-competence Among Five Ethnic Groups of Preschoolers in the United States," 653.
68. M. J. Sala, *"The Conflict between Collectivism and Individualism in Adolescent Development: Asian-Indian Female Decision-Making in Regard to Cultural Normative Behavior,"* (PhD dissertation, Loyola University, Chicago, 2002).
69. *India West*, June 29, 2012.
70. Segal, "Asian-Indian Families," 339.
71. G. Inman, M. G. Constantine, and N. Ladany, "Cultural Value Conflict: An Examination of Asian-Indian Women's Bicultural Experience", in *Asian and Pacific Islander Americans: Issues and Concerns for Counseling and Psychotherapy*, ed. D.S. Sandhu (New York, NY: Nova Science Publishers, 1999).
72. Segal, "Cultural Variables in Asian-Indian Families," 238.

73. Jambunathan, Burts, and Pierce, "Comparison of Perception of Self-competence among Five Ethnic Groups of Preschoolers in the United States," 654.

74. Phillip Abrams, "The Historical Sociology of Individuals: Identity and the Problem of Generations," in *Historical Sociology*, ed. Phillip Abram (Ithaca, NY: Cornell University Press, 1982), 255.

75. Ibid.

76. George, *Coconut Generation*, 38–39.

77. Ibid.

78. Prema A. Kurien, "Being Young, Brown, and Hindu: The Identity Struggles of the Second Generation Indian Americans," *Journal of Contemporary Ethnography* 34, no. 4 (August, 2005): 434–369.

79. Y. L. Espiritu, *Asian American Men and Women Love, Labor, Laws* (Thousand Oaks, CA: Sage Publications, 1997); M. Zhou, "Are Asian Americans Becoming 'White'?" *Contexts* 3, no. 1 (Winter, 2004): 29–37.

80. Dasgupta, "Gender Roles and Cultural Continuity in the Asian-Indian Immigrant Community in the United States." 956.

81. Balasubramaniam. *The Relationship between Ethnic Identity, Self-Concept and Acculturation in Asian-Indian Adolescence*, 25.

82. Ibid.

83. Min Zhou. "Are Asian Americans Becoming White? 31.

84. R. Gawle, "Desi Chameleon: Gen X Indian Americans Need the Right Blend of East and West," *India Abroad*, November 22, 2002; Hedge, 318.

85. Hedge, M. Hanson, E. Lynch, and K. Wayman, "Honoring the Cultural Diversity of Families When Gathering Data," *Topics in Early Childhood Special Education* 10, no.1 (Spring, 1990): 112–131.

86. Dasgupta, "Gender Roles and Cultural Continuity in the Asian-Indian Immigrant Community in the United States," *Sex Roles. A Journal of Research* 38, nos. 11/12 (November, 1998): 953–975; A. Portes and R. Rambaut, *Legacies: The Story of the Immigrant Second Generation* (Berkley, CA: University of California Press, 2001; R. S. Johal, "The World is Ours: Second Generation South Asians Reconcile Conflicting Expectations," (Masters thesis, York University, 2002).

87. V. Balasubramaniam, "The Relationship between Ethnic Identity, Self-Concept and Acculturation in Asian-IndianAdolescents," (PhD diss., University of Houston, 2005), 24.

88. Ronald Takaki, *Strangers from a Different Shore: A History of Asian Americans* (Toronto, CA: Little Brown & Co., 1998), 215.

89. George, *Coconut Generation*, xv.

90. Radha S. Hedge, "Translated Enactments: The Relational Configurations of the Asian-Indian Immigrant Experience," in *Reading in Cultural*

Contexts, eds. J. Martin T. Nakayama and L. Flores (Mountain View, CA: Mayfield, 1998), 318.

91. Chen, "Shaping a Philippine-Chinese American Identity," *Filipino Reporter,* July 24, 1997.
92. Laura Uba, *Asian Americans: Personality Patterns, Identity and Mental Health* (New York, NY: Guildford Press, 1994).
93. Tom, in an interview with the author, Dallas, TX, February 25, 2011.
94. Thomas Kulanjiyil, "Landscape: Mental Health Needs of South Asian-Indians," in *Caring for the South Asian Souls: Counseling South Asians in the Western World,* eds. Thomas Kulanjiyil and T. V. Thomas (Bangalore: Primalogue Publishing & Media, 2010), 26.
95. Robert T. Carter, *The Influence of Race and Racial Identity in Psychotherapy: Toward a Racially Inclusive Model* (New York, NY: John Wiley & Sons, Inc., 1995), 51.
96. Chen, "Shaping a Philippine-Chinese American Identity," 19.
97. J. H. Taylor, *The Halfway Generation: A Study of Asian Youth in Newcastle Upon Tyne* (Atlantic Highlands, NJ: Humanities Press, 1976).
98. Ibid.
99. Ravindra S. Johal, *The World is Ours: Second Generation South Asians Reconcile Conflicting Expectations,* 5.
100. Jamie Matthew, "Trials: Children of Post-1965 Indian Immigrants" (fifth article of a five-part summary series) http://thekkattil.net/documents/1093377989_content.pdf (accessed December 12, 2012).
101. Interviews with the author on various dates.
102. Ravindra S. Johal, *The World is Ours: Second Generation South Asians Reconcile Conflicting Expectations,* 36.
103. Ibid.
104. Sharma, *Walking a Cultural Divide,* 55–56.
105. Leela Cherian, "Hitting Out: Violent Behaviors in Asian-Indian American Homes" in *Caring for the South Asian Soul: Counseling South Asians in the Western World,* eds. Thomas Kulanjiyil and T. V. Thomas (Bangalore: Primalogue, 2010), 48.
106. Ibid.
107. K Ahmed, "Adolescent Development for South Asian American Girls." *in Emerging Voices: South Asian American Women Redefine Self, Family and Community,* ed. S. R. Gupta (Walnut Creek, CA: Alta Mira Press, 1999), 37–49.
108. P. Arora, "Imperiling the Prestige of the White Woman: Colonial Anxiety and Film Censorship in India," *Visual Anthropology Review* 11, no. 2 (June 1995): 18.

109. Arpana G. Inman, Nicholas Ladany, and Madonna G. Constantine. "Cultural Value Conflict: An Examination of Asian-Indian Women's Bicultural Experience," 32.

110. Monica McGolderick, ed., *Revisioning Family Therapy: Race, Culture and Gender in Clinical Practice* (New York, NY: The Guildford Press, 1998), 370.

111. Paul G. Herbert, *Anthropological Insight for Missionaries* (Grand Rapids, MI: Baker Book House, 1985), 213.

112. Ibid.

113. Ibid., 212.

114. Dasgupta Shamita Das, "Gender roles and cultural continuity in the Asian-Indian Immigrant Community in the United States," *Sex Roles: A Journal of Research* Vol. 38, no. 11/12 (June, 1998): 953–975.

115. G. Bhatacharya, "Drug Use among Asian-Indian Adolescents: Identifying Protective/Risk Factors," *Adolescence* 33, no. 129 (1998): 169–84.

116. Romolo Dugsin, "Conflict and Healing in Family Experience of Second-Generation Emigrants from India Living in North America," *Family Process* 40, no. 2 (Summer 2001): 233–41.

117. Bhatacharya, "Drug Use Among Asian-Indian Adolescents: Identifying Protective/risk Factors", 177.

118. Ruban G. Rumbaut and Alejandro Portes, *Ethnicities: Children of Immigrants in America* (London, UK: University of California Press, Ltd., 2001), 44–69.

119. S. Jambunathan and K. P. Counselman, "Parenting Attitude of Asian-Indian Mothers Living in the United States and in India," *Early Child Development and Care* 172, no. 6 (December, 2002): 659.

120. Terry Arendel, *Contemporary Parenting: Challenges and Issues* (Thousand Oaks, CA: Sage, 1997), 16.

121. Sodowsky Gargi Roysircar and Carey John C., "Relationships between Acculturation-Related Demographics and Cultural Attitudes of an Asian-Indian Immigrant Group," *Journal of Multicultural Counseling and Development* 16, no. 3 (July, 1988): 117–136.

122. Vanaja Dhruvarajan, "Relationships between Acculturation-Related Demographics and Cultural Ethnic Cultural Retention and Transmission among First Generation Hindu Asian-Indians in a Canadian Prairie City," *Journal of Comparative Family Studies* 24, no. 1 (Spring, 1993): 63–79.

123. Das and Kemp, "Between Two Worlds: Counseling South Asian Immigrants," 23–24

124. Ibid.

125. Baptiste. "Family Therapy with East Indian Immigrant Parents Rearing Children in the United States: Parental Concerns, Therapeutic Issues and Recommendations." 347.

126. Segal, "Cultural Variables in Asian-Indian Families," 240.
127. Ibid.
128. Ibid.
129. Romolo Dugsin, "Conflict and Healing in Family Experience of Second-Generation Immigrants from India Living in North America," *Family Process* 40, no. 2 (Summer, 2001): 233–241.
130. Segal, "Cultural Variables in Asian-Indian Families," 239.
131. Dugsin, "Conflict and Healing in Family Experience of Second-Generation Immigrants from India Living in North America," 235.
132. Mallika Chopra, *100 Promises to My Baby* (Emmaus, PA: Rodale Inc., 2005).
133. R. Shams and R. Williams, "Differences in Perceived Parental Care and Protection and Related Psychological Distress between British Asian and Non-Asian Adolescents," *Journal of Adolescence* 18, no. 3. (June, 1995): 329–348.
134. Shamita Das Dasgupta "Gender Roles and Cultural Continuity in the Asian-Indian Immigrant Community in the United States," 966.
135. Baptiste, "Family Therapy with East Indian Immigrant Parents Rearing Children in the United States," 351–357.

CHAPTER 3

Cultural Identity and Intergenerational Conflicts

SOURCES OF INTERGENERATIONAL CONFLICTS: MAJOR OBSERVATIONS

In the previous chapter I examined some of the sources of and differences between the cultural values of first and second-generation Indian immigrants. Based on the literature review and on my own observations and experience, I offer here a description of some of the sources of intergenerational conflicts, first from the perspective of first-generation Indian immigrants and then from the perspective of second-generation immigrants. These identified sources of conflict and instruments used to measure intergenerational conflicts among other ethnic communities, such as Korean and Chinese immigrants, shaped the survey instrument used to measure intergenerational conflicts among the Asian-Indian immigrant community in the United States. The result of this survey is reported in Chap. 4 (also see Appendix).

Drawing on my pastoral, educational, and pastoral counseling experience, I have identified the following points as the major factors that create intergenerational conflicts in the families. Some of the points are also noted by family therapist David Baptiste. My observations are primarily from two perspectives, as there are multiple generations involved in these conflicts, such as the first-generation parental perspective and the second-generation immigrant perspective, as briefly explained in the following section.

© The Author(s) 2017
V. Jacob, *Counseling Asian Indian Immigrant Families*,
DOI 10.1007/978-3-319-64307-6_3

Fear of Losing Children to the American Culture

Generally, most Asian-Indian immigrant parents tend to be optimistic about the United States and the many opportunities it offers to them and to their children. However, they fear that their children, who are exposed to the American culture and absorb it as a means for their survival, will abandon the family/cultural values of their birth. This creates in parents the strong fear of potentially losing their children to the United States culture, for the first-generation parents often equate conformity to their traditional cultural values with family loyalty. Consequently, children's departure from the visible markers of the family's ethnic identity, parental cultural expectations, and values is perceived by parents as undeniable proof that they have lost their children to the United States culture, which strikes at the heart of the family's value system. This generates in first-generation parents the fear of a family's death, as they are unable to retain and pass on their cultural values to the next generation. For those parents, family means holding their family members together for a meaningful life by means of their idealized ethnic cultural values. When this does not happen, the parents are irritated, frustrated, and feel disrespected, rejected, abandoned, and isolated as they lose their children, family pride, and family's reputation in a strange community and country.

Loss of Parental Authority over Children

In the Asian-Indian cultural understanding, even today parents are living for the sake of their children. Even though there may be several adjustment problems between husbands and wives, couples typically stay married— not only to avoid the social stigma of divorce, but also for the sake of their children. Parents sacrifice their time, talent, and treasure for the material and educational growth of their children. Many parents hold more than two jobs in order to educate and enhance their children's lives. This sacrificial life of parents also forces them to set high standards and expectations for their children. However, such Asian-Indian parents rearing children in the United States become aware of two very painful post-immigration facts of life: in the United States there are vastly different rules for parenting children, and the new rules significantly lessen their general authority over their children. As a result, these parents often feel "less like a parent" raising children within the United States cultural context, often wondering if they are in charge of their children or their children are in charge of them.

Though Asian-Indian fathers tend to experience the greatest difficulties with the loss of their absolute authority over their children, both mothers and fathers complain that parental authority appears to be less important to children in the United States than in their specific native country. The young South Asians who are insulated and overprotected from the culture at large (but have grown up in a more egalitarian cultural context, questioning authority and expecting logical reasoning for parental actions) may be judged by the older generation as rebellious.[1] In this context parents consciously or unconsciously become angry toward and frustrated about the American culture. They feel that the American culture is loose, free, and not fit to discipline children. The reaction to this feeling is an increased inclination toward and closeness to ethnic culture and an irrational, unconscious, and unresolved anger toward the American culture.

Loss of Authority to Discipline Children

Many Asian-Indian parents feel constrained in terms of their authority over and right to discipline their children "appropriately" consistent with the usual and acceptable modes of disciplining children in their native country. Invariably, parents discover that rules for disciplining children are among the many rules that are different for parenting children within the United States cultural context. In their native country, many Asian-Indian parents used disciplinary practices that, by United States standards, are considered harsh and even abusive (e.g., some forms of physical and verbal punishments, such as inculcation of guilt and shame). Consequently, disciplinary methods acceptable and appropriate in their native country to achieve the desired disciplinary outcomes are unacceptable and inappropriate in the United States. Therefore, Asian-Indian parents believe that the "American expectations and rules" disregard and devalue their indigenous cultural beliefs, rules, and expectations for family interactions (such as disciplining children) and leave them without effective means of disciplining. This experience leads the Asian-Indian parents to be overwhelmingly cautious in disciplining their children in the United States because of their unfamiliarity with other disciplinary methods and their fear of breaking the law.

Loss of Authority in Selecting Children's Mates

Asian-Indian immigrant families in the United States represent a diversity of dialects, religions, and cultures. But based on their common Indian cultural values, a majority of Asian-Indian parents see it as their responsibility to select mates and decide who their Asian-Indian children will marry. Consequently, the loss of authority in selecting their children's mates is one of the more troubling concerns for most Asian-Indian immigrant parents in the United States. Arranged marriages continue to be the norm in India, though the cultural practice of arranged marriages among Asian-Indians is in transition due to globalization and the influence of Western media and culture. Notwithstanding the decline in the practice, a majority of Asian-Indian parents, irrespective of the family's caste and religious affiliation, continue to endorse arranged marriages for their young adult children. In this regard, Yao reports that the Indian-American parents she interviewed in Texas continued to arrange their children's marriages even though at the time of interviews many of the families had lived in the United States for more than a decade.[2]

Among Asian-Indian immigrants, caste and religious affiliation are intimately related to the practice of arranged marriages. Potential marital partners rarely, if ever, are chosen from a different religious sect. In this regard, in Asian-Indian communities, if there are few or no eligible candidates (by religion and class) with whom to arrange a marriage for a child, parents, along with their marriageable children, may visit their native country to seek a spouse. Some parents may even "import" a potential spouse for a child from their country of origin. This tends to be truer in the case of wives than husbands.[3] In the United States, however, most Asian-Indian adolescents and young adults object to and reject arranged marriages. Instead, they insist upon selecting, dating, and eventually marrying someone of their own choosing, based on the American notion of romantic love.

Parents complain that children's refusal to accept an arranged marriage is a rejection of them and their values and negatively reflects upon them as parents within the Asian-Indian community. Parents also reference the progressively increasing divorce rate among younger Asian-Indian immigrants, worrying about their children's ability to "make a good marriage." When children insist on "self-arranged" marriage, it is a source of gossip and is reported among the parental community, even in their native villages. This, in turn, brings great social stigma, shame, and guilt upon their entire family. As a result, immigrant parents lose face in their community.

LOSS OF FAMILY FACE DUE TO CHILDREN'S UNCONVENTIONAL BEHAVIORS

Within the Asian-Indian community, parents are held responsible for their children's behaviors, and poor behavior on their children's part reflects negatively upon them as their conventional beliefs and social community norms hold that children are responsible to enhance family pride by honoring their parents through appropriate behaviors and outstanding accomplishments. For many Asian-Indian parents, their primary reference group continues to be family and friends in India and in the Indian immigrant community social groups. Vijay Prasad, author of *The Karma of Brown Folk,* suggests in an interview that

> The high standards are reinforced by relentless parental and community pressure to conform. South Asian young people, who don't conform to the myth, deny their parents' access to the power centers of the community: joining the chamber of commerce, becoming a leader in the temple or heading a community organization. The pressure on the child is enormous and the parents suffer the embarrassment of their children not being the performing animals of their community.[4]

Consequently, when children behave unconventionally (e.g., reject an arranged marriage, become Americanized, etc.), parents invariably complain that such behaviors dishonor them as "Asian-Indian parents" and devalue their standing as "Asian-Indians" within the Asian-Indian community. This makes the Asian-Indian parents feel that they are bad parents and irretrievably shamed, which leads to a sense of low self-worth, rejection, isolation, abandonment, and failure in life. Many parents have asked me in despair, "Why should I live after being a failure in life to save my children?" These concerns contribute to inter-generational stresses and conflicts that fuel parents' intense need to control their children's behaviors, especially out-of-culture behaviors.

Out-of-culture behaviors are behaviors that deviate from the usual and customary community norms and culturally specific behaviors of a group of people. According to Baptiste, behaviors such as changes in dietary habits (a strict Brahmin's eating steak, a Muslim eating ham) marrying across caste and race, intercaste marriage, females wearing clothing that is deemed to be too sexy, teenage and unwed pregnancy, over-aged unmarried children (especially females), cohabiting, and children becoming "too

Americanized" are all deemed out-of-culture behavior.[5] Typically, Asian-Indian families in the United States, both recent and settled immigrants, irrespective of their religion, live in communities heavily populated by fellow Asian-Indians. Members of these "Asian-Indian communities" provide active social support for each other as they navigate the post-immigration transitional/adjustment period, and often function as surrogate support networks in lieu of the pre-emigration extended family support networks that were disrupted when the family immigrated to the United States. Additionally, community members function as unofficial arbiters of appropriate, expected, and acceptable cultural and moral standards by which community members, in particular parents, are evaluated.

Accordingly, community members are often confronted with an unwritten, but expected standard of acceptable/appropriate conduct required for members to remain in "good standing" as Asian-Indians or, more importantly, "good Asian-Indian parents." Intentionally or not, the social interactions and public behaviors of families in these communities, including children, often are evaluated relative to a family's perceived social class (including caste) and status. Predictably, children, especially young adults, often complain of feeling restrained and being caught in a bind—parents wanting them to succeed in America, but simultaneously wanting them to remain in all ways Asian-Indian.

Family Dignity Over Individual Autonomy

When a second-generation immigrant is found not fitting into the normative frame of their parents' culture, it is gossiped about, discussed, and spread among the Asian-Indian community and damages parents' worth as it is measured by their children's education, success, and adherence to Indian values.[6] This experience, in turn, insults, isolates, disrespects and ostracizes the first-generation parents in the social, religious, and political communities where they lose face. Then, the first-generation immigrants impose and reinforce their cultural values on their children, exerting parental authority to save the family's reputation. Consequently, most second-generation immigrants remain outside the dominant system—the culture and community of their parents. This labels them as rebellious and they feel taunted and rejected. Rather than finding ways to connect and relate to others, many of them withdraw into their personal space, suffering rejection and isolation. They often find alternative ways to exist and create their own internal world of fantasies and revenge as they are not welcomed into the space of either the dominant American society or of their parents' immigrant society. This leads to greater levels of confusion, emotional stress, frustration, depression, and identity crisis for these "rebels."

Those who are emotionally disconnected often distance themselves physically, moving away from their parental homes and community. This act of "moving out and moving at a distance"[7] creates an enormous stress for parents, as unmarried family members moving out and "moving at a distance" from the parental home without proper reasons (e.g., education, job, or marriage) is further cause for gossip and stigmatization. If a young adult moves out of his/her parental home before marriage, it is typically perceived as a sign of a family clash. When first-generation parents exert parental authority over their children to establish family dignity and save their face in the community, second-generation immigrants often get offended and aggravated. The second-generations often withdraw into an inner world where they become both the insider and the outsider, with complete control over that inner world and not allowing anyone to invade that space.

Due to the rejection they experience by the larger society that leads to their reclusive behavior of exclusion inside their own space, they become precisely the figure that they hate in the dominant culture. Thus, they restrict the access of others to their inner space and enlarge it by engaging with their own ideas and fantasies, creating enemies within their space. In other words, family—the core value and center of the identity of the first-generation immigrants—often does not function as a strong support system to second-generation Asian-Indian immigrants as they try to resist peer pressure and learn from the family. The futility of reaching into the cultural space of their parents leads them, naturally, to withdraw into their peer group or into their own personal space. This is where the importance of a meaningful relationship with a pastoral counselor/therapist comes in a therapeutic space of communication.

THE SURVIVAL MECHANISM OF SECOND-GENERATION ASIAN-INDIANS

The chief pursuits of first-generation immigrants are economic advancement and providing opportunities for their children. Hence, they are found emotionally distant from the dominant host culture and more attached to their home culture. But the existence of the second generation brings about a series of painful adjustments and the constant juggling of two worlds as bifurcated between the land of their parents and the land of their birth. They are pulled in one direction at home and another at school. They barely speak their ancestral language in their homes. They learn about America at school and about India at home. At school they learn about the American ideals of freedom and individualism while at home they are taught about duty and role expectations.

The language predicament, academic difficulties, alienation from American peers, perception based on skin color, lack of confidence, need for affirmation, parental expectation, cultural and religious norms, finding friends, choosing a career, finding love/a spouse, a God worth following, and a faith community of which to be a part all make their lives extremely challenging. These experiences differentiate them from the rest of their kind.

However, these second-generations are both different and the same. They are different from their parents, relatives, and from their peers. They often seem identity-less and squeezed in between Indian and American cultures, living in between the dominant Western and immigrant cultures. They are at the periphery, the margin, and this creates an identity crisis for them. Since they are born and living between two or more cultures, their unique social environment forms different characteristics and behaviors.

At the same time, they are also like other Indians. As Lartey rightly points out, like every other human person, second-generations in certain aspects are like all others, like some others, and like no others.[8] I think it is better to acknowledge and affirm their uniqueness rather than emphasize their differences so that they may not be pushed further outside into the marginal space of the dominant societies.

People who hold power and play with the power dynamics often create a normative frame and decide who the insiders are and who the outsiders are, which makes the second-generation immigrants "emotional refugees." This is true both in the dominant Western culture and in the immigrant culture. When these "power holders" often describe the second generation as "rebellious," they ignore that their experiences are adaptive and part of a larger experience. Living in the marginal space of culture and society negatively affects identity; it impairs one's own sense of self, causes low self-esteem, and leads to further self-alienation and self-marginalizing. It limits the person's ability to explore possibilities and to connect and interact by putting them in a static place. Thus, their life remains stagnant as they are unable to open themselves to numerous potential directions and multiple ways. When parents see this happening with their children, some first-generation Indians seem to detach helplessly, which is often interpreted as "adults who don't care." Others go to the opposite extreme and excessively interfere in the lives of their children, causing young people to lose respect for adults, reject their values, and ultimately swing wildly towards radical narcissism.

The second generation seems to exhibit a double minority syndrome. They suffer from double marginalization, first on account of their ethnicity and secondly due to generational differences. They become a minority within a minority in the multiethnic, multicultural world of the United States. The model minority syndrome is also negatively affecting the emerging generations. It sets both unrealistic expectations and artificial precedents to emulate. This only aggravates the unpleasant tension between the generations. Further, the inability to handle failure and attain goals prescribed by parents and community increases the pain of failure. This results in perpetual conflicts, extreme rebellion, physical abuse, absconding from home, and, in certain cases, teenage suicide.[9] Counselors and psychotherapeutic rooms are safe spaces for these people and can allow them emotional catharsis and help them achieve relational development.

Issues Relating to Ethnic Identities

When people from different cultures interact, their internalized beliefs are re-examined from the perspective of the dominant culture. Generally, those encounters threaten one's sense of belonging to a particular ethnic group, raises questions about cultural loyalties and casts many doubts about one's social and psychological support systems. One may feel caught between two conflicting worlds, behaving in one way at home and in another way outside. This results in a person having two totally different identities. This fragmentation of identity becomes the source of severe psychological pain. According to Augsburger,

> The uprooting of the village person leads to fragmentation of the personality as well. The movement from the solidarity of an organically connected community to the isolation of an urban metropolis leaves persons with a sociocentric self-organization consciously (and to a far extent unconsciously) incomplete, isolated from their sources of life, severed from their essential values.[10]

For Asian-Indians, the change in essential values is felt more in the migration to countries that have a culture that promotes individualistic focus.

Acculturative Stress

In the process of acculturating, both first- and second-generation immigrants are negatively affected.[11] While parents worry more about cultural erosion, their children suffer from cultural confusion. If parents are strangers in the stores and public places, their children are strangers at home. In the process of renegotiating identities in acculturation, peoples' identities never remain intact. Rather, they either become hybrid or hyphenated. Sandhu, Portes, and McPhee identify at least six major elements of acculturation: perceived discrimination, homesickness, perceived hate, fear, stress due to culture shock, and guilt for leaving loved ones behind.[12] Adaptation to societal norms, cultural values, and daily behaviors of the prevailing group constantly cause inevitable psychological stress and problems for members of acculturating groups.[13] As a result, threats to cultural identity, feelings of rejecting one's cultural values, powerlessness, feelings of marginality, a sense of inferiority, loneliness, hostility, perceived alienation, hopelessness for the future, perceived estrangement from one's native group, and discrimination become major mental health concerns.[14]

Poor Communication Pattern

Societal structure, perceived understanding, cultural identity, and bias prevent adequate and necessary intercultural dialogue between parents and children, as well as with the larger society. As a result, many second-generation immigrants are lonely, even amidst people, and are isolated within a community. The first-generation parents who came to the United States with a dream of economic prosperity and better living are often engaged with their work. Many people work multiple shifts in order to provide for their family and children. For the first-generation immigrants, earning money and meeting the physical and educational needs of their children are the primary concerns. In the midst of their busy life and consumed by the desire to provide materially for their children, these parents often forget or ignore their children's emotional needs and fail to engage in open communication required for developing and maintaining meaningful relationships. In that context, communication often becomes one-sided.

Discussions on many of the psychological and emotional needs are often excluded from home life. For instance, American children learn about safe sex in schools and parents often talk about sexual health with their children. This is not customary in Indian families. Parents or elders do not talk about sex with children. It is a common belief that HIV/AIDS is the problem of gays, sex workers, and drug-users. Since they are sure their children do not use drugs and do not have sex before marriage, first-generation parents think it is not necessary to talk about sexually transmitted diseases with their children. Moreover, since drugs, AIDS, premarital sex, and homosexuality are considered taboo subjects, no one wants to raise such topics during conversation.

Asian-Indian parents believe that children can be protected from sexually transmitted diseases if they are taught family values and ethics. Many of the first-generation Indians believe that if they do not talk about what is taboo, children will not think about taboo matters. Thus, communication regarding taboo issues, such as sex and sexuality, normally does not occur at home.

LOVE AND CARE: DIFFERENT LEVELS OF UNDERSTANDING

Second-generation Indian immigrants who are different from their parents, their other American peers, and their relatives back in India defy any standard categorization. Yet, they are so much like their parents and others. This difference and sameness can be seen, as well, in their understanding of love. First-generation Asian-Indians often equate love and care in terms of meeting children's physical, educational, material needs, and ensuring their financial security. But for second-generations, though it is a part of caring, love and care for them is more than having their material needs met. They love the relationship with their parents and are looking for a meaningful connection with them. Since they do not have a role model at home, they look outside the home for shaping of their identity, even while they are still very young. Often the tension between the parents also becomes a struggle for second generations to have adequate understanding about the value of family that their parents portray to their children.

I do not blame the first-generation parents for their limited understanding of love and care because their concept of love has been developed from their own experiences growing up in the financially weak families of their childhood in a poorer country. However, this is not the experience of second-generations. For them, everything is available—except the physical proximity and love of their parents. Therefore, they interpret love and care in terms of quality time that is spent with their family. These different levels of understanding may help therapists to better understand and counsel this community.

There are additional reasons for the intergenerational conflicts within Asian-Indian families. They can be summarized as follows:

Differences in Cultural Identity: For first-generations, identity is ascribed and caste-related identity is imposed. For second-generations, identity is achieved; family and caste-related identity is rejected.

Communality vs. Individuality: First-generations are more communally minded, while second-generations are more individually minded. While the former see individuals in terms of social hierarchy and interpersonal relationships governed by formal and elaborate rules, the latter view all persons as equal and interpersonal relationships as informal and flat without any complexities. While first-generations emphasize extended families and interdependence, second-generations prefer nuclear family, privacy, and independence. While the former emphasizes collective responsibilities and collective achievements, the latter emphasizes personal responsibility and individual achievement.

Caste and Religion versus Class and Spirituality: For first-generations, while social behaviors are caste and religion related, they are class related for the latter. For first-generations, while roles are well defined and gender-based, it is flexible and loosely defined for second-generations. For first-generations, while religion plays a dominant role in everyday life, for second-generations it is less religious and more spiritual. For the former, while religious rituals play a crucial role in daily life, for the latter, rituals are mostly secular and religious rituals are less important. While first-generations tend to be fatalistic and superstitious, second-generations tend to be critical, rational, and requiring more logical explanations.

Emotional Restraint and Indirect Communication vs. Expression and Direct Communication: While first-generations keep emotions in check, second-generations tend to freely express their emotions and feelings. First-generations are more goal and status driven, while second-generations are more relationship driven. While the former values uniformity, the latter values diversity. For the former, leadership is based on position and role. For the latter, leadership is based on trust and relationship. For first-generations, decision-making is directive, mostly made by those who hold power in the group with the rest expected to follow through. For second-generations, decision-making is participatory and democratic in nature, with the consideration given to all input and the involvement of everyone appreciated.

While the former use internet for information, the later use it for relation-ship. Among first-generations, communication with others is often indirect and contextual, formal, and planned. But for second-generations, it is usually direct and to the point, informal, and spontaneous.[15]

We must understand the Asian-Indian immigrants in light of these characteristics if we are to provide them meaningful counseling/therapy. It is important to remember that the Asian-Indian population in the United States has split in terms of generational and cultural character. First-gener-ation immigrants preserve more of their home-country flavor and traditions, while their children born in the United States share only a certain part of their parents' culture and are more assimilated into American culture. This, obviously, often causes conflicts within families.

The family-first concept of Indians plays a pivotal role in promoting and maintaining cohesiveness and stability in the family. Ironically, the extended family network is both a boon and bane for Asian-Indian Americans. The obligation to put family needs above one's own personal needs is a source of psychological affliction for second-generation immigrants. But for the first-generation immigrants, the extended family support system is seen as critical protection against mental health issues. For Asian-Indians who have a hierarchical order of relationship, respect for the elderly is crucial. Most of the first-generation Indian immigrants in United States believe that it is necessary to bring honor to the family even at the cost of sacrificing personal freedom and pleasure, and in this process, the emotional expressions are generally inhibited.

Even in psychological pain, children are expected to suppress their strong emotions in obedience to parental authority and family honor. The value of honor is so strongly ingrained in Asian-Indians that even discussing personal psychological problems with mental health practitioners is considered a "disgrace" for the family. However, in sharp contrast, dramatic and painful value conflicts emerge when American-born children defy and reject their ancestors' way of living. Children are torn between the demands of becom-ing Americanized and the desire of their parents that they adhere to the values of their ancestors.

Most of the second-generation immigrants express their opinions freely and have disdain for their cultural heritage. They often think their parents' expectations are unreasonable and at odds with the American way of living. It is observed that second- generations often make rude and nasty remarks about the national origin of their parents, pointing out that their parents think like people from underdeveloped or "Third World" countries, failing to acknowledge that they are here in the United States because of their parents.

Many cultural values crucial to the first generation, such as bringing praise and honor to the family by practicing filial piety, expressing deference to elders, and making personal sacrifices for family members, have become meaningless for second-generation Indian immigrants in United States. This widened gulf between the values of parents and children is emotionally and psychologically painful, and becomes fossilized or accumulated over time in the immigrant families. Conflicts that result due to the chasm between first-generation and second-generation values lead to further family dysfunctions.

These and other problems that Asian-Indians face in the United States are compounded by the unavailability of the village/community/extended family setting they enjoyed back home in India, even in the urban areas. Most Asian-Indians have expressed dismay at the lack of communally-centered communities of healing, expecting to find in the United States structures similar to those found in the same denomination they were members of in India. The impact of that void is compounded when they cannot find therapy "friendly" to them as most is self-centered in its approach. Thus, the primary function of psychotherapy/pastoral counseling must be the facilitation of healthy and meaningful relationships with oneself, others, and God by reducing the stress among this community and improving individual and family functioning.

OVERVIEW

- Personality development from an Asian-Indian perspective is relational and grounded in collective communal identity.
- The community is a valuable source and place where care and healing can take place.
- From the perspective of first- and second-generation Asian-Indians, there are reasons for intergenerational conflicts.
- The second-generation Asian-Indians face a survival struggle at home and in the mainstream American society.

NOTES

1. Sam George, *Coconut Generation: Ministry to the Americanized Asian-Indians* (Niles, IL: Mall Publishing Co., 2006), 113.

2. E. L. Yao, "Working Effectively with Asian Immigrant Parents," *Phi Delta Kappa* 70, no. 3 (November, 1988): 223.
3. S. P. Wakil, C. M. Siddique, and F. A. Wakil, "Between Two Cultures: A study in Socialization of Children of Immigrants," *Journal of Marriage and the Family* 43, no. 3 (November, 1981): 929–940.
4. J. Blake, "South Asian Atlantans Feel Burden of Model Minority Myth." *Atlanta Journal Constitution,* February 3, 2002, http://www.modelminori ty.com/joomla/index.php?option=com_content&view=article&id=222: south-asian-atlantans-feel-burden-of-model-minority-myth-&catid=41: identity&Itemid=56 (accessed November 19, 2012).
5. Baptiste, "Family Therapy with Asian Indian Immigrant parents Rearing Children in the United States: Parental Concerns, Therapeutic Issues and Recommendations," 353.
6. Dugsin, "Conflict and Healing in Family Experience of Second-Generation Immigrants from Indian Living in North America," 236–237.
7. The phrase "moving at a distance" in this book means not following parental and community cultural values. For instance, in Indian culture, when two people meet together, they inquire about each member of the other's family. At a family or community function, if their children do not participate as a part of the communal cultural practice, everyone will inquire as to the reason and, thus, parents or other members of the family who attend the function will be placed in an embarrassing situation.
8. Lartey, *In Living Color,* 34.
9. George, *Coconut Generation,* 56. Also see Sunita Shorabji, "Suicide Amongst Indian Americans: We're Stressed, Depressed, But Who's Listening?" *India West News paper,* July 12, 2013, http://www.indiawest.com/news/12062-suicide-amongst-indian-americans-we-re-stressed-depressed-but-who-s-listen ing.html?utm_source=Newsletter+-+2013+-+July+12&utm_campaign=DNL +-+July+12%2C+2013&utm_medium=email (accessed July 16, 2013).
10. David W. Augsburger, *Pastoral Counseling across Cultures.* (Philadelphia, PA: The Westminster Press, 1986), 84.
11. D.S. Sandhu, P.R. Portes, and S.A. McPhee, "Assessing Cultural Adaptation: Psychometric Properties of the Cultural Adaptation Pain Scale," *Journal of Multicultural Counseling and Development,* 24, no. 1 (January 25, 1996):15–25.
12. Ibid.
13. T.A. Kulanjiyil, "Landscape: Mental Health Needs of South Asian Indians," in *Caring for the South Asian Soul,* ed. T.A. Kulanjiyil and D.V. Thomas (Bangalore: Primalogue), 22.
14. Sandhu, Portes, and McPhee, 22.
15. George, *Coconut Generation,* 100–101.

CHAPTER 4

Presentation and Interpretation of the Empirical Data

INTRODUCTION

In this chapter, my major goal is to report, analyze, and interpret the results of the survey data which are coded and tabulated in the Appendix. The presentation and interpretation of the data in this chapter are also employed to test the factors presented in Chap. 1 that contribute to intergenerational conflict in Indian immigrant families.[1] The survey instrument is designed on the basis of the literature reviewed, cultural values of Asian-Indians described in Chaps. 2 and 3, the sources of conflicts identified, and instruments used to measure intergenerational conflicts among other ethnic communities, such as Korean[2] and Chinese[3] immigrants. The questionnaire was set in such a way as to test in-depth and quality communication in intrafamily relationships, mutual acceptance of culture, cultural values, beliefs and practices, valuing one culture over another, integration of cultural values among the multiple generations of the Indian immigrants in the United States, and awareness programs initiated by sociocultural and religious centers.

The questionnaire is divided into six sections:

1. Intra-Family Relationships between First- and Second-Generation Immigrants
2. Communication, Mutual Acceptance, and Respect of Cultural Values
3. Overvaluing of Ethnic Culture and Cultural Values
4. Intergenerational Conflict and Individual/Family Functionality

© The Author(s) 2017
V. Jacob, *Counseling Asian Indian Immigrant Families*,
DOI 10.1007/978-3-319-64307-6_4

5. The Role of Sociocultural and Religious Institutions in Educating How to Manage Cultural Struggles and Acculturation
6. Demographic Details and Multi-Ethnic Identity

In order to give a better sense of the survey respondents, the demographic data will be discussed first, though it appeared at the end of the survey. Responses from the other sections will be presented as they appeared in the survey.

Intra-Family Relationship Between First- and Second-Generation Immigrants

The purpose of this section of the questionnaire is to understand the family dynamics in an intergenerational and multicultural context. It is specifically designed to assess how the family relationships between husband/wife and parents/children operate when different cultural generations are living together under the same roof. Therefore, questions in this section are arranged in such way as to highlight the actual family experience under investigation.

It is generally assumed within popular culture that good parents raise good children. This notion is confirmed by Heinz Kohut's theory of self-psychology, which asserts that unity among parents helps children to idealize their parents and develop a healthy self.[4] Unity and intimacy among husbands, wives, and children can be assessed in various ways. One of the measures used in this research is open and transparent communication between parents and children. In traditional Asian-Indian culture, communications in families are often one-sided and parents often make decisions. The empirical data in this study confirms that the same pattern is followed even today by the majority of first-generation Asian-Indian immigrants who live in the First-World nation of America (Table 1).[5] Since conversations are one-sided and the decision-making process is considered parental business, when children raise questions, parents often equate that with questioning their authority. Therefore, it is common in Asian-Indian families for parents to discourage the asking of questions. The data in this research confirm this observation (Table 2).

It is observed that parental generations whose personhood has been formed and developed in the Indian cultural context naturally give more importance to traditional Indian cultural values and practices, even though they live in the Western world (Table 4). The term "too traditional" here is used to describe those parents who primarily value traditional Indian cultural elements over American/Western cultural values and practices in their daily lives. It is observed that parental emphasis on traditional Indian cultural values and practices sets the stage for intergenerational conflicts in the family.

Another disparity in the thought process of multiple Asian-Indian immigrant generations is the parental belief that their children do not understand life-situations the way they themselves do. In other words, first-generation parents believe that their second-generation children are not as capable as their parents are of thinking critically (Table 5). However, second-generation immigrants who are born, raised, and socialized in the American individualistic and consumer culture believe that it is their right to share their opinion in the family or in the community (Table 6). As a participant observant, I had several opportunities to talk with Asian-Indian parents and what I understood from those conversations is that most first-generation immigrants believe that it is inappropriate for children to interfere when their elders talk about something important. Again, the bottom line or underlying truth is their belief that "children are not matured or experienced enough to understand life-situations as their parents do." Some of them also believe that it is a matter of disrespect if youngsters share their opinion without parental permission. This is also a contributing factor to intergenerational conflict and family dysfunction.

Many first-generation immigrants believe it is unnecessary for their children to know everything that goes on in the family. Many parents conceal serious matters, such as parental disputes and arguments, from young adults. First-generation immigrants operate this way because they believe that if children are not exposed to bad things, they will not do bad things. However, they ignore the fact that children learn things not only at home, but from many other sources, including the larger culture in which they reside. For instance, though parents may argue and attack each other in private, their children easily detect this from parents' body language, silence, and gestures. This is also the case with initial discussions on certain important family matters.

For the most part, children are not involved in decision-making process in Asian-Indian families. Typically, decisions are communicated to children after they have already been made (Table 8).

In terms of mutual respect, the data reveal that all members in their families are mutually respected (Table 3). However, additional data (presented in Table 4) show that it is not a respect that unconditionally accepts a person's worth, values, beliefs, and practices. Rather, it is a sort of respect for persons that are a part of the family. In other words, the "mutual respect" that is indicated by the respondents in this research is only the respect that is accorded persons who are part of the family, not respect for an individual's total personality, which includes their faith, beliefs, cultural values, practices, and cultural identity.

Some first-generation immigrants think that their children will be spoiled if love is openly expressed to them. Thus, most first-generation immigrants discourage open expressions of love/using loving language with their children. This may be because many parents do not show physical or verbal signs of affection/open love to their children. For some parents, it is even difficult for them to say to their children, "I love you" (Table 9). Though love can be expressed in various ways, the love expressed through loving language and physical signs are easy to understand. Such expressions of love can be important to the development of self, as noted by Heinz Kohut, who asserts that one should feel acceptance, love, and respect in the family in order to develop a healthy self.[6]

While the parental community takes care of children on the premise that children are unable to understand life-situations as their parents do, children often claim that they have sufficient knowledge to take care of themselves. Obviously, parents and children do not agree on this matter. In the Asian-Indian culture, children are always treated as children, even when they are legally adults and mature enough to understand life. The parental notion that their children will never understand as they do is culturally derived (Table 5).

This thinking provides another clue leading to the conclusion that first-generation immigrants are emotionally fused with their children and think their children should always be dependent on them. The data in Table 7 support this stream of thought. From the perspective of second-generation immigrants, it may be that their parents' refusal to accept that their children are competent to make good decisions and take care of themselves contributes to their identity crisis. However, first-generation immigrant parents cling to the belief that their children cannot care for themselves out of fear of children becoming independent and being lost in the American culture.

Saving face in public is a major concern to the Asian-Indians. First-generation immigrants generally do all they can to save face in their communities. To avoid social stigma they often exercise their authority over their children to discipline them and keep them from doing something contrary to Indian values and traditional cultural practices. For instance, in

Indian culture, the name and fame brought by one member in the family is the name and fame of the entire family; similarly, the entire family also shares the shame and guilt brought in by one member. Therefore, most parents believe that it is their responsibility to keep the family free of social stigma, even at the expense of their family's unity and harmony (Table 10).

Questions regarding familiarity with American culture produced contradictory responses (Table 11). Since no further attempts were made to clarify to what extent the respondents are familiar with American culture, it is not possible here to state to what extent and with which aspects of American culture the first-generation immigrants are familiar. Based on my experience with several first-generation immigrants and the data presented in Tables 27 and 50–56, I suggest that many first-generation immigrants are "one-sided" in their familiarity with American culture. This is to say that though first-generations may be familiar with some aspects of American culture (e.g., lack of parental control in child-rearing, lack of interdependence among parents and children, allowing dating, accepting teenage pregnancy, divorce, lack of submission, lack of respect to elders, etc.), they eschew them in favor of traditional Indian culture and practices. Many first-generation parents believe that the aforementioned attitudes *are* "the American culture" and they are afraid to expose their children to that "American culture" that is familiar to them. However, they conveniently ignore/refuse to admit that they are more or less perpetuating the cultural practices of their families and relatives in India today in an effort to preserve the culture from the influences of globalization, modernization, and media culture.

Another practice that leads to intergenerational conflict and/or family dysfunction among Asian-Indian immigrant families is the setting of unrealistic expectations for their children by first-generation parents. The majority of parents expect that their children will behave like typical, "proper Indians." Whenever this expectation is not met, parents become frustrated, irritated, and agitated, feeling that they are bad parents. This emotional state can escalate and cause frustration and aggression within the family (Table 12).

Showing respect to parents and the elderly is practiced in various ways among Asian-Indians. Implicit forms of children's obedience to parents include talking humbly to elders, not yelling or shouting or raising their voices to parents and elders, not talking back, standing up when adults enter the room, and receiving parents and elders with due respect when they come home. Asian-Indians parents teach their children to address older males as "uncles" and older females as "aunties." Addressing an older person by first or last name is always considered disrespectful. When a guest, especially an older person, visits one's home, it is customary for the entire family, including the children, to come out and greet the guest, receiving them with a warm welcome. First-generation immigrants in the United States expect their children to observe such cultural practices.

However, second-generation immigrants living in the dominant American culture do not readily meet this expectation and often choose not to practice the actions of respect. A majority of second-generations hold the belief that only people who deserve respect should be shown respect. The data in Table 14 substantiate this claim. Second-generation young adults adopt the values of the dominant culture and tend to consider everyone as equal. Thus, addressing a person by their last name is, for the second-generation immigrants, evidence of respect for that person. Moreover, the mainstream culture does not teach second-generation immigrants to simply accept that respect and authority are rightly ascribed to a person by virtue of their age. These very different attitudes regarding respect create huge tension between generations living under the same roof. The data from my research show that both first- and second-generation immigrants agree that Asian-Indian parents demand their children always show respect for elders (Table 13).

I have experienced, first-hand, family conflict associated with the issue of respect for elders. I was invited by a family to be a special guest for lunch after preaching in their church during the Sunday Service. While I was sitting in their living room, I overheard the father of that family yelling at his son because he did not come out of his room to properly receive me when I arrived at their house. For the father, his son's not coming out from his room to greet me was a matter of disrespect. After a while, the son reluctantly joined us and we had a good conversation. At the end of the conversation, he apologized to me, saying, "Pastor, I ignored you not because I have some problem with you, but I thought I would let my dad receive you as you are his friend." Later, as I continued my conversation with the father, I tried to discuss the differences between his and his son's cultural understanding, reminding the father that I was a stranger to his son and the father's guest. I suggested that it was the son's intention to give his father space to be with his friend and to offer privacy to his father and the guest. Thus, not being aware of the reasons for a particular behavior (in this case failing to properly "show respect") caused friction between first- and second-generation family members.

While the policy of the second generation is to 'give and take' respect as it is earned, the first-generation policy is to expect respect for parents and elders, whether or not the respect is reciprocated or merited (Table 14).

Like other people of color, second-generation immigrants also face racial discrimination in every area of their lives. However, the level of emotional pain that the second-generation immigrants experience can be different from that of the first-generation immigrants. Second-generation immigrants born, raised, socialized and educated, speaking the same language with same accent, and mostly thinking and acting like their American counterparts are often regarded as "others" in their own land. They are rejected in their own land by those members of the dominant, larger society. When they return to their parental community, they are also rejected, as they are not fully Indian. They are discriminated against as a minority in both dominant society and in their parental community. The triple emotional pain of rejection, discrimination, and isolation that this group experiences from their American counterparts due to their skin color and from their parental community due to their cultural difference can be much more severe than that experienced by first-generation immigrants.[7]

The data in Table 15 offer some idea of the emotional distress second-generations suffer due to discrimination by their American counterparts and in the Asian-Indian immigrant community.

Still, being aware and being understanding are two very different positions when it comes to empathizing with others. There is no guarantee that those who claim to be aware of the peer pressure their children face actually understand what this means for them. Neither does it necessarily lead parents to empathize with their children.

Asian-Indian parents feel it is their responsibility to exercise control in every area of their children's lives. Thus, it is common for Asian-Indian parents to place restrictions on their children, even after they become young adults, for instance, regarding talking on the phone with friends, especially with an opposite gender (Table 16). Here, again, is a case of misunderstood intentions causing friction and tension among multiple generations.

Asian-Indian parents also exert influence over their children's choice of friends. It seems that, indirectly, they try to keep their children from associating with friends from cultures other than the Indian . This may be due to a fear that their children will pick up Western cultural values and become lost to American culture (Table 17).

Another area where Asian-Indian parents restrict their children's choice is regarding the clothing they wear. Most first-generation immigrants strongly encourage clothes that do not expose the body parts of their children, and set other rules about their children's attire. However, adolescents and young adults are often influenced by the media in terms of what is stylish and trendy and choose their dress by what clothes are readily available and deemed popular. Fashions that are revealing or show off the body are widely advertised and promoted in popular culture. Second-generation immigrants may feel peer pressure to wear the same kind of clothes that their non-Indian friends wear. This creates significant stress and conflict within Asian-Indian families as the second-generation immigrants contend with their parents' restrictions regarding clothing choice and peer pressure to dress in a certain way (Table 18). Thus, another source of intergenerational conflicts in the Asian-Indian family is identified.

In the traditional Indian cultural context, irrespective of religion and caste, a family devotion or prayer time is observed in most families, usually in the evening. It is generally an unwritten rule that all family members should be at home before darkness falls (typically, 7:30 p.m.) for this devotion. In some homes, when the parents are still engaged at work, it is the children's duty to lead and conduct the family devotion. Following family prayer and dinner, children usually study and the elders go to bed. Even today, despite the negative impact of modernization and globalization, this devotional practice continues to be observed in most Indian families.

It is common in many Asian-Indian immigrant families in the United States for mothers to work a night shift and fathers to work a day shift, rarely seeing one another. Still, they believe or assume that every member of the family, especially the children, will be at home by a certain time in the evening. Table 19 shows that all second-generation respondents indicated that their parents insist on their being home every day at a certain time and that the first-generation respondents overwhelmingly agree that they expect their children to return home each day at a set time. During my interviews with second-generation immigrants, I was often surprised to be asked why their parents insist that they be home at a set time, maybe 8:00 or 8:30 p.m. I have suggested that perhaps first-generation parents are still in the unconscious mode of expecting the traditional evening family devotion and assume that their children automatically know of that expectation. A concern for their children's safety and security is likely to be another reason for an early curfew.

In this section, intrafamily interactions were examined using responses to 19 questions. It is very evident that there are strong differences between the perceptions and perspectives of the first- and second-generation immigrants. These differences in perspectives and values, especially in the terms of ascribed authority and parental control, create tremendous stress and tension in Asian-Indian family life.

Communication, Mutual Acceptance, and Respect to Cultural Values in the Family

Strange cultural context, busy life situations, stressful jobs, responsibilities, and financial commitments to families and extended families often diminish the amount of quality time spent together for many immigrant families living in the United States. Spending quality conversational time with family members can help reduce the stress level the family is experiencing and to make life more meaningful in the midst of all the challenges Asian-Indian immigrants face (Table 20).

In addition, empathic listening can be a mark of healthy families. Active and empathic listening is healing in every case, especially in the context of emotional and psychological pain. For a majority of families lack of quality conversational time means a lack of active and empathic listening (Table 21). This difference in perception between first and second generations may be the result of a generation gap, with each generation having different expectations about and understandings of conversation, and the meaning of active listening not being the same for first- and second-generation immigrants.

In traditional Indian culture, dinnertime is often a time for conversation. Parents, grandparents, and children together enjoy dinner, usually immediately following family prayer/evening devotion. In the immigrant context, though most first-generation immigrants insist that their children return home before late evening, they still often fail to spend conversation time with their children during the dinner hour. Moreover, many second-generation immigrants who prefer American food (Table 83) come home having dined outside the home. Because of all these challenges, first-generation immigrants, even those who uphold traditional cultural values, are often unable to practice those values in the home (Table 22).

As noted earlier, children are often discouraged from questioning their parents (Table 2). The expectation that children listen, obey, and follow their parents' instructions at home, is also the expectation for children at school (Table 23). The considerable discrepancy in these figures may be due to different levels of understanding of what it means to encourage asking questions, and to what extent. Second-generation immigrants might be comparing their parents with the circumstances of their white, middle-class counterparts' parents, while first-generation immigrants might be comparing their parenting practice to their own childhood experience and their parents' attitude towards asking questions.

The questionnaire reveals that just 33 percent of second-generation immigrants regard their parents as free and outgoing in associating with their children. Similarly, only 27 percent of first-generation respondents indicate that they are free and outgoing in terms of associating with their children. My intimate conversations with some second-generation respondents reveal that the phrase "free and outgoing in associating with their children" and "being encouraged to raise questions" are positive indicators of and factors for emotional connection, feelings of like-mindedness, and being 'modern' in terms of thought pattern and actions. Though first-generation immigrants may have lived in the United States for two or three decades or more, the majority of that group agrees that they are not free and outgoing, particularly as compared to their Caucasian or African-American counterparts (Table 24).

Attitudes towards the quality of association between parents and children were also tested with a question about interracial marriage. One hundred percent of respondents in both the first-generation and the second-generation immigrant groups do not believe that the first-generation parental community looks favorably on interracial marriages (Table 25). This disapproval is likely for various reasons (e.g., cultural priority, concerns about sexual assault, and the high divorce rate) discussed in Chap. 2 of this book. Another example of restricted family conversation between parents and young adult children is matters of sex and sexuality. Since sex and topics related to sexuality are taboo in Indian family conversations, such topics are often avoided, as "dirty" subjects. As mentioned in detail in Chap. 2, parents may hold the assumption that if subjects such as love, kissing, sex, and sexuality are not discussed at home, children will not think about or do these "bad" things. All the respondents, both first and second-generation immigrants, agreed that there was no open communication about kissing, hugging, sex, and sexuality between parents and children (Table 26). This is another example of the attitude of a lack of openness or not being "free and outgoing."

In addition to sex, sexuality, and related topics being taboo, physical touching beyond a handshake between opposite genders is also taboo in the value system of most first-generation Asian-Indian immigrants. Though many first-generation immigrants who have lived in the United States for several decades hug their American friends as a survival technique, hugging rarely occurs between Indians or other Asians. However, for second-generation immigrants, hugging is a matter of greeting and acceptance. Kissing and expressing love in public are common in the United States culture. These different understandings among generations regarding acceptable practices concerning the physical expressions of affection often create intergenerational conflicts in the family. The data collected for this study reveal that 100 percent of second-generation respondents agree or strongly agree that their parents do not approve of children kissing or expressing love with their boy/girlfriend in public. All first-generation respondents also agree or strongly agree that such practices in public or in front of other people are unacceptable (Table 47).

As previously noted, respect of parents and elders is expressed in various ways in Asian-Indian culture. In terms of family communication, one of the important ways to express respect for parents is through implicit obedience and not talking back. Back-talking to parents and elders is definitely considered disrespectful by all first-generation respondents in this study, and all the second-generation respondents confirmed that their parents strongly believe that talking back is disrespectful (Table 28).

Demand for obedience to parents and elders, is very strong among Asian-Indians. Whenever there is a difference of opinion in the family, parents' opinions and words are final. The data collected for this research reveal that 100 percent of second-generation respondents agree or strongly agree that their parents/grandparents expect their children always to obey them. Similarly, 100 percent of first-generation respondents expect their children to obey them even if their children's opinion, suggestions, or interests differ from their parents'. The data indicate that parents expect obedience in all things (Tables 29 and 70). This unrealistic expectation is another major source of intergenerational conflicts and family fights.

Any action that contradicts family values and brings shame, guilt, and/or isolation on the family in the given community is considered disrespectful behavior. Therefore, each member of an Asian-Indian family is trained and cautioned not to bring shame upon the family by violating family values and community interests. All the second-generation respondents in this study agreed that their parents expect them not to bring shame on their family, and all the first-generation respondents confirmed that they hold that expectation (Table 30).

During their own upbringing, Asian-Indian parents themselves often experienced restrictions, controls, and litanies of what and what not to do. They internalized those rules and now apply them to their children.

However, first-generation parents are often aware that child-rearing practices and the disciplining of children are quite different in the United States than in India. For instance, corporal punishment by parents in India is not considered child abuse, but in the United States it may be a serious crime, depending on the severity of the corporal punishment.

When second-generation immigrants compare themselves with their non-Indians counterparts, they often feel that their parents place a lot of restrictions and conditions on them. This leads them to believe that their parents do not accept them unconditionally. Responding to a question on unconditional acceptance from parents, all second-generation respondents indicated that their parents ought to accept them as they are, while just 70 percent of first-generation parents indicated that they accept their children for whatever they are (Table 35).

Most Asian-Indians value education for their children and see it as being of prime importance. Parents often hold down two to three jobs in order to provide advanced education for their children. Asian-Indian parents tend to focus on education as being of primary importance in the early adolescent and teenage periods of their children's lives. Consequently, many parents hold that academic life is more important than social life for their children during that time. Parents in several families that I worked with did not allow their college-aged children to work part-time, even though the families were struggling financially, fearing it would negatively affect their education. Parents such as these believe that their children's sole responsibility during these years is to focus on their education and do well academically. The parents' responsibility is to be sure their children have access to a good education and to provide for the children's educational needs.

The pressure to do well in school often means that parents will limit distractions that might hinder their children's academic achievement, distractions such as friends, social activities, and extracurricular activities at school. Ghazala Bhatti, who studied Asian children's home and school environments, discovered that parents attributed no relevance to sports in the school day, and claimed that sports should not be given any priority over the basic skills of reading and writing.[8]

As children get older, they are expected to spend more time studying than socializing.[9] The data collected for this study support this view, with 63 percent of first-generation respondents seeing a social life as not very important for their children aged 17–20. Only 4 percent of second-generation respondents shared their parents' perspective (Table 32).

The academic pressure immigrant children endure due to unrealistic expectations set up by their parents is detailed in Chap. 2 of this study. A significant majority (66 percent) of second-generation respondents in this study agreed that their parents' academic expectations for them always exceeded their performance. In support of this perception, all first-generation respondents agreed that their academic expectations for their children were always high (Table 33). For instance, one of my second-generation respondents, during a personal interview, sarcastically told me, "my parents in my childhood were always more worried about the one or two marks I used to lose than the 98 or 99 marks I used to gain on the exam." It is true that most of the children with whom I spoke (either on the phone or in person) earned high grades in their education. Yet, many of them felt that they did not reach the level of their parents' expectations, which resulted in personal dissatisfaction and low self-esteem.

The high educational aspirations and goals parents set for their children are often considered "unrealistic expectations" and are misunderstood by second-generation immigrants. A major reason for this extreme emphasis on education is the experience of first-generation immigrants. The majority of the first-generation Asian-Indians who enjoy the benefits and blessings of the United States today are doing so primarily because of their education. Most first-generation immigrants worked and studied hard, performed well academically, and became accomplished professionals, such as engineers, doctors, nurses, and business people. It was often their professional success that brought them to the United States. In other words, first-generation immigrant parents may believe that their educational success is the sole source of all the blessings that the second-generation immigrants enjoy in the United States today. Therefore, it is natural for them to believe that education is the foundation of all success in life. The empirical data collected in this study confirms this; it shows that 100 percent of second-generation respondents agreed that their parents link educational success with life success, and all the first-generation respondents believed educational success to be a major part of achieving life success (Table 45).

In some cases, the siblings of parents in this study were unable to come to the United States or enjoy the benefits of this land because they did not study or complete advanced education in India. Though some less-educated men and women were able to come to the United States through the sponsorship of their accomplished siblings, the sponsored immigrants often suffer unemployment, which can lead to other family difficulties.

It should be noted that there is a "down side" to the extreme emphasis first-generation immigrant parents place on educational achievement for their children. I will call this *down side* "false family pride." Because in Indian culture one family member's achievement and success is the entire family's achievement and success, at least a minority first-generation immigrant parents often choose educational majors for their children without considering their children's intellectual capacity and emotional strength. As a result, children may be forced to pursue an "esteemed" profession, such as medicine, engineering, or law, for the sake of the family's prestige and social status. Though the parents may have the money to afford the education required for one to become a doctor, lawyer, or engineer, a child's intellectual and emotional capacities may not allow him or her to successfully complete their studies. Dropping out of college/professional training school brings great shame upon the family and results in tremendous guilt and low self-esteem for the child who fails to achieve the expected degree. Further, it results in family stress, intergenerational conflict, and family dysfunction. I personally encountered a few young adults living with great shame, guilt, and low self-esteem, addicted to drugs and alcohol because they could not fulfill their parents' wishes in regard to their education.

Parents and children need to realize that educational success does not necessarily guarantee life success. Neither is academic achievement the sole reason one is successful in life. Rather, a successful person is usually accomplished and well developed in many aspects of his/her life. I have seen many first-generation Asian-Indian immigrants who focused primarily on financial security, social dignity, and family prestige through educational success fail tragically in the area of meaningful relationships, peaceful family life, and emotional/psychological health. Though education certainly plays a role in a successful life, romanticizing educational success and holding it up as the sole reason for a successful life, without taking a holistic view, leads to a one-sided vision, unrealistic goals, intergenerational conflict, family dysfunction, and other failures in life.

Indian culture is allocentric, meaning it is family and community oriented, with interdependence considered essential and insisted upon for healthy growth. First-generation immigrant parents, whose personhood was formed and developed in a communal culture, constantly and consistently believe that individual autonomy is unhealthy and that interdependence is better than individual autonomy (Table 27). Belief in the allocentric nature of personhood, interdependence, and different views regarding family interest and personal interest can also lead to intergenerational conflict. While an emphasis on family interest is the byproduct of communal culture, an emphasis on individual interest is the byproduct of an individualistic culture. The pertinent question here is whether it is fair or unfair to sacrifice personal interest for the sake of family interest? While 92 percent of second-generation respondents agree that it is unfair to sacrifice personal interest for the sake of family interest, 100 percent of first-generation respondents believe it is reasonable and fair to do so (Table 34).

Most first-generation immigrants live for the sake of their family, especially for the sake of their children. For example, several families I encountered have marital conflicts, and at least a handful of those families, husbands and wives have been sleeping in separate bedrooms for years. Yet, they live in the same house without seeking divorce or legal separation for the sake of their children. Though the dysfunction of these families may affect family members in different ways, parents stay together to maintain the status quo in the community. These parents sacrifice their freedom and live in the same house to protect children from the social stigma attached to children of divorced parents. Thus, parents sacrifice their personal interests for the sake of the family interest. In such a cultural context, it may seem reasonable for the parents to expect their children also to sacrifice some personal priorities or interests that conflict with the family interests. However, it becomes difficult and often unacceptable to second-generation immigrants to do so, as the American culture in which they are born, raised, and socialized does not generally expect such personal sacrifice for the good of the group.

For first-generation immigrants, loving their children means meeting their children's material, educational, and financial needs. Most parents are willing to hold two or more extra jobs in order to meet their children's needs. However, for second-generation immigrants love means something more than providing for those basic material needs. They expect more physical proximity with their parents, physical and verbal signs of affection, and physical touching. Based on the data collected for study, 100 percent of second-generation respondents value love with more physical touching and verbal signs of affection over merely having housing, food, education, and material needs provided for them. However, 73 percent of first-generation respondents disagreed with the statement that meeting educational and material needs of their children is more important than showing mere love. Interestingly, 39 respondents out of that 73 percent scribbled in a little space found at the end of the question that "both are equally important." Nonetheless, more than one-fourth (27 percent) of the first-generation respondents did believe that meeting the educational and material needs of their children has greater priority than showing overt love in words (Table 36).

In the traditional Asian-Indian culture, as a part of their ascribed authority, parents usually do not wait for children's permission to enter into their rooms. The survey shows that 97 percent of the second-generation respondents indicated that they are not okay with their parents entering their rooms without their permission, whereas 57 percent of first-generation respondents said that they do not wait for their children's permission to enter their children's rooms (Table 37). This suggests that the majority of first-generation immigrants still unconsciously exercise their internalized, culturally acquired behaviors in the lives of their second-generation children without realizing that the children hold different opinions about the behaviors. It also reveals that though first-generation immigrants have been physically present in the United States for decades, they are still greatly influenced, emotionally and psychologically, by Indian cultural values, which they still practice.

Another aspect of parental control is evidenced when children have prolonged telephone conversations with the opposite gender. As reported earlier, parents often exert control over the length of their children's phone conversations,   particularly when the friend is of the opposite gender. Responding to the question about parents' complaints over the length of their children's phone conversations with opposite-gender friends, 87 percent of the second-generation respondents agreed that their parents are not okay with them having lengthy telephone conversations with friends of the opposite gender. Similarly, 88 percent of the first-generation parent respondents agreed that they disapprove of these long conversations (Table 38). Parent's restrictions on lengthy telephone conversations with so-called boyfriends/girlfriends may be due to a fear that protracted talks may lead to dating.

Dating is socially unacceptable among Asian-Indians, and those parents never encourage their children to date—neither Indians or non-Indians. Responding to the question regarding parental encouragement for dating Indians or non-Indians, 100 percent of second-generation respondents agreed that their parents never encourage dating, whether with Indians or non-Indians. Similarly, 100 percent of first-generation respondents agreed that they do not encourage their children to date (Tables 39 and 62).

Parental control, briefly discussed in regard to other survey questions, is one of the many unique cultural practices of first-generation Asian-Indians that makes these parents different from their counterparts in Western cultures. Almost every Indian parent believes that it is always their duty and responsibility to correct, give advice, and guide their children because children are not as knowledgeable as their parents. This survey used for this study indicates that 90 percent of second-generation respondents agree that their parents advise them regarding what to do with their life, even though they want to make their own decisions. First-generation respondents unanimously concur, with 100 percent indicating that they often advise their children about what to do with their lives (Table 31). From my conversation with several Asian-Indian parents I learned that they believe it is their responsibility to make decisions for their children. Though parents have good intentions in taking responsibility for making their children's decisions, that practice often becomes a source of intergenerational conflict within the family.

As noted earlier, Asian-Indian parents who exercise control in every area of their children's life decide, in many cases, who should be their children's friends, how long they should talk to their friends on the telephone, and how they are to behave in the community and at home. In addition to choosing friends, parents also feel a responsibility to oversee the time children spend with their friends. To a question related to parental permission for children to socialize with their friends, 48 percent of respondents among the second-generation group agreed that their parents rarely allow them to socialize with their friends. Among the first-generation respondents, 47 percent indicated that they do not restrict children in socializing with their friends (Table 48), but the data mean that more than half of the first-generation respondents do exercise parental control to restrict their children's socializing with their friends.

Parents who use their ascribed authority make most of the major decisions on choice of educational majors, careers, spouses and many other important matters for their children. According to the empirical data from this research, all the second-generation respondents agree that it is their parents who make decisions about major life-events as mentioned above. However, only 55 percent of respondents among the first-generation immigrants concede that they are the ones who make major decisions for their children. Note that, 48 of that 55 percent of respondents are fathers (Table 41).

This points up the fact that it is fathers in the Asian-Indian community who often initiate decision-making and take disciplinary actions. Here again, parents exercising control over their children and making decisions for them regarding major events often create intergenerational conflict in the family. Even though parents often make these major life-decisions, none of the respondents among the first or second generations feel that children are the parents' property (Table 42). For instance, prolific writer and well-known, eloquent speaker, Oscar Ravi Zacharias, explains clearly how his father dominated him in his childhood. Yet, he believes that it was his father who helped him to achieve many of his goals.[10]

The majority of Asian-Indian parents encourage their children to speak the mother tongue at home. Though most second-generation immigrants speak a little of their parent's vernacular language, most of them do not read or write it. The empirical data collected for this study show that a significant majority of second-generation (79 percent) and first-generation (83 percent) respondents agree that parents encourage their children to speak the vernacular at home (Table 40).

Gender discrimination among Asian-Indian parents towards their children is reported in various contexts. Female infanticide, female genocide, and female fetus abortion were practiced in India for many years. However, practices such as female fetus abortion and neonatal sex discrimination tests have been legally prohibited in India for many decades. In this study, 68 percent of second-generation respondents disagree that their parents treat them differently based on their gender and 92 percent of first-generation respondents agree that they do not treat their children differently because of their gender (Table 44). However, 31 percent of second-generation respondents report that they are uncertain about whether or not they are treated differently than their siblings of a different gender. The uncertainty surrounding this issue may be due to the fixed gender roles and male domination that are commonplace among Asian-Indians.

Another area of misunderstanding between first- and second-generation Asian-Indian immigrants is in the matter of child-rearing, disciplining, and judgment. What first-generation immigrants often consider as correcting and disciplining is perceived by second-generations as judgment. According to the data collected as part of this research, 100 percent of second-generation respondents agree or strongly agree that their parents "judge" them according to their Indian standards, and 96 percent of first-generation respondents believe that they "discipline" their children based on their understanding of appropriate child-rearing practices (Table 46). The data also direct our attention to the necessity of open dialogue between the generations living together in the family home. This experience also helps us understand how different cultures shape the identity and worldview of each group of people in a given culture, and how it influences the way they think and understand.

Asian-Indian parents try their best to meet all the educational, material, and financial needs of their children, endeavoring to provide everything they need. All first-generation respondents agree or strongly agree that it makes them happy when they provide their children things that they could not enjoy in their own childhoods. Thus, observing parental control and parental actions, all the second-generation respondents agree or strongly agree that their parents re-live their childhood through their children (Table 49).

OVERVALUING OF ETHNIC CULTURE

The data in this section reveal how ethnic culture is valued or overvalued in the family where several generations of culture are living together. When one culture is intentionally or irrationally valued over another, the "other culture" is automatically "put down" in a subtle or indirect manner. This research indicates that 57 percent of second-generation respondents reported having always been told that Indian culture and lifestyle is the best, while 61 percent of first-generation respondents always believe this to be true (Table 50). Among the second-generation immigrant respondents, 50 percent always, and 50 percent occasionally, are advised to maintain Indian culture at home and in the community, while 71 percent of first-generation respondents always, and 29 percent occasionally, advise their children to do so (Table 51). Though it is theoretically easy for the first-generation immigrants to advise their children to uphold Indian cultural values while living in the United States, practically it raises many challenges, stresses, confusions, and intergenerational conflicts within the family.

Placing a high value on Indian culture may lead parents to compare their own children with the children of friends, measuring their talents, gifts, intellectual capacity and smartness—which is not a good practice as each person is different and unique. When a child is judged based on such criteria, parents deliberately ignore the dignity and worth of the personhood of the child. The data collected for this research study reveal that 4 percent of respondents among second-generation immigrants always, and 18 percent occasionally, believe that their parents compare them with other Indian children around them. However, only 14 percent of parents agree that they occasionally do so (Table 58).

The majority of first-generation immigrants who believe that Indian culture and lifestyle are best also believe that American culture is very permissive and lacks parental control. In this study, according to the second-generation immigrants, 56 percent of their parents always, and

42 percent occasionally, think the Indian culture/lifestyle is preferable to the permissive American culture, with 27 percent of first-generation parents always, and 69 percent occasionally, believing that American culture is very loose and lacking parental control (Table 53). This is where we need to reconsider the data in Table 11 in light of parents' familiarity with American culture. A comparison of the data in Table 11 with the data in Tables 55 and 56 will enable us to understand that the first-generation parental community's claim that they are familiar with the American culture is very biased (Tables 27 and 65).

It is evident from this analysis that the majority of first-generation immigrants who overvalue the ethnic culture and life style also exalt the Indian dress code as a modest way of dressing. Based on the response of second-generation immigrants, 16 percent of their parents always, and 47 percent occasionally, believe that the Indian dress code is the modest way of dressing, while 9 percent of first-generation respondents always, and 43 percent occasionally, believe so (Table 54).

Another major area of intergenerational conflict, as discussed briefly in this chapter is the issue of dating. Among the many reasons that are raised against dating, one of the major reasons is religious or spiritual. According to the data, 41 percent of respondents among the second-generation group always, and 24 percent occasionally, are taught that dating is against the family's spiritual beliefs and faith tradition, while 41 percent of respondents among the first-generation group always, and 36 percent occasionally, believe that dating is against the family's spiritual belief and faith tradition (Table 52). Most parents fear that dating involves sexual assaults, unwed pregnancies, abortions, and many other moral issues associated with dating. Therefore, most of the Christian parents, as well as many non-Christian parents, believe dating is against their spiritual beliefs and faith tradition. Further, the "spiritual belief" that the parents promote may not necessarily be organized religious belief. It can also be their personal moral understanding. My research found that 93 percent of respondents among second-generation immigrants never, and 7 percent rarely, are encouraged by their parents to date, while 96 percent of respondents among the first-generation group never and 4 percent rarely encourage their children to date (Table 62).

Sex, sexuality, and sex-related topics are taboo and usually avoided during Asian-Indian family conversations (Tables 26 and 47). For this reason, there is no sex education for children either in the Indian families or in Indian schools. According to the observation of the second-generation respondents, 61 percent of their parents are never, and 39 percent are rarely, happy about the sex-education curriculum used in the United States public schools, while 69 percent of first-generation respondents report they are never, and 31 percent are rarely, happy with the sex-education curriculum in public schools (Table 57).

As mentioned earlier, in most cases regarding marriage, Asian-Indian parents prefer marriage between couples of the same caste, religion, and culture. Anything against this age-old practice creates conflict in the family. In this study, 96 percent of respondents among the second-generation group think that their parents will always have problems if they marry a non-Indian male or female, while 91 percent of respondents among the first-generation group agree that they will never be happy if their children marry a non-Indian male or female (Table 59).

There may be several reasons for first-generation immigrants discouraging interracial marriages for their children. One reason is the fear of divorce. Most Asian-Indian immigrants, particularly first-generation immigrants, believe that the reason for the low divorce rate among Indians (both in India and in the United States) is due to the conservative ethnic culture. According to the second-generation respondents, 90 percent of their parents always, and 10 percent occasionally, believe that the low divorce rate among Indians is because of the Indian culture. One hundred percent of the first-generation respondents believe that to be true (Table 60).

The Asian-Indian culture in general, and most first-generation Asian-Indian immigrants in particular, consider and promote interdependence as the healthy way of growth and condemn independence and individual autonomy as being unhealthy. This view is supported by 97 percent of the first-generation respondents who always (and the remaining 3 percent occasionally) believe that individual autonomy and independence is Western and unhealthy. However, based on the observation of the second-generation respondents, 71 percent of their parents always, and 27 percent occasionally, agree that individual autonomy and independence is Western and unhealthy (Table 55). Similarly, 36 percent of the first-generation respondents never and 64 percent rarely believe that the American culture is good for their children to practice. According to the observations of second-generation respondents, 55 percent of their parents never and 45 percent rarely think that is so (Table 56). Regarding the parental community's attitude towards American culture, 87 percent of second-generation respondents observe that their parental community is occasionally too judgmental about American culture, while 80 percent of first-generation respondents also agree that they are occasionally judgmental of the Western culture (Tables 27 and 65).

Due to the feeling that Indian culture and life is the best and American culture is not good to imitate or adopt, many Asian-Indian parents consider sending their children back to India, especially during their teenage years. Responding to a question regarding sending second-generation immigrants back to India during their teen years, 44 percent of second-generation respondents always, and 50 percent occasionally, think that their parents would have sent them back to India during their teen age if the opportunity presented itself. In the same way, 54 percent of first-generation respondents always, and 39 percent occasionally, preferred to send their children back to India during their teenage years (Table 61).

Another matter that can be disruptive to family harmony, though it may seem less important, is food preference. While first-generation immigrants prefer Indian food, the majority of second-generation immigrants prefer American food. According to the data, 88 percent of second-generation respondents always, and 12 percent occasionally, prefer American food. None of the first-generation respondents always prefer American food, though 77 percent occasionally prefer it (Table 63).

First-generation elderly Indian immigrants (those in their 60s and 70s) often think India is the better place for them to live. Reasons for this attitude may be freedom to speak in their vernacular, frequent opportunities to meet their relatives and friends, and the availability of traditional and herbal medications without health insurance, and many other conveniences. However, elderly Indians are forced to stay here for the sake of their children and grandchildren. Many of them are simply babysitters to their grandchildren after being retired from highly ranked professional positions. The data from this research support this view, as a huge majority among the second-generation group (91 percent) indicates that their parents think India is the better place to live (if there is sufficient money), while 94 percent of first-generation respondents also hold that belief (Table 64).

Based on the research for this book, while 79 percent of second-generation respondents always believe that the second-generation immigrants are different from their parents, only 43 percent of first-generation respondents always believe that to be the case (Table 66). This understanding of sameness often does not allow the parents to accommodate any difference in the second-generation immigrants, for instance, difference in cultural beliefs, values, and practice, because they believe that "since he/she is my son/daughter he/she should do exactly what I do and the way I do it."

This demand for similarity in thinking prevents any profitable critical thinking.

Emphasis on one's own cultural values, beliefs, and practices is common among every cultural community. However, when someone puts an irrational emphasis on one's ethnic cultural values, beliefs, and practices in a culturally pluralistic family or society, it disrespects and offends others who hold/ observe different beliefs, values, and practices. According to the data collected for this book, while 61 percent of second-generation respondents observe that their parents put too much emphasis on Indian cultural values and traditions, 73 percent among the first-generation respondents agree that they put too much emphasis on Indian cultural values and traditions (Tables 4 and 67).

Intergenerational Conflict and Individual/Family Functionality

The data in this section help us understand and assess the level of intergenerational conflict and individual/family functionality within the Indian immigrant community living in the United States. Some of the issues examined in previous sections, such as issues of respect and parental authority, are re-examined in terms of their contributions to family conflict and dysfunction.

It has been previously noted that talking back to parents and elders is always considered as a matter of disrespect, especially for first-generation immigrants. Adherence to this behavior is mandatory for children. But the second-generation immigrants who are raised and socialized in the domi- nant American culture are encouraged to question things that are unclear and illogical. Many second-generation immigrants who do not understand the responses and reactions of their parents (which are culturally condi- tioned) may question and talk back to their elders. As a result, family conflict and dysfunction may intensify. The empirical data collected in this research show that 72 percent of second-generation respondents agree that they talk back to their parents/grandparents whenever there is a clash with them, and 59 percent of respondents among the first-generation immigrants observe that to be true. Since it is a matter of disrespect and shame, many parents may not disclose that their children back-talk them, though they actually do (Table 68). However, 46 percent of second-generation respondents and 84 percent of first-generation respondents agree that the second-generation immigrants ignore their parents/grandparents when they impose their views on them (Table 69).

As a part of their parental authority, Asian-Indian parents may not hesitate to raise their voice when they are angry with their children. Neither are they afraid of using corporal punishment to discipline their children. While more than one-third of the respondents (35 percent) among the second-generation immigrants in this study agree that their parents yell and shout at them, a slightly higher percentage (38 percent) among the first-generation immigrants agree that they are occasionally forced to do so (Table 71).

When parents yell and shout at their children who are born and raised in mainstream American culture, the children react in various ways. One of the ways children react is to shut themselves inside their rooms, isolating themselves from others. As the data show, 86 percent of second-generation respondents and 80 percent of first-generation respondents state that the second-generation immigrants lock themselves in their rooms after a fight with their parents/grandparents (Table 72). This would indicate that they choose to cut off communication with other family members and distance themselves from others to show their dislike for not being spoken to in a civil manner. Further, this study reveals that 65 percent of second-generation respondents and 64 percent of first-generation respondents report that the second-generation immigrants stay overnight with their friends after a clash at home (Table 73). According to the data collected in the research for this book, constant family fights and intergenerational conflicts also reduce the appetite. Among second-generation respondents, 92 percent, and 94 percent of first-generation respondents, indicated that second-generation immigrants do not eat at home for days after a family-fight (Table 74). The empirical data from this research reveals that 100 percent of second-generation respondents agree (82 percent) or strongly agree (18 percent) that they do not talk to their parents for days after a clash/fight at home, while 94 percent of first-generation respondents also agreeing that is true (Table 75). Further, 98 percent of respondents among the second-generation group and 100 percent of the first-generation respondents agree with the statement that the normal family routine/behavior is disrupted for days, even weeks, after there is a fight at home between parents and children (Table 87). It shows that the intergenerational conflicts lead the individual and family to a stage of dysfunction.

Though the second-generation immigrants isolate themselves, and distance themselves emotionally and physically from their family and parental community, staying overnight with friends, not eating at home for days, and cutting off communication with the family following a family fight, 91 percent of second-generation respondents and 94 percent of the first-generation respondents disagree that the second-generation immigrants move out from their parental home as a result of family fights (Table 76). As shown in Table 42, although the immigrant generations undergo several difficult situations due to cultural differences at home, none of the respondents (either among the second-generations or first-generations) believes that children are a parent's property. This would suggest that, despite intergenerational conflicts and related difficult issues, family provides a sense of belonging, security, and protection for the Asian-Indian immigrant community in the United States.

Imposing parental cultural values often leads to intergenerational conflicts. A large majority of the second-generation respondents (91 percent) agrees that they get angry and argue with their parents/grandparents when parents impose their cultural values and beliefs on them, while 78 percent of first-generation respondents agree that this upsets their children (Table 77). Further, 59 percent of second-generation respondents and 66 percent among the first-generation respondents agree that second-generation immigrants get angry and destroy things at home when they are judged and/or disciplined by Indian standards (Table 78). However, according to data from this research, 97 percent of second-generation respondents and 88 percent of first-generation respondents disagree that constant conflict at home leads to use of drugs, tobacco, and/or alcohol (Table 79). Only 1 percent of respondents from both second- and first-generation immigrants agree that the second-generation immigrants get in trouble with the police after fights in the home (Table 80).

There are several symptoms that indicate clinical depression in a person. One of those symptoms is lack of appetite (not eating) or overeating. The data collected in this research reveal that 87 percent of second-generation respondents and 70 percent of first-generation respondents agree that the appetite of the second-generation immigrants is poor and they do not like to eat after family fights (Table 81). Further, while 76 percent of second-generation respondents agree that they feel depressed when they are judged by Indian standards, 68 percent among the first-generation group report they observe the same behavior in their children (Table 82).

It is natural that affirmation and appreciation develop self-acceptance and self-worth, while constant criticism and negativity develop frustration, lack of relational skills, and low self-esteem. The data in this research support this fact, with 98 percent of second-generation respondents indicating that everything they do is a painful effort as they are constantly judged by Indian values and principles and 78 percent among the first-generation group agree that they often hear their children making that claim

(Table 83). Further, 47 percent of second-generation respondents agree that they feel worthless when they are constantly judged by Indian values and principles, with 29 percent respondents among the first-generation group agreeing that they sense that among their children (see Table 84). The data collected in this research reveal that 100 percent of the respondents among both the first- and second-generation groups agree that the second-generation immigrants feel frustrated and dejected (sad) when they are judged and disciplined by Indian values and principles (Table 85).

However, the first-generation respondents, even at the expense of their children feeling sad, angry, depressed, having bouts of no appetite, and enduring family dysfunction, are more concerned about maintaining their social reputation, prestige, and upholding Indian values. According to the data, 100 percent of second-generation respondents agree that their parents are more concerned about saving face and family reputation in public rather than helping their family and all the first-generation respondents agree that saving the family image in public is their first priority (Table 86).

To prevent the stigma that occurs when family fights become public, first-generation immigrants often try to minimize the issue of family fights, saying they are common in all families. According to this study, 97 percent of second-generation respondents agree that first-generation immigrants pretend that family fighting is common and that there is nothing to worry about, and 100 percent of first-generation respondents support their children's observation and agree that they accept family fighting as a common occurrence (Table 88). Asian-Indians usually do not take their family issues to persons outside the family for fear it would become gossip and spread throughout the community. Therefore, due to fear of social stigma, seeking professional help from a therapist outside the family is rare among the Asian-Indians. The data from this research reveal that all the respondents from both the first- and second-generation groups agree that their families do not seek professional help even when there are constant fights and arguments at home (Table 89).

Parents whose personhood is formed and developed in the Indian cultural context often expect their children who are born, raised, and socialized in the Western culture to behave like proper Indians. This unrealistic expectation often leads to intergenerational conflicts and family dysfunctions. The data collected in this research show that all the second-generation respondents agree that their parents expect them to be a good man/woman, behaving like a "proper Indian," with a significant majority of 87 percent of first-generation respondents believing that being good children means behaving like a proper Indian (Table 90).

It is a well-known fact that constant conflicts and criticisms distance people emotionally and physically. This is very true in the case of the second-generation immigrants. For second-generation Asian-Indian immigrants, family fights not only cause them to distance themselves emotionally from their parents, it also makes them withdraw from their parental community. It seems that second-generation immigrants often equate their parents with the parental community. Their aversion to being judged by their parents' standards is often projected onto their parental communities as well. The empirical data in this study reveal that a significant majority (95 percent) of second-generation respondents agree that they rebel against their parents and parental community when they are constantly judged by traditional Indian standards. The first-generation respondents express this fact in a different way, with 81 percent stating that their children always have some aversion to and reservation regarding the Indian community (Table 91).

Another factor that contributes to intergenerational conflict is the negative reaction of first-generation immigrants to their children choosing a boyfriend or girlfriend for themselves. All the second-generation respondents in this study observed that their parents think it is unnecessary for them to have a boyfriend/girlfriend prior to their marriage, with 100 percent of first-generation respondents agreeing with their children's observations (Table 92). This attitude of their parents may be one reason why many children hide their boyfriend/girlfriend relationship from their parents. All the second-generation respondents in this research agree that they do not share anything about their girl/boyfriend with their parents, with 82 percent of first-generation respondents agreeing that is true (Table 93). The research data further indicate that only 25 percent of second-generation respondents and 29 percent of first-generation respondents agree that children discuss with parents the peer pressure they face (Table 94). Similarly, 97 percent of second-generation respondents agree that they hide most of their emotional needs from their parents, though only 16 percent of first-generation respondents claim that their children never hide their emotional needs from the parents (Table 95).

Due to different stress factors, cultural influences, stressful jobs, and various other reasons, parents fail to be role models for their children. That failure does not help the second-generation immigrants with regard to their identity development. This study found that only 42 percent of second-generation respondents observe that their parents get along well and never fight with each other, with 77 percent of first-generation respondents asserting that they get along well/never fight with their spouses (Table 96). I believe that for some first-generation immigrants, sharing details of intergenerational conflicts, family conflicts and intimacy issues between husbands and wives with a person outside the family (i.e., this author), made them uncomfortable and prevented many of them from responding honestly to some of the survey questions.

It has already been reported that it is the parents who control most of the affairs and make the major decisions in Asian-Indian families. The research data reveal that 76 percent of second-generation respondents observe that it is their parents who control most of their family affairs, while 58 percent of first-generation respondents believe that to be true (Table 97). Further, 28 percent of second-generation immigrants agree that their fathers are authoritarian, 37 percent believe that their mothers are equally domineering/controlling. Thirty-four percent of first-generation fathers (17) are uncertain about who is the authoritarian figure in the family and 66 percent (33) disagreed with their children's observations. Seventy-two percent of first-generation mothers (36) were uncertain about who is the authoritarian/domineering/controlling parent and 28 percent (14) disagreed with their children's observations (Tables 98 and 99). Only 37 percent of second-generation respondents and 50 percent of first-generation respondents agree that a happy relationship exists between parents and children (Table 100). Again, the definition of "happy relationship" could be different for first-generation and second-generation immigrants.

It is evident from the data that the conflicting cultural values, beliefs, and practices between the first- and second-generation immigrants are major reasons for the intergenerational conflict and family dysfunctions. First-generation immigrants expect the second-generation immigrants to follow the cultural practices and uphold the cultural values and beliefs of the parents, and to behave the same way as their parents. Given that 100 percent of second-generation respondents agree that they cannot blindly obey their parents' principles and values, and that 100 percent of first-generation respondents agree that their children choose not to obey traditional Indian cultural values and practices they implement at home (Table 101), it is evident that their expectations for their children are unrealistic. Further, this study shows that only a minority among the second-generation group (9 percent) and a slightly higher percentage (14 percent) among the first-generation group agree that the second-generation immigrants try to behave like a proper Indian at home and in the community (Table 102). When the parents think that their children need to behave like proper Indians, the children believe that it is practically impossible to accommodate their parents. This is a deeply held conviction on the part of the second-generation respondents. Biju, a 21-year-old study participant, asked me, "Uncle, how is it possible for me to behave and act like my dad? His first 32 years he lived in India, but I did not live in India for 32 days of my 21 years. Then how can my dad expect me to behave like a proper Indian?" This is one of the major stress factors for both first- and second-generation immigrants.

In this research, the vast majority of respondents among the second-generation group (98 percent) agree that their parents judge them according to Indian cultural values and standards and 72 percent of respondents among the first-generation group also agree with this view (Table 103). However, in their understanding, first-generation immigrants do not characterize their behavior as "judging" but feel they are "disciplining" their children (Table 46).

Religious and Social Institutions: Education, Cultural Struggles, and Acculturation

The data collected in this section of the survey help us understand the role that religious institutions and social institutions play to make the immigrant communities aware of their cultural struggles, stress related to acculturation, and the need for acculturation. Among the study samples, 33 percent of respondents from both first- and second-generation respondent groups attend Indian churches/temples/mosques that conduct services in English (Table 104). The remaining 67 percent from both first- and second-generation respondents attend churches/temples/mosques that conduct services in an Indian vernacular language (Table 105). The data also reveal that no respondents either from the second-generation or from the first-generation group attend American English church/ temple/ mosques (see Table 106).

Though all the respondents from both first- and second-generation groups attend churches/temples/mosques, only a minority (27 percent) of the second-generation group and 33 percent of the first-generation group agree that their churches/temples/mosques speak about the cultural struggles of immigrants (Table 107). Other churches/temples/mosques either ignore that issue or conveniently avoid it and do not see the need to offer education and awareness programs addressing those struggles. While

89 percent of second-generation respondents and 71 percent of the first-generation group agree or strongly agree that their church/ temple/ mosque often teaches that Indian culture is the best (Table 108), the majority of churches/ temples/ mosques do not address the issues of immigrant struggles. Thus, they rarely help the immigrant community to simultaneously live meaningfully in both cultures (i.e., the ethnic culture and the dominant American culture). According to the data, 15 percent of second-generation respondents and 4 percent of first-generation respondents agree that their churches / temples/ mosques help immigrant families to live simultaneously in both American and Indian cultures in a meaningful way. However, the percentage of second-generation respondents that agrees with this statement is almost four times greater than the size of the first-generation respondents (Table 109).

Religious and community centers, as teaching agents, have the moral responsibility to educate the immigrant community about the cultural struggles and the process of acculturation. The data from this study show that 62 percent of second-generation respondents and 35 percent of first-generation respondents disagree that their church/ temple/ mosque conducts any seminars, workshops, or conferences on the sociocultural struggles of Indian immigrants in the United States. While 33 percent of first-generation respondents answered this question in the negative, 32 percent are uncertain about how to answer the question (Table 110). These two groups together constitute 68 percent, which is mirrored in the second-generation responses. Further, the data make it clear that 55 percent of second-generation respondents and 41 percent of first-generation respondents agree that their churches/ temples/ mosques do not encourage debate or discussion on issues immigrants face (Table 111). Another 20 percent of second-generation respondents and 25 percent of first-generation respondents are uncertain how to answer the question.

Most Asian-Indian parents neither encourage dating nor marry their children outside of their religious, cultural, and language communities. However, due to the changes brought by globalization and reactions to traditional cultural elements, a few second-generation immigrants break this age-old custom and marry outside their caste, class, culture, race, and ethnic group. Such marriages are often regarded as socially unacceptable, as they bring social stigma and stress to the family. In that context, 85 percent of second-generation respondents and 74 percent of first-generation respondents disagree that their churches/ temples/ mosques teach about interracial marriages (Table 112).

Acculturation is the process by which people learn different aspects of a culture that is not theirs and learn to incorporate parts of the culture into their daily living so as to survive in their new environment. For new immigrants, this is a major part of living a meaningful life. In my opinion, sociocultural and religious centers should play a critical role in making new immigrants aware of what is involved in acculturation. However, in answering the question about church's/ temple's/ mosque's role in teaching about the process of acculturation, 84 percent of second-generation respondents and 74 percent of first-generation respondents disagree that their church/ temple/ mosque teaches the need for acculturation (Table 113).

It is interesting that none of the second-generation immigrants born and raised in the United States subscribe their membership to an American English church/ temple/ mosque. Even though this group is thrice marginalized, they find it comfortable and meaningful to practice their spirituality/faith with their Asian-Indian friends. According to the data collected for this study, 67 percent of churches/ temples/ mosques attended by second-generation respondents and 64 percent of churches/ temples/ mosques of first-generation respondents do not always listen to the concerns of second-generation Indian immigrants (Table 114). A cross-analysis of the demographic details of the study samples reveals that the minority of churches/ temples/ mosques that do listen to the concerns of second-generation immigrants are Indian-English and not those that conduct services in an Indian vernacular.

Various research studies, along with my experiences in ministry, validate the experience of second-generation immigrants that they are different from their parents in the United States and their cousins in India. However, how we perceive the difference is a matter of serious concern. Instead of seeing the difference in a positive way, often this difference is seen as an "otherness" that disqualifies them as members of the community. Second-generation immigrants experience this "otherness" both in their parental community and also in the larger dominant American community. While they are "others" in American society because of their skin color, they are "others" in their parental community due to their language and the Western cultural practices they espouse. Because of this negative notion of "otherness," second-generation immigrants feel rejected by both communities. This leads me to suggest that if the second-generations' "otherness" could be recognized as strength, regarded as a capacity to link both Indian and American communities, and considered as potential for bridge-building, their lives would be more meaningful and rewarding.

There is another danger associated with blindly subscribing to the oppo-site extreme (i.e., considering that they are the same as first-generation Indian parents or their cousins living in India). This will definitely do more harm than do good to the second-generation immigrant community. This is where the intercultural principle of "Trinitarian" formation of human personhood comes into play. For Kluckhohn and Murray, that principle states that every human being is in some respects (1) like all others, (2) like some others, and (3) like no others.[11] Data in this research reveal that only 44 percent of second-generation respondents believe that the church/ temple/ mosque they attend has two different views about the first- and second-generation immigrants. But 74 percent of first-generation respondents believe that their churches/ temples/ mosques do have two different views about the first- and second-generation immigrants. Again, no other tool could be used to assess the nature of these two different points of view (Table 115). However, if the community has a different, positive view of second-generation immigrants, that different view will be guiding, sustaining, and reconciling to them.

As mentioned earlier, a vast majority of the second-generation immi-grants are unable to read and write their parental vernacular language, though they can speak it to some extent. It is often difficult for them to understand the vernaculars, particularly if someone speaks quickly. Yet, the data in this study reveal that 65 percent of churches/ temples/ mosques of the second-generation immigrants and 63 percent of churches/temples/ mosques of the first-generation immigrants always use an Indian vernacular to teach and preach (Table 116). Churches/ temples/ mosques that conduct services in English are more convenient to the second-generation immigrants. The majority of respondents among both first-generation (57 percent) and second-generation (55 percent) immigrants agree that the second-generation immigrants fully understand the English accent used by Indian teachers/ preachers in their church/ temple/ mosque (Table 117).

Since second-generation immigrants are different from their parents, their emotional, cultural, and spiritual needs are also different. Churches/ temples/ mosques and other sociocultural centers are the most important places where Indian communities gather to fill their emotional, spiritual, and cultural needs. At those gatherings, they appear in Indian dress, use an Indian language, and express their cultural values and traditions. However, even in those places, the emotional, cultural, and spiritual needs of the second-generation immigrants are often not fully met as the centers may not seriously consider the needs of second-generations. According to the data collected in this study, 81 percent of second-generation respondents believe that their church/ temple/ mosque does not consider their emotional, spiritual, and cultural needs, and one-fifth (20 percent) among the first-generation respondents also agree with that statement (Table 118). Those churches/ temples/ mosques that ignore the emotional, spiritual, cultural needs and concerns of second-generation immigrants are striving to somehow impart Indian cultural values to them and make them proper Indians in the United States. The data indicate that 56 percent of second-generation respondents and 62 percent of first-generation respondents agree that the churches/ temples/ mosques in their area try to make the second-generation immigrants proper Indians (Table 119). At the same time, 74 percent of second-generation respondents and 90 percent of first-generation respondents believe that their churches/ temples/ mosques are only concerned about the spiritual issues of their members and do not worry about the sociocultural and emotional issues that Indians face (Table 120).

As Table 115 demonstrates, the opposite extreme of seeing second-generations as "the other" in a negative sense is to view them exactly the same as their parents whose identity and self/personhood has been developed in the Indian culture. This study found that 58 percent of second-generation respondents and 48 percent of first-generation respondents agree that their churches/ temples/ mosques consider second-generation immigrants as simply Indians, the same as Indians born and raised in India (Table 121). Due to the extremes of sameness on the one hand, and perceived negativity of their "otherness" and negligence of their various needs on the other, 67 percent of second-generation respondents agree or strongly agree with the statement that their current churches/ temples/ mosques cater primarily to their parents, not to them. However, 81 percent of first-generation respondents believe that their church/ temple/ mosque is both for them and for their children (Table 122). Even after being aware that the second-generation immigrants are unable to fully understand their parental languages, only 14 percent of churches/temples/mosques of the second-generation immigrants and 26 percent of the first-generation immigrants have separate services in English (Table 123).

The analysis and the interpretation of the research data support the literature reviewed and the observations identified in Chaps. 2 and 3. The empirical data indicate that the Asian-Indian community is split into two generations and that there is a cultural value conflict that results in family dysfunction because first- and second-generations understand, value, and practice two opposing sets of cultural values. While first-generation parents behave based on Indian cultural values, second-generation immigrants' behavior is informed by mainstream American culture. This leads to intergenerational conflict and family dysfunction.

In Chap. 5, these issues are examined from the psychological perspectives of Sudhir Kakar and Heinz Kohut. Using the theoretical frameworks of Kakar and Kohut, I analyze the ways in which each culture shapes the personhoods of people and how it helps us understand the internal world of others when they behave in different manners. Kakar's collective self and Kohut's cohesive self will be examined, along with their other theoretical concepts for the purpose of developing a psychotherapeutic model for Asian-Indian immigrants in the Western cultural world.

NOTES

1. Since the cultural values, beliefs, and practices of Asian-Indians are narrated in detail with adequate supports of various historians in Chap. 2, limited quotations are used in this chapter.
2. Jee-sook Lee, "Intergenerational Conflict, Ethnic Identity and Their Influence on Problem Behaviors among Korean American Adolescent" (PhD diss., University of Pittsburg, 2004).
3. Xiaoyan Fan, "Protective Factors against Intergenerational Conflict in Chinese Immigrant Families: A Pilot Study" (PhD diss., Loyola University Chicago, 2012).
4. Heinz Kohut, *The Restoration of the Self* (New York: International Universities Press, 1977).
5. Table numbers refer to tables in the Appendix (pp. 000–000).
6. Heinz Kohut, *Analysis of the Self* (New York: International Universities Press, 1971), 50, 64.
7. Sam George, *Understanding the Coconut Generation: Ministry to the Americanized Asian Indians* (Niles, Illinois: Mall Publishing Co., 2006), 55.
8. Ghazala Bhatti, *Asian Children at Home and School* (London: Routledge, 1999), 64.
9. Narindar Singh, *Canadian Sikhs: History, Religion, and Culture of Sikhs in North America* (Ottawa: Canadian Sikhs' Studies Institute, 1994), 28.
10. Oscar Ravi Zacharias, *Walking from East to West: God in the Shadows* (Grand Rapids, MI: Zondervan, 2006).
11. C. Kluckholn and H. Murray, *Personality in Nature, Society and Culture* (New York: Alfred Knopf, 1948).

CHAPTER 5

Relationship, Culture, Community and Personhood

INTRODUCTION

The data related to intra-family relationships among multiple generations and intergenerational conflict discussed in the previous chapters provide the raw material for the next step—the development of an appropriate model of pastoral care that effectively addresses the particular forms of intergenerational and intrafamily conflict experienced by Asian-Indian immigrant families in the United States. The model seriously considers the cultural experiences of these people in order to prevent misunderstanding, misdiagnosis, and mistreatment. It draws on both Indian and Western behavioral and social science resources, specifically the work of Sudhir Kakar and Heinz Kohut, in the development of a model of pastoral psychotherapy. This model will, hopefully, also be effective for Asian-Indian immigrants in other Western countries where the dominant culture significantly differs from Asian-Indian culture and who encounter the same types of family conflicts experienced by Asian-Indian immigrant families in the United States.

The first part of this chapter briefly explores Sudhir Kakar's psychoanalytic understanding of the development of self in the Indian context. The major focus of this section is the role of family dynamics and their relationship to personality development. In other words, Kakar examines the role of family-centered Asian-Indian culture in shaping a healthy personhood in the given context. The role of relationship between mother and infants, good mother, bad mother, origins of identity in the patriarchal culture, psychosocial matrix of childhood, and culture and collective sense of identity are

© The Author(s) 2017
V. Jacob, *Counseling Asian Indian Immigrant Families*,
DOI 10.1007/978-3-319-64307-6_5

the major concepts central to an understanding of Kakar's psychological theory of personhood used here.

The next section discusses Kohut's understanding of the self from the perspective of a psychoanalytic psychology of the self. A central focus is the role of primary relationship and the power of empathy. Some of the major concepts central to an understanding of Kohut's psychological theory of the self, discussed in detail in this section include the psychology of the self as it relates to self-objects, mirroring, idealizing, narcissism, empathy, introspection, and transference. This section also shows how this psychology of the self can be appropriately adjusted to respond to the cultural norms of Asian-Indians.

Finally, I discuss the implications of Kohut's psychological theory of the self for the Asian-Indian understanding of the "communal self" in relation to Kakar's concept. My major focus is on those nuances of Kohut's psychoanalytic psychology of self that highlight the role and impact of relationships on the development of a cohesive self for the purpose of developing a model of pastoral psychotherapy (based on those nuances) for Asian-Indian families immigrating to the United States.

KAKAR: BIOGRAPHICAL SKETCH AND MAJOR WORKS

In order to fully understand Kakar's theoretical formula and its relevance to the development of a model of pastoral psychotherapy for Asian-Indian immigrant families, it is helpful to know something of his personal and clinical background. Sudhir Kakar, born in 1938, is a psychoanalyst and writer living in Goa, India. He constructed his understanding of personality to suit the Indian context. While the fundamentals of his theory are primarily derived from Erik Erikson, the applications are tailored for the Indian context and meet the needs of Indian people. Distinguishing Kakar is his sensitivity to the Indian cultural context and his attempt to explain concepts and categories of Erikson's theory, which were developed in the context of Europe and the United States in familiar Indian terms.

In *The Indian Psyche*,[1] Kakar gives a personal introduction to his early life, his later conviction to become a psychoanalyst, and his subsequent training. He reminisces about his happy childhood during the early 1940s when he lived in West Punjab, where his father worked for the British Raj as a magistrate in the civil administration. His life was centered on friends of his age, comprised mostly of children of their servants. He used to play especially with girls whom he was attracted to, with whom he enjoyed "the secret delight of sexual games."[2] Until he was six years old, the only son of doting parents, he was the center of every one's attraction. But when his sister was born, his parents' attention shifted away from him and he felt what he experienced was now less than love.[3]

His father came from a well-to-do family of merchants and contractors who lived in a typical Indian extended family. He was also brilliant in studies and received a scholarship to do graduate study in economics and political studies at Lahore. He loved the Indian way of life and was proud of his ancient culture. But he was also ready to identify with his British co-workers to fight against the decay of an Indian society, which was riddled with black magic and superstitions. His mother, on the other hand, came from a family that was more Westernized and had studied at sophisticated English-medium schools.

His mother's family was not a traditionally extended one like his father's. Kakar confessed that watching flickering images at a movie theater in Lahore owned by his grandmother's family was one of the things he enjoyed most as a child. He says watching a love scene brought him "closer to unraveling the secret of adulthood, which every child yearns to understand."[4] However, his childhood came to an end with the partition of India in 1947, resulting in significant losses for the family and the breaking of family ties.

Thus, began the shift for Kakar from life in an extended family to study at successive Christian missionary institutions. His father advised him to study mechanical engineering at Ahmedabad in Gujarat, where he came into contact with his mother's sister Kamala, who was the head of the psychology division of a research institute. Through her strength and influence Kakar first encountered the Western world. He started reading European writers and thinkers, especially the philosophy of Bertrand Russell, and was fascinated by Sigmund Freud's works on psychoanalysis. He finished engineering when he was 22 and began another career in shipyard training in West Germany, where he made use of his newfound freedom from his conservative Indian family and indulged in drinking and womanizing.[5]

However, he became very homesick at that time and longed for the life of Indian towns. He also confessed that he discovered India while living in the West and he really came to understand its history and culture through the eyes of Western scholars.[6] Kakar completed his graduate studies in economics at the University of Mannheim in West Germany, returned to India in 1964, and worked at the newly established Indian Institute of Management at Ahmedabad. He soon left this unsatisfying job and confessed that he suffered from severe identity crisis. Thereafter, he first came into contact with Erik Erikson at Harvard and, later, when Erikson came to India in the late 1960s for a few months to research his book on Mahatma Gandhi.[7]

Kakar, like his mentor Erikson, believes that every human individual has the potential of attaining hope, purpose, wisdom, and other moral virtues, and that individuals need not suffer conflict, anxiety, and neurosis because of instinctual biological forces. He also says that individuals are capable of determining each situation in a constructive way and, even though they fail at one stage, they are ready for change at a later stage.[8] With their increasing independence and the ability to respond to different crises, individuals are endowed with the potential to direct growth throughout their lives. He believes that personality is determined more by learning and experience than by heredity. Psychological experiences and not instinctual biological forces are the determinant factors for individual development. Therefore, the ultimate goal of the individual is to develop a positive ego identity that encapsulates all the basic strengths which includes hope, love, and wisdom.[9]

Development of Personality

In his writing, Kakar interchangeably uses the terms identity and personality. He utilizes Erikson's concepts of stages of "psychosocial growth," from the infant depending on the nurturing care of the mother to the young adult's sense of identity and emotional stability. To Kakar, "identity is meant to convey the process of synthesis between inner life and outer social reality, as well as the feeling of personal continuity and consistency within oneself, which occurs at the same time in some kind of confirming community."[10] This identity is not just confined by the individual but is also influenced by the historical and cultural milieu. He says that it is this search for identity that marks the turning point in the individual's development. He uses traditional Hindu concepts and categories to explore the psychological development of the individual, and herein lies Kakar's unique contribution to psychoanalysis: his pioneering application and usage of the Hindu worldview to explain the insights of Erikson.[11]

For Kakar, identity has other connotations and perspectives that extend beyond the individual and the social to include the historical and cultural. This concept is ideally suited to integrate the kinds of data—cultural, historical, and psychological—which must be included in a description of the Indianness of Indians: "the network of social roles, traditional values, caste, customs, and kinship regulations with which the threads of individual psychological developments are interwoven."[12] Kakar's discussion of human development in India is organized around yet another basic developmental line or sequence, "one which describes the arc of growth in terms of the individual's reciprocity with his (sic) social environment, where for a long time the members of his immediate family are the critical counter players."[13]

Mother and Infants

Kakar, like Kohut, believes that the nature of an individual's first relationship—with the mother—profoundly influences the quality and dynamics of social relations throughout his/her life.[14] It is within this dyad that a person first learns to relate to the others and begins to develop his/her capacity to love in its wider sense. It is here that the individual originates as a social being. Kakar says,

> During the first few months of life, the infant lives in a psychological state that has variously been termed undifferentiated, non-differentiated or unintegrated. All these terms mean the same as in this stage there is no clear and absolute distinction between conscious and unconscious, ego and id, psyche and soma, inside and outside, I and what is not-I. Through constant exchange with the mothering person does the infant begin to discriminate and differentiate these opposites, which are initially merged, and thus to take his/her first steps on the road to selfhood.[15]

The infant's development and relationship with the mother that nurtures it are optimal only when that relationship becomes a kind of psychological counterpart to the biological connection of pregnancy. This optimal condition can be termed variously as mutuality, dual unit, reciprocity, or dialogue. All these terms convey that what is good and right for one partner in the relationship is good and right for the other. The reciprocity between mother and infant is a circular process of action-reaction–action in which, ideally, the mother welcomes her infant's unfolding activities and expression of love with her own delighted and loving responses, which in turn stimulate the baby to increase his/her effort and to offer his/her mother further expression of gratification and attachment. This mutuality is, by far, the single most important factor in enabling an infant to create a coherent inner image of a basically reassuring world and to lay the foundation for a true self. Without a true self, he/she is often likely to become a bundle of reactions that resignedly complies with, or is in constant struggle against, the outer world's infringements. Kakar believes that as it is found in most societies "it is the mother who helps her infant to deal with anxiety without feeling devastated and to temper and manage the inevitable feelings of frustration and anger."[16]

The Good Mother

The term "infant" is often used for a baby who cannot yet walk. However, the actuality of childhood and identity development in India suggests that the psychosocial quality of infancy extends through the first four or five years of life. This period is the span of time in which feeding, toileting, and rudimentary self-care are provided. It is also the time in which capacities such as walking, talking, and the initial capacity for reasoning begin to become evident.

This extension of the definitions of infancy and toddlerhood is not arbitrary. Kakar believes that the first developmental stage of childhood, characterized by a decisive and deep attachment to the nurturing mother— by dependence upon her for necessities and the pleasures of succor and comfort, and by the crisis of trust in the benign intentions of others towards oneself—is prolonged in such a way that the second and third developmental stages seem not to take place subsequently but are compressed into one.[17]

Thus, Indian children do not psychologically move away from their "first all-important other"—their mother—in their life until between the ages of three and five. During this period of prolonged infancy, the Indian child is intensely and intimately attached to his/her mother. "This attachment is an exclusive one, not in the sense of being without older and younger sibling close in age who claim and compete for the mother's love and care, but in that the Indian child up to the age of four or five exclusively directs his demands and affections towards his/her mother in spite of the customary presence in the extended family of many other potential caretakers and substitute mothers."[18]

This attachment is manifested in and symbolized by the physical closeness of the infant and his/her mother. Even up to the fifth year, if not longer, it is customary for Indian children to sleep by their mother's side at night. During the day, mother carries the youngest or the one most needing attention astride her hip, keeping the others within arms' reach as she works inside or goes outside. The Indian infants' experience of their mother is a powerful one as they are constantly held, cuddled, crooned, and talked to. Their contact with her is of an intensity and duration that differentiate it markedly from the experience of infancy in Western worlds. Quite often the infant is picked up, breast-fed, and comforted, even at the slightest whimper of distress. Therefore, "it is by no means uncommon to see an old grandmother pick up a crying child and give him/her her dried-up breast to suck as she sits there, rocking on her heels and crooning over him/her. The intensity of the infantile anxiety aroused by inevitable brief separations from the mother is greatly reduced by the ready availability of the other female members of the extended family."[19]

From the moment of birth, an Indian infant is greeted and surrounded by direct, sensual body contact and by endless physical ministrations. The emotional quality of nurturing in traditional Indian families serves to amplify the effects of physical gratifications. According to Kakar,

> An Indian mother is inclined towards a total indulgence of her infant's wishes and demands, whether these be related to feeding, cleaning, sleeping or being kept company. Moreover, she tends to extend this kind of mothering well beyond the time when the infant is ready for independent functioning in many areas. Thus, for example, feeding is frequent, at all times of the day and night and on demand. And although breast feeding is supplemented with other kinds of food after the first year, the mother continues to give her breast to her child for as long as possible, often up to two or three years: in fact, suckling comes to a gradual end only when there is a strong reason to stop nursing, such as second pregnancy.[20]

Similarly, without any push from the mother or other members of the family, Indian toddlers, in general, take their own time learning to control their bowels, and proceed at their own pace to master other skills such as walking, talking, and dressing themselves. A young child's wishes are fully gratified and his/her unfolding capacities and activities accepted as far as the parents' means permit. Though this experience of gratification may not be always with open delight, it definitely happens with affectionate tolerance. "Given the experience of his mother's immediacy and utter responsiveness, an Asian-Indian child generally emerges from infancy to childhood with a staunch belief that the world is benign (non-threatening) and that others can be counted on to act on his behalf. The child has come to experience his/her core self as loveable: I am lovable for I am loved."[21] This experience of extended infancy provides Indian children a secure base from which to explore their environment with confidence. This confidence in the support and protection of others, together with the vivid memory of maternal ministrations, provides the basic modality for the social relations throughout the life cycle. In other words, most of the first-generation Asian-Indian immigrants approach others with an unconscious sense of their own lovability and with an expectation that trustworthy benefactors will always turn up in times of difficulty. Suspicion and reserve are rare in these persons.

Many character traits ascribed to Asian-Indians in Chap. 2 of this book are a part of the legacy of this particular pattern of infancy:

> Trusting friendliness with a quick readiness to form attachments and intense, if short-lived, disappointment if friendly overtures are not reciprocated, willing to reveal the most intimate confidence about one's life at the slightest acquaintance and the expectation of a reciprocal familiarity in others and the assumption that it is natural both to take care of others and to expect to be cared for.[22]

This is the core of the Indian personality in terms of confidence in the safeguarding supportiveness of others and trusting in the fundamental benevolence of the environment.

The Bad Mother

In India, the anxiety that may fester around the theme of separation stems at least partly from that moment in later infancy when the mother may suddenly withdraw her attention and her presence from her child. Child-rearing in India, during infancy, is varied. Some mothers may scold, and at times will discipline with corporal punishment. Many mothers may threaten their children when the child repeatedly insists that she should go away, leaving the child, or frightening a child with a ghost or goblins in the mango tree or coconut tree. Some mothers might also threaten to lock the child in a dark room. Briefly, threats, abandonment, and isolation are deemed common methods of character development, along with corporal punishment. "These are apprehensions that urge an Indian child to 'be good.' Yet, these punishments are threatened or carried out in a context of reliable mothering and family affection. They do not immobilize development, but recede into the depths of the psyche, a flickering trace of the dark side of the Indian inner world."[23]

Kakar argues that if there is dis-ease in the mother–infant relationship, it stems not so much from styles of maternal reprimand and punishment, and not from the duration and intensity of the connection between mother and infant, but rather from the danger of inversion of emotional roles—a danger which all too frequently becomes a reality, particularly in the case of the male child.[24] An Indian mother tends to perceive a son as a kind of savior and to nurture him with gratitude and even reverence, as well as with affection and care. For a range of reasons, the balance of the nurturing may be so affected that the mother unconsciously demands that the child serve as an object of her own unfulfilled desires and wishes, however antithetical they may be to his own wishes (especially in the case of a boy as her savior). The child feels compelled, then, to act as her savior. Faced with her unconscious intimations and demands he may feel confused, helpless, and inadequate, frightened by his mother's overwhelming nearness and yet unable (and partly unwilling) to get away.

In his fantasy, her presence acquires the ominous visage of the bad mother. According to Kakar, "images of the bad mother are culturally specific. To a large extent, they are a function of the relationship between the sexes in any society. In patriarchal societies, they reflect the nature of the mother's own unconscious ambivalence towards the male child. For instance, aggressive, destructive impulses towards the male child are a distinctive probability in societies which blatantly derogate from and discriminate against women."[25]

INFANCY AND EGO: ORIGIN OF IDENTITY IN A PATRIARCHAL CULTURE

In the Indian cultural context, the main emphasis in the early years of childhood is not encouragement of the child's individuation and autonomy but rather avoidance of frustration and the enhancement of the pleasurable mutuality of mother and infant.

By and large Indian children are neither pressed into active engagement with the external world, nor are they coerced or cajoled to master the inner world represented, temporarily at least, by his bodily process. Thus, with respect to elimination, the toddlers in India are exempt from the anxious pressure to learn to control their bowel movements according to a rigid schedule of time and space.[26]

This does not mean that no attempts are made to train toddlers in cleanliness. At about the age of three a child may indeed be taken outside in the morning, seated in a hollow made by his mother's feet and coaxed to relieve himself. What is relevant here is that such attempts are not systematic instructions or *a priori* rules. Therefore, "such attempts rarely become the occasions for a climactic battle of wills in which the mother suddenly reveals an authoritarian doggedness that says her nurturing love is, after all, conditional,"[27] as is often the case in the West. In the traditional Indian culture, most of the Indian children learn to control their bowels by imitating older children and adults in the family. Kakar observes that this relaxed form of toilet training can contribute to the formation of specific personality traits such as a relative feeling of timelessness, a relaxed conscience about our swings of mood, and a certain low-key tolerance of contradictory impulses and feelings, not only in oneself, but in others as well.[28]

In India, the process of ego development takes place according to a model that differs sharply from that proposed by Western psychologists. Indian mothers consistently emphasize "the good object" in their behavior. It is simply because Indian mothers tend to accede to their children's wishes and inclinations, rather than try to mold or control them. Thus, Indian children do not have a gradual step-by-step experience of the many small frustrations and disappointments that would allow them to recognize a mother's limitations, harmlessly, over some time. Rather her original perfection remains untarnished by reality, a part of the Indian iconography of the Indian inner world. This shows that the "detachment from the mother by degrees that is considered essential to the development of a strong, independent ego, since it allows a child almost imperceptibly to take over his/her mother's function in relation to himself/herself is simply not a feature of early childhood in India."[29] Kakar believes that a child's differentiation of himself/herself from his/her mother (and consequently of the ego from the id) is structurally weaker and comes chronologically later than in the West with this outcome: "the mental process characteristic of the symbiosis of infancy plays a relatively greater role in the personality of the adult Indian."[30] Further, says Kakar,

> In these, the so-called primary mental process, thinking, is representational and affective; it relies on visual and sensual images rather than the abstract and conceptual secondary process thinking that we express in the language of words. Primary process perception takes place through sensory means – posture, vibration, rhythm, tempo, resonance and other non-verbal expression, not

through semantic signals that underlie secondary process thought and communication. Although every individual's thinking and perception are governed by
his idiosyncratic mixture of primary and secondary processes, generally speaking,
primary process organization looms larger in the Indian than the Western
psyche.[31]

Compared to Western children, an Asian-Indian child is encouraged to
continue in a mythical magical world for a long time. In this world, objects,
events, and other persons do not have an existence of their own, but are
intimately related to the self and its mysterious moods. The projection of
one's own emotions on to others, the tendency to see natural and human
'objects' predominantly as extensions of oneself, the belief in spirits animat-
ing the world outside, and the shuttling back and forth between secondary
and primary process modes are common features of daily conversations. The
emphasis on primary thought process finds cultural expression through
many Indian folk-tales in which we see birds and trees speak and animals
converse with each other. Clinically, the persistence of primary processes in
an individual's thinking and perception has been associated with psychopathology, in the sense that it suggests the persistence in adult life of an
infantile mode of behavior. However, according to Pinchas Noy, "in
many kinds of normal regression, such as reveries and day dreams, artistic
activity, and creative endeavor, primary processes govern the sphere of
thoughts without signs of regression in other aspects of the individual's
life."[32]

The contradictory aspects of the maternal presence can coexist in the
young child's psyche without disturbing each other, for it is a feature of
primary mental processes characteristic of infancy that contradictions do not
cause urgent conflicts pressing for resolution. "It is only later, when the ego
gains strength and attempts to synthesize and integrate experience, that
conflicts erupt and ambivalence comes into its own, and that the negative,
threatening aspects of earliest experience may be forcibly repressed or
projected onto the external world."[33]

Taken into the child's ego, the "good mother's" maternal tolerance,
emotional vitality, protectiveness and nurturing become the core of every
Indian's positive identity. Alongside this positive identity, however, and
normally repressed, is its counterpart: the negative identity that originates
in experiences with the demanding, sometimes stifling, all-too-present
mother. Whatever the contours of the negative identity, they reflect certain
defenses against the "bad mother" who may have been most undesirable or

threatening, yet, who was also most real at a critical stage of development. According to Kakar,

> In conditions of psychological stress and emotional turmoil, the negative identity fragments tend to merge in a liability to a kind of psychological self-castration in a predisposition to identify with rather than resist a tormentor, and in a longing for a state of perfect passivity. Although the inner world of Indians is decisively influenced by both the good and the bad versions of the maternal-feminine, the adult identity consolidation of men (sic) is of course not to be cast exclusively in these terms. For identity is constituted not only out of early feminine identifications, but also later masculine ones, all of them rearranged in a new configuration in youth. Expression of the maternal-feminine in a man's (sic) positive identity, the adaptive aspect, is neither deviant nor pathological but that which makes a man (sic) more human.[34]

The seeds of a viable identity require the fertile soil of a compatible family structure and a corresponding set of cultural values and beliefs. In India, the child learns early that emotional strength resides primarily in his/her mother, that she is where the action is. The cultural parallel to the principal actuality of infancy is the conviction that mother-goddesses are reservoirs of both constructive and destructive energy. Therefore, the primary themes of Indian identity, emerging from the infant's relationship with his/her mother, are inextricably intertwined with the predominant cultural concerns of India. These concerns, both individual and social, govern, inform, and guide the Asian-Indian inner world in such a way that they reverberate throughout the identity struggles of a lifetime.[35]

PSYCHO-SOCIAL MATRIX OF CHILDHOOD: THE FAMILY

With psychological identification with the family group being so strong among Asian-Indians, not only an actual break but even the loosening of the family bond may be a source of psychic stress and inner conflict for family members. A separation from the family, for whatever reason, not only brings a sense of insecurity, but also means the loss of significant others who guarantee the sense of sameness and affirm the inner continuity of the self. Psychiatric observations in India on the occurrence of certain kinds of mental disturbances following a break from the family amply bear this out.[36] Other than psychological explanations, there are deeper reasons for the importance of family in a person's life, such as economic realities and consideration of social prestige. In a country like India, where there is no social security, unemployment compensation, or old age benefit, it is the family that provides temporary relief when a member is facing a financial struggle. The family and extended family provide life insurance for most people in crisis. Socially, a person's worth and recognition of his/her identity are intimately bound up in the reputation of his/her family. When a man or woman approaches a major life transition, particularly marriage, the character of the family weighs heavily on the scales of his/her fate.

Just as family, and extended family, is the primary field and foil for an Indian individual's developing sense of identity, caste is the next circle in his/her widening social radius. Family and caste are the parameters of Indian childhood. Caste here does not mean the caste system of the four major castes and subcastes. Rather, it means the caste's values, beliefs, prejudices, and injunctions, as well as its distortions of reality become part of the individual's psyche and the content of the ideologies of their conscience. Because of this, much of the individual behavior and adaptations to the environment that in Westerners are regulated or coerced by the demands of the superego, is taken care of in Indians by a communal conscience. In contrast with the Western superego, the communal conscience is a social rather than an individual formation: it is not inside the psyche. In other words, "instead of having one internal sentinel, an Indian relies on many external "watchmen" to patrol his/her activities, especially his/her relationships in all the social hierarchies."[37] The greater authority of the codes of the communal conscience, as opposed to the internalized rules of the individual superego, creates a situation in which infringements of moral standards become like situations "when no one is looking." Such situations normally arise when the individual is away from the watchful discipline of his/her family, caste, and village groups.

Culture and Personality

The culture of any particular society, which surrounds us from the beginning of life, envelops us like the very oxygen we breathe and, without which, we do not grow into viable human beings. A person's identity—of which the culture he/she has grown up in is a vital part—is what makes a person recognize himself/herself and be recognized by the people who constitute one's world. Identity is not something that people choose, rather something that seizes them. Therefore, it can be said that the cultural part of our identity is wired into our brains. The culture in which an infant grows up constitutes the software of the brain, much of which is already in place by the end of childhood.

Different cultures shape the development of their members in different ways. For instance, in India, ideal psychological wholeness or maturity is quite compatible with an ego which is relatively passive and less differentiated against the Western thinking of healthy self as differentiated, individuated, and autonomous. Given this, Kakar argues that an ideal psychological maturity that presumes to translate experiences and practices of one society into universal norms for others should give us pause or make us stop.[38] Kakar further depicts the influence of culture in a person's life in the following statement:

> Culture is so pervasive that even when an individual seems to break away from it, as in states of insanity, the 'madness' is still influenced by cultural norms and rituals. Even in a condition of extreme stress, the individual takes from his (sic) culture its conventions or traditions in implementing and giving form to an idiosyncratic disorder, the culture providing, as it were, the patterns of misconduct.[39]

Quoting Heinz Hartmann, Kakar further notes,

> It is now generally accepted that the newborn infant brings with him (sic) an innate capacity or readiness to adapt into the culture in which, he (sic) is received. His (sic) innate potential for growth, for learning, for relationships, can normally be expected to unfold in culturally appropriate ways in the course of interaction with the world around him (sic).[40]

Accordingly, a mother's response to her infant depends not only upon her emotional stance towards motherhood deeply rooted in her own life history, or upon the inborn constitution of her child, but also upon her culture's image of the role of motherhood and of the nature of a child.[41] To put it briefly, the development of the ego cannot be comprehended except in its interdependence on the society into which an individual child is born, a society represented in the beginning by the mother and other culturally sanctioned caretakers.[42]

Collective Sense of Identity

The sense of one's identity is neither completely conscious nor unconscious, although at times it may appear to be exclusively the one or the other. Identity in the Indian context cannot be confused with the concepts of role or character, although there may be an overlap of all three. Identity also cannot be completely characterized in terms of self-conception and self-esteem. A disturbance in the sense of identity is not the same as role conflict or a conflict in values, although occasionally it may be manifested as either. At the same time, when we consider the identity of an individual, personal growth and communal change cannot be separated, nor the identity crisis in individual development, from the contemporary crisis in the historical development of the individual's group. Kakar believes that the term "identity crisis" no longer carries the forebodings of an impending pathological disaster. Rather, it is accepted as designating a necessary turning point, a crucial moment, when development must move one way or another, marshalling resources of growth, recovery, and further differentiation.[43]

Many of the salient aspects of the Indian society, like family-centeredness, religion, regional affiliation, language, and caste/class play a crucial role in the development of the self-concept, an individual self being formed and developed within the communal self. The collective sense of identity characterizing the individual's significant social groups, such as caste, class, nation, or culture, gets transmitted into the infant's earliest body, entering the very core of the Indian ego and, thus, becomes inextricably intertwined with a personal sense of identity which emerges from the earlier accrued identifications.[44] Individual accomplishments are valued only if they improve the well-being and/or status of one's family or community. The guiding principle is that the collective identity affirms preservation and enhancement of the well-being of the group. Every person in a group is expected to uphold the collective identity over individual identity. They are even expected to subjugate their own inclinations and make personal sacrifices if needed. In such conflicting situations, everyone always regards the collective self over the personal self.[45]

Caste and gender further accentuate the issue of identity development in Indian society. As Kakar points out,

> The daughter of a Hindu family hardly ever develops an identity of her own. She is expected to remain chaste and pure and upon reaching marriageable age, she is seen as economic liability because of dowry. On entering her

married home, her status changes. She is seen as a wife, as a daughter-in-law, as a sister-in-law in the new home. And then as a mother, a grandmother and should her husband predecease her, as a widow. In the new home, she buries her past and new identity is ascribed to her. No permanent identity, but ever changing identity from her changing role.[46]

It is clear that identity is less achieved and more ascribed; ascribed by birth, family, community, caste, status, and religion. The ascribed identity tends to restrict choices open to the individual. According to this notion, one's identity, to a large extent, tends to be the reflection of familial and social norms and expectations. Personal interests, goals, welfare, and glory are secondary to that of the family. In order to attain harmony within the family, it is essential for an individual to surrender or merge into his or her family, resulting in the loss of his or her individuality. It is precisely this location of identity in the core of both, the individual and communal culture, its emergence from the interplay of the psychological and social, the developmental and the historical, which makes the concept difficult to comprehend. And yet it also gives it its power and promise for fruitful interdisciplinary work.

Kakar's theory is developed in the Indian cultural context, where the communal self is emphasized over the individual self, interdependence is stressed over independence, and family interest over individual interest. Though the parental community, first-generation immigrants, is living in the United States, their perceptions, outlook, worldview, and cultural values are still based on the culture in which their identity is formed and shaped. Since second-generation immigrants are born, raised, and initially socialized with their first-generation parents, the parental values become a part of their identity. In other words, the experience of the second-generation immigrants cannot be isolated from their parental cultural experience. Therefore, when the second-generation immigrants seek therapy, they can never be understood as an entirely different group of people separated from their parents, simply because the second-generation's level of cultural assimilation far exceeds the level of their parent's acculturation.

In this context, Kakar's theory helps us understand the unique nature of Asian-Indian immigrants—both first and second 'cultural generations'—and to develop a therapeutic counseling model for them as many of them are facing intergenerational family conflicts. Further, it helps us understand the importance of family therapy and its primary principle that every group is a unit, and a part cannot be isolated from the whole without understanding the experience of the whole. Kakar's theory helped me to develop my five-stage psychotherapeutic counseling model for the Asian-Indian immigrants living in the multiple cultural spaces of the Western world.

HEINZ KOHUT

The next theorist who contributes to my five-stage therapeutic counseling model for the Asian-Indian immigrants in the United States is Heinz Kohut. Kohut describes the human self as formed and developed in the context of relationship. This theory seriously considers family when it talks about human identity and self. While the implications of Kohut's psychological theory of the self is engaged with the Asian-Indian understanding of the "communal self," the importance of this information is considered for developing my model of psychotherapy for Asian-Indian immigrants in the United States. To better understand the theoretical stance of Kohut, we need to understand his personal clinical background.

Biographical Context

Heinz Kohut was born in Vienna, Austria, in 1913. He was the only child of his Jewish parents, Felix and Else. His father was a pianist who, after four years of service on the eastern front in World War I, went into the paper business. Heinz was home-schooled for the first four years of his life as his mother hired tutors for him. He later studied medicine at the University of Vienna and graduated in 1938. Because of Hitler and the Nazis' takeover of Austria in the spring of 1938, Kohut found himself in danger and left in 1939 for England where he stayed in a camp while waiting for a visa to go to America. He arrived in America in 1940 and went to the University of Chicago. According to Siegel,

> In retrospect, one wonders about the wellspring of Kohut's originality and its final focus on narcissism. I would speculate that his creativeness was a compensatory response to some early deprivations that had threatened the cohesiveness of his budding self. One major deprivation was the absence of his father during World War 1. I do not know the exact dates for his father's military service, but Kohut had been born in May 1913. For Kohut's father, the war had been a catastrophic interruption of his career as a concert pianist and he was unable to pursue his musical aims after he returned. One can easily

imagine the father's depression and the son's disillusionment in the now returned father, who must have been a distantly admired hero during his military service.[47]

This insight of Siegel helps us understand how his biographical background may have influenced his conceptualization of the idealizing self-objects and how he mainly attributes them to the male figure in the child's parental relationship.

Little Heinz was close to his mother and remained so for many years. However, his mother was a somewhat distant woman who was overly involved in her own social life, often leaving Heinz in the care of servants and tutors. Though Heinz was the only child to his parents, he was privately tutored at home without being sent to public school, which later made it difficult for him to feel at ease in large groups, even as an adult.[48] From this context, one can speculate on basic psychological traumas sustained during Heinz's childhood. Added to that trauma, Kohut was suddenly torn out of his circle of non-Jewish friends during late adolescence and young manhood as a result of the growing influence of the Nazi movement aimed at Austrian youth. As a troubled young man, Kohut went to meet with August Aichhorn for analysis.[49] We can see how that therapy and the childhood experience of Kohut might have helped him to develop the theoretical concepts of the important role that mothers play in the development of a cohesive self and the role of mirroring. This biographical background also illuminates Kohut's perspective on narcissism.

Kohut served as a neurologist at the University of Chicago. He was drawn to psychiatry and developed a love for psychoanalysis. He was trained at the Chicago Institute of Psychoanalysis between 1944 and 1947, where he joined the faculty as a training analyst the following year.[50] Kohut was married to Elizabeth Meyer on October 9, 1948, and had one son, Thomas.

Kohut's Clinical Context

According to Paul Ornstein, Kohut's clinical context can be understood in three defining periods: 1950–1959, 1960–1965, and 1966–1977.[51] Ornstein points out that in the first period, Kohut is applying what we may refer to as a critical correlation of the psychoanalytic theory to literature and music. In the second period (1960–1965), Kohut is applying methods he considered from his first period to problems in psychoanalysis. This period sees Kohut moving from the unconscious human dynamics as he begins to reconsider introspection, empathy, and the different forms of transference. In the third period (1966–1977), according to Ornstein, Kohut saw the fruits of the previous two periods, birthing a major breakthrough as he brought about what ended up growing into a new psychoanalytic approach to narcissism that defined Kohut's self psychology. This presentation of Kohut by Paul Ornstein is more logical and seems to be the best way of understanding the birth of Kohut's psychology of the self in a logical and simple way.[52]

According to Siegel, Kohut's early papers contain repeated themes.[53] The first is his intense interest in Freud's metapsychology, with a particular focus on genetic, dynamic, and psychoeconomic points of view. A second theme is Kohut's interest in narcissistic issues, expressed in his concern about vulnerable people and their struggle to regulate tension and maintain psychic cohesion. A third theme concerns the method of data collection in the analytic situation. Therefore, it is clear that Kohut was influenced by Freud's ego psychology, challenged by his practice and interest in narcissism, and shaped by his experience in practice. The way Siegel has organized Kohut's work makes it more practical, correlational, and simple, in its sense.[54]

Kohut is considered the founder of self psychology, a system in which the self is a key concept and refers to the conscious reflective personality of a person. Self psychology shares in common with object-relation theory—the idea that self is formed in relation to other objects (meaning, usually, other people). However, Kohut found limitations in classical psychoanalytical theory's explication of the self and eventually moved away from it. Though Kohut started his clinical work using the prevalent Freudian psychoanalytic approach in both his teaching and practice, self psychology differs from Freud's classical drive theory in many aspects, from the structures of the self to pathology and its cures. Unlike the classical drive model, where neurotic patients were viewed as having an intact structure—id, ego, and superego—in self psychology, narcissism and disorders of the self imply that the very central structures of the personality are defective. Classical Freudian drive theory explains pathology in terms of repressed, unresolved conflicts of an Oedipal nature where successful therapy means achieving freedom from instinctual conflicts. In contrast, Kohut explains that narcissism and disorders of the self result not from repressed drives, but from defects in the psychological structures of the self developed from childhood. Therefore, successful therapy involves healing the deficits by acquiring new structures.[55]

KOHUT'S UNDERSTANDING OF THE 'SELF'

In order to fully understand Kohut's concept of self, it is necessary to understand some of the key concepts of his theory. Kohut, in *Restoration of the Self*, states,

> The present volume transcends my previous writings on narcissism in several directions. In the earlier contributions, I presented my findings concerning the psychology of the self mainly in the language of classical drive theory. In comparison with my earlier contributions, the present work expresses more explicitly my reliance on the empathic-introspective stance, which has been defining my conceptual-theoretical outlook ever since 1959. This step – the full acceptance of the consequences of the fact that the psychological field is defined by the observer's commitment to the introspective-empathic approach – led to a number of conceptual refinements, indicated by termino-logical changes, as exemplified by my use of the term "self-object transfer-ence" instead of the formerly used term "narcissistic transference."[56]

In this quotation, we see the development of Kohut's understanding of the self and how he sought to bring theory and clinical observation together for the construction of his therapeutic practices. Kohut emphasizes almost everywhere that empathy is at the center of his therapeutic approach as much as it is the basis of understanding human development and a way that transforms how we understand narcissism. Kohut further states that

> The present book is not a technical or theoretical monograph detachedly written by an author who has achieved mastery in a stable and established field of knowledge. This book is a report of an analyst's attempt to struggle toward greater clarity in an area that, despite years of conscientious effort, he was unable to understand within the available psychoanalytic framework – even as amended by the work of modern contributors.[57]

Having thus understood Kohut's journey, we now need to discuss the themes that are the major concepts of Kohut's self psychology so as to understand Kohut's view of human self.

Narcissism

The term narcissism originates from Greek mythology and is used to refer to the fact that humanity has the propensity to libidinal object love or libidinal energy directed exclusively toward oneself. Freud can rightly be understood to have drawn the term narcissism from his understanding of the Greek myth as indicating an exclusive self-absorption and apply it to his psycho-analysis. According to Wagon,

> The modern concept of narcissism is not quite as modern as it may seem. Narcissus, according to Greek mythology, was the son of the river god Cephissus and the nymph Lariope. His exceptional physical beauty was much admired and made him the desire of many. Yet in that slender form was the pride so cold that no youth, no maiden touched his heart. Narcissus mocked his admirers, among them the nymph Echo, and rejected every potential lover. Finally, the goddess Nemesis heard the vengeful prayers of those scorned by the proud young man, and caused Narcissus to fall in love with his own reflection in a pool.[58]

This legend further states that Narcissus was so enamored of himself he even tried to give kisses to his own image. He kept admiring his own reflection in the pool and ended up dying because he could not even drink water for fear of disturbing the "other" he was seeing in the water. He died, and the myth says a flower that bears his name sprang up where he died. In psychoanalysis, the person who has the self as a love object is considered to be narcissistic. Such persons are self- absorbed and unable to love or relate with others.[59]

Kohut makes it clear in the following statements how his focus on narcissism differs from that of classical psychoanalysis:

> When we turn to the narcissistic personality disorders, however, we are no longer dealing with the pathological results of unsatisfactory solutions of conflicts between structures that are in essence intact, but with forms of psychological malfunctioning arising in consequence of the fact that the central structures of personality – the structures of the self- are defective. And so, in the narcissistic personality disorders, our description of the process and goals of psychoanalysis and of the conditions that characterize a genuine termination (under what circumstances we can say that the analytic task has been completed) must therefore be based on a definition of the nature and location of the essential psychological defects and on a definition of their cure.
>
> The nuclear psychopathology of the narcissistic personality disorders (corresponding to the repressed unresolved conflicts of the Oedipus complex of the structural neuroses) consist of 1) defects acquired in childhood, in the psychological structure of the self, and 2) secondary structure-formations, also built up in early childhood, which are related to the primary defect in one or two similar, but, in certain crucial respects, different ways.[60]

Here, Kohut presents a psychoanalysis that emphasizes and facilitates the analysis of the relational aspects of the structures of the self. Kohut is building his case that the disturbances that are evident in narcissistic disturbances cannot be accounted for by the drive theory postulated by Freud's psychosexual approach because there is more to the growth of the self (revealed in the clinical setting) than just sexual drives. This, therefore, raises the importance of looking at the relationship of the child in relation to primary caregivers. Kohut also proposes that disturbances in childhood are not limited to the very early stages of human development as claimed by Freud, but such realities can also occur at a much later time than was held to be the norm in Freud's day.

Kohut's departure from Freud on the understanding of narcissism can be clearly understood in terms of his appreciation of the influence of parental attitudes on the formation of the self of the child. Kohut claims that while innate determinants contribute to the development of the child and narcissism, the child's interplay with his/her environment is of utmost importance and warrants special attention.[61] Kohut contends that his focus of clinical attention is on the relational aspects of the child's development:

> If I were asked what I consider to be the most important point to be stressed about narcissism I would answer: its dependent line of development, from the primitive to the most mature, adaptive, and culturally valuable. This development has important innate determinants, but the specific interplay of the child with his environment, which furthers, or hinders the cohesion of the self and the formation of idealized psychic structures, is well worth further detailed examination, especially with the aid of the study of the varieties of the narcissistic transferences... I shall add only one small point to the results I have previously reported, namely, that the side-by-side existence of separate developmental lines in the narcissistic and in the object-instinctual realms in the child is intertwined with the parents' attitude toward the child (i.e., that the parents sometimes relate to the child in empathic narcissistic merger and look upon the child's psychic organization as part of their own), while at other times they respond to the child as to an independent center of his own initiative (i.e., they invest him with object libido).[62]

He also reveals that there are separate lines of development in the psychic development of the narcissistic child, and these directions deal with both the instinctual and the relational developmental dimensions. Here, Kohut's point of thought is that the Freudian approach is limited to instinctual developmental focus of the narcissistic child and it ignores the second line of development. The additional developmental dimension is relational and focuses on the interaction with the primary caregivers. What Kohut's theory is advocating here is a reconceptualization and reframing of narcissism that calls for looking at both the positive and the negative.[63] Kohut is proposing to see narcissism as a necessary form of development that calls for healthy relating through empathic response by an empathic attuned self-object, which may be in real early life or in therapy.

Briefly stated, Kohut argues that narcissism must be visualized not only from its emphasis on drive theory put forward by Freud, but it must also be envisioned from its relational perspective or, for example, the environmental context or influence. In other words, he argues that narcissism has two independent lines of development that are never to be viewed as antagonistic. Rather, they should be viewed as complementary and, hence, comprehensive. He argues further that the development of narcissism should be gleaned from the evidence available and, hence, be embraced with acceptance and an affirmative attitude, both in theory and practice.

He then reveals his struggle, torn as he was between the classical psychology learning group with which he had worked, and the new psychology of the self group that wanted him to give them more information. He finally saw the need to push forward and refine those aspects of classical psychology that needed to be revised or ignored. Thus, he says,

> But once I had recognized that this step was indeed necessary, that it involved neither an abandonment of the viewpoints of science, in general, nor of those of scientific depth psychology, in particular, I could proceed to confront the essentials of the intellectual task. Specifically, I had to outline a theoretical structure that would be adequate to fulfilling three demands, which I will now set down in the order of their increasing importance: 1) the new psychology of the self must remain in an unbroken continuum with traditional psychoanalytic theory to preserve the sense of the historical continuity of the group self in the psychoanalytic community; 2) the new theoretical system must, at this point in the development of psychoanalysis, not disregard the fact that the classical theories, especially as expanded in the form of modern ego psychology, though applicable only in a restricted area, are neither in error nor irrelevant; 3) the new theory, while clear, must not be dogmatic and definitive, but open to change and capable of further development.[64]

The three points Kohut mentions in this quote are critically important as I seek to develop a relevant method of care that will be appropriate for Asian-Indian immigrant families in the United States. The third point is particularly important as it challenges me not to accept the existing theories and methods as dogmatic and definitive. It helps to seek to understand Kohut on the one hand, and seek to develop the tools that will be relevant to the context of the persons who need care on the other. In his clinical observations, Kohut saw that persons who invest others with narcissistic libido are experiencing those others narcissistically, that is, as self-objects. To a narcissistic person, a self-object is an object or person undifferentiated from the individual who serves the needs of the self.

Kohut does not view narcissism as necessarily pathological, unlike traditional psychoanalytic theory. Rather, he formulates the concept of narcissism in such a way as to show how it actually plays a role in psychological health. Instead of instincts, Kohut emphasizes normal narcissism as a sign of psychological health. Kohut believes that narcissism has its own line of development so that ultimately no individual becomes independent of self-objects. He further theorizes that a non-responsive self-object could lead one to feel helpless and empty, with lower self-esteem and with narcissistic rage.[65]

SELF AND SELF OBJECTS: UNDERSTANDING HOW THE SELF DEVELOPS

Kohut understood that the development of self neither occurs in isolation, nor from drives. Rather it occurs in relationships. The infant is born in a human environment but without a self. However, the child's self forms as its parents act and respond to the child, where interplay between the infant's innate potentials and the parents' responsiveness takes place. Parents serve as the child's self-objects, performing what the child cannot do for him/herself. As the child grows, he/she starts to internalize those functions, provided an adequate responsive environment is offered. In such an environment, the nuclear or the core self develops into a cohesive self. In the epilogue of his book, *The Restoration of the Self*, Kohut acknowledges that an attempt at a concise definition of the self is nearly impossible because of the nature of what he refers to as the self. He labors to clearly speak his heart in these revealing words:

> My investigation contains hundreds of pages dealing with the psychology of the self – yet it never assigns an inflexible meaning to the term self, it never explains how the essence of the self should be defined. But I admit this fact without contrition or shame. The "self" is not a concept of an abstract science,

but a generalization derived from empirical data. Demands for a differentiation of "self" and "self-representation" (or, similarly, of "self" and a "sense of self") are, therefore based on a misunderstanding. We can describe the various cohesive forms in which the self appears, can demonstrate the several constituents that make up the self and explain their genesis and functions. And we can, finally, distinguish between various self-types and can explain their distinguishing features on the basis of the predominance of one or the other of their constituents. We can do all that, but we will still not know the essence of the self as differentiated from its manifestations.[66]

In the previous discussion, Kohut helps us understand his psychology of the self and opens the door for us to make it applicable in different contexts. Here, Kohut does not define "self." Rather, he describes his understanding of the psychology and the constituents of the self. He states how the "self" functions as revealed through his clinical work with persons dealing with narcissism. Kohut's understanding of the self is presented mainly from his experiences with narcissism and how the persons he encountered in clinical practice helped him to understand the structures of the self. The structures of the self are central to an understanding of Kohut's psychology of the self.[67]

Kohut uses the term self to refer to a "specific structure in the mental apparatus" or as the "center of the individual's psychological universe."[68] For Kohut, the self is not merely a concept. Rather, he understands the self broadly, more in terms of awareness and experience. The self is a unit, cohesive in space and enduring in time, which is the center of the initiative and the recipient of impressions.[69] This makes the self take on the active agent, performing functions that were traditionally ascribed to the ego, the locus of all relationships. This formulation allows Kohut to bypass the tripartite model and to introduce his new notion of the bipolar self.[70]

THE STRUCTURES OF THE SELF

When considering the structures of the self, Kohut takes the drive theory further and highlights the role of caregivers of children as central to the psychology of the self. According to Kohut,

> The differences between the traditional and the self psychologically informed therapeutic approaches to classic transference neuroses and relate to their different conceptions of the basic pathogenesis. The classical position maintains that we have arrived at the deepest level when we have reached the

patient's experience of his impulses, wishes, and drives, that is, when the patient has become aware of his archaic sexual lust and hostility. The self psychologically informed analyst, however, will be open to the fact that the pathogenic Oedipus complex is embedded in an oedipal self-object distur- bance that beneath lust and hostility there is a layer of depression and of diffuse narcissistic rage. The analytic process will, therefore, not only deal with oedipal conflicts per se but also, in a subsequent phase, or more frequently, more or less simultaneously, ... focus on the underlying depression and the recognition of the failures of the child's oedipal self-objects, given that the flawed self-object matrix is the breeding ground for the pathogenic Oedipus complex in childhood.[71]

Regarding Kohut, Siegel states, "Retaining the self as his central focus, he conceptualizes the drives as breakdown products of a fractured self. Kohut suggests that when disrupted, the child's affection and assertiveness fracture into the 'drive elements' of sexuality, aggression, and destructive hostil- ity."[72] Kohut's argument, as I understand it, is that the drive theory will only be scratching the surface if the dynamic of the childhood relationships with the primary caregivers is not considered as the bedrock of the devel- opment of a cohesive self.

In *The Search for the Self*, Kohut writes, "Let me present my argument in the briefest form by drawing the outlines of a separate development of single drives and functions, on the one hand, and of the self, on the other hand."[73] Here, Kohut connects Freud's drive theory and his understanding of the self from a perspective that calls for more attention to the role of the caretakers of the child and how their level of reactivity to the needs of the child impacts the child's development.

The second line of development he proposes marks the cornerstone of Kohut's self psychology. Kohut says,

It is my impression[74] that, from early on, the child's empathic environment reacts to him with two sets of responses: one is attuned to his experience of single parts of his body and of single bodily mental functions, and another is attuned to his beginning experience of himself as a larger, coherent and endur- ing organization (i.e., to himself). If careful observation of parental (especially of maternal) attitudes toward the baby should confirm this impression, one could take this finding as support for the theory of the existence of a primitive self at the very early stages of life. The fact, furthermore, that the baby reacts with rage to the unempathetic responses from the side of the early environment may also be interpreted as supporting the theory of a rudimentary self at the very beginning of life – narcissistic rage, it may be argued, presupposes an active and reactive self which insists on control over a dimly sensed self-object. . . . Suffice to say that reliably cohesive and enduring self-experience seems to be acquired by gradual steps. When the self is finally well established, it takes its position, as a superordinated structure, above the experiential world of single parts and functions.[75]

The development of the self that Kohut sees happening in childhood can be understood in terms of mirroring and idealizing relationships of the child- primary caregivers' dynamic. He sees the importance of these functions of the parents/parenting as crucial to the development of a cohesive self. Basing his theory on clinical work with persons who were narcissistic, Kohut designated the mirroring role to the mother and the idealizing role to the father. He saw these two relationships as important in helping the development of the self. He states,

It seems very likely, for example, that, while traces of both ambitions and idealized goals are beginning to be acquired side by side in early infancy, the bulk of nuclear grandiosity consolidates into "nuclear" ambitions in early childhood (perhaps mainly in the second, third, and fourth year), and the bulk of "nuclear" idealized goal structures are acquired in later childhood (perhaps mainly in the fourth, fifth, and sixth years of life). It is also more than likely that the earlier constituents of the self are usually predominantly derived from the relation with the maternal self-object (the mother's mirroring acceptance confirms nuclear grandiosity; her holding and carrying allows merger-experiences with self-object's idealized omnipotence), whereas the constituents acquired later may relate to the parental figure of either sex.[76]

He further explains that Freud's biological tenet of this essential bisexuality of humans might be rephrased in psychological terms when re-evaluated against the background of a bipolar self that is derived from male and female self-objects.[77]

Self-Object

Kohut defines self-objects as those persons or objects that are experienced as part of the self or that are used in the service of the self to provide a function for the self.[78] The rudimentary or the basic self merges with the self-object and has its needs satisfied by the actions of the self-object.[79] The self-object is not an objective person or a whole object but only has meaning in regard to the experiencing person.

"**Mirroring**" can be defined as a confirming response that the child receives from an empathic self-object. This satisfies the need for acceptance by an adult that confirms to the child that they are being valued as another human being whereby the child internalizes that acceptance and it becomes a structure that grows or is the bedrock of their acceptance of self-worthiness. This process of internalizing the mirroring of the maternal self-object is what is called transmuting internalization, which means the borrowing of the self-object's valuing of the child's self-worthiness into the structure of the child. It leads into self-acceptance and assertiveness.[80]

The "**idealization**" that Kohut sees as another important aspect of the development of the child responds to the need of the child to merge with the strength and omnipotence of the idealized parent. Mainly this is associated with the male parent. This aspect helps the child in the development of the self to establish, together with the other, a balanced sense of self.[81] It has been said that the failure of one of the parental empathic responses to the child that is needed for the development of a nuclear self can be compensated for by an empathic response in the other.

Transmuting Internalization

Internalization in psychoanalysis is a method of healing or rebuilding the psychic structure of one's inner world. Kohut conceived of a similar process of internalization, transmuting internalization. This is the process by which aspects of the self-object are absorbed into the child's self. However, when the parents or the other self-objects fall short of or delay gratification of a child's needs, and if the frustration is tolerable and not traumatic, this optimal frustration compels a child to take in aspects of the self-object in the form of specific functions. The child loses some of the magical expectations that are narcissistic and gains some particle of inner structure. The inner structure of the child then performs some functions that the object previously performed for him/her, such as comforting, mirroring, or controlling tension.[82] The transmuting internalization refers to the depersonalizing shift from the personality of the object, which performs the function, to the function itself.

Empathy

For Kohut, "the best definition of empathy – the analogue to my terse scientific definition of empathy as 'vicarious introspection'[83] – is that capacity to think and feel oneself into the inner life of another person."[84] It is our lifelong ability to experience what another person experiences, though usually and appropriately to an attenuated degree. Under normal circumstances, this ability will change in specific ways along an individually developed variable, but on the whole predictable, developmental road.[85] For Kohut, the importance of empathy in the development of self is the most important aspect of the creation of a strong sense of being.

It is important to understand that while Kohut, in his writing, may have led us to believe in the strict gender roles in relations to mirroring and idealizing, his emphasis is more on the importance of the role of empathy from the parenting environment than it is about the mother and father. He also responds to the issues of the "absence" of the mother and "insufficiency" of mothering that leads to fixations in childhood due to excess gratification, saying,

> It may not make any difference whether it is the child's biological mother who is the provider. It may not even make a crucial difference whether one or several people are involved in the mothering, as you would say, or in the empathic environment of the child, as I would say . . . one must think not simply in terms of "mothering" and "mother," but in terms of the total complexity of an environment and whether it is positive or negative.[86]

These statements confirm his claim that the environment in which the child is brought up shapes the child's understanding of him/herself. Kohut's psychology of the self came about via his work with adults who were dealing with problems of narcissism. It was in the clinical setting of counseling that he sought to understand the genesis of the woundedness of the persons who sought therapy that revealed to him the vicissitudes of the environment of persons' childhood years. As he came to understand these problems, Kohut discovered that there was need to cure this wounding by recreating healthy responses in therapy that would allow the analysis and lead to having a cohesive self.[87] Briefly stated, for Kohut, it is through an empathic relationship that self develops, both in the parent-child interactions and in the therapist-client relationship. In both cases, empathy is combined with warmth to provide understanding in an accepting environment. In a warm and responsive environment, the self will develop empathy for itself and others. Growth may be reactivated in the empathic atmosphere of the therapeutic setting.

Bipolar Self

A "nuclear" or "core" self is formed through the responsiveness of self-objects. The nuclear self is made up of two parts: the grandiose-exhibition-istic self and the idealized parental image. Together, the grandiose self and the idealized parental image are known as the bipolar self. The former self becomes established by relating to a self-object that empathically responds to the child by approving and mirroring this grandiose self. The latter is the child's idealized parental image, which is established by relating to a self-object that empathically responds to the child by permitting and enjoying the child's idealization of the parents.[88] Both involve a form of merging experience with the self-object. The grandiose self refers to the child's self-centered view of the world and his/her deluding in being admired and praised. The idealized parental image is antithetical or contradictory to the grandiose self in which it implies that someone else is perfect. The child experiences a merger with that idealized object: you are perfect and I am a part of you.

Both parts of the nuclear self are to be empathically responded to by a self-object. Through numerous repetitions, the self-object responds to the child's mirroring and idealizing needs, which are the aspects of the grandi-ose self that the child exhibits and the idealized image he/she admires. The failure on the part of the self-object to mirror the growing self and to foster idealization that can lead to the fragmentation of the self or the loss of vitality by the immature self. The emergence of self is the result of the inborn potential of the child and the empathic relationship between parent and child. The parents or the self-objects respond to the child's mirroring and idealizing needs. The subtle failure of responsiveness by the self-objects that are not traumatic help the emergence of the nuclear self. The nuclear self emerges through a process of transmuting internalization by which the self-objects and their functions are replaced by the self and its functions.

As the self becomes a cohesive self through integration, risk of fragmen-tation gradually recedes. In a healthy personality, grandiosity becomes modified to allow the pursuit of realistic goals and provides energy, ambi-tion, and self-esteem.[89] The idealized objects are increasingly viewed with realism and, eventually, the child withdraws from idealizing and the self now takes over the functions previously performed by the idealized objects.[90]

FRUSTRATION: A PATH FOR INTEGRATION

Frustration plays a key role in the building up of self-structures and becoming a cohesive self. From the earliest developmental stage, the child has a sense of omnipotence and perfection of being merged with the primary caretaker, usually the mother. To preserve this part of the original experience of perfection, the child establishes a grandiose image of his/herself: the grandiose self that is a stage of development in which everything good is regarded as a part of the infant and all badness is outside the infant. The child tries to maintain this original perfection by assigning to the adult absolute perfection by forming an idealized parental image.

However, because the parents are not perfect, their response or lack of response will bring about minor, non-traumatic failures for the child. A close and empathic bond is a necessary environment if non-traumatic failures are to be used to build the self, rather than to fragment it. In such an environment, the child can take on the comforting, tension- reducing task bit by bit that had been done for him/her. It is the type of optimal failure that leads to structure-building of the self.

EMPATHY AND THE CURE OF THE SELF

For Kohut, psychopathology is due to the structural deficit that occurs when early self-objects do not empathically respond to the child. Such failures will lead to a fragmented self where feelings of emptiness, hopelessness, and low self-esteem will transpire. To fragment is to have a structural regression, a shift to a simpler, archaic mental organization. More serious fragmentation is experienced as a sense of coming apart, a loss of continuity in the self, or loss of cohesiveness in one's thoughts and actions.

Empathy is the mode of observation in which the therapist observes and understands the client's subjective experiences and communicates the understanding in an interpretive form to the client. Therefore, for Kohut, empathy is not simply a therapeutic agent. It is also a method to collect data about the client. Siegel states,

> Vicarious introspection, Kohut's definition of empathy, is the way one can learn about inner experiences of another. Empathy is *the* data-gathering tool in psychoanalysis and, Kohut argues, an experience or an act may be considered to be psychological *only* when it is observed via introspection and

empathy. Any other mode of observation lies within the physical field. . . .
Empathy is the tool that gathers psychological information.[91]

Further, Kohut claims that the cure of persons hinges upon the analyst's
ability to connect with the counselee through empathic attunement that
allows the restructuring of the injured self into a healthy self.[92] Therefore,
Kohut does not see empathy as God's gift bestowed only on a few elect, but
something many can achieve.[93] The centrality of empathy in therapy is that
it seeks to remedy the aborted development of the healthy cohesive self that
was affected in childhood through the non-empathic failures of the
mirroring and idealizing self-object. The cure which the self needs in
psychotherapy can be understood by revisiting the psychopathology that
precipitated the need.

The cure of the self in Kohut's self psychology is achieved through the
mode of empathy that is seen as both a research tool into a deeper understanding of the vicissitudes of childhood empathic failure, as well as an
apparatus for reconstituting, or reconstructing, the supportive structures
of the development of the cohesive and healthy self. Kohut takes the
dynamic on the parental self-objects in the successful development of a
cohesive self in early childhood to model a therapeutic model that sees the
therapist as a person offering a second chance of developing a cohesive self
in the adult child. He explains the importance of self psychology by
highlighting that it allows the analyst to operate differently in the therapeutic approach that he/she takes. Kohut claims that self psychology has
supplied analysis with new theories which broaden and deepen the field of
empathic perception and relating that recognizes that healthy transferences
and transmuting internalization are key to the cure of the self.[94]

Empathy in self psychology allows the analyst to collect undistorted
data.[95] There is also an understanding of the reactivated childhood transference dynamics as a positive development that can lead to cure rather than
be merely defensive responses. The transference that occurs in therapy is
seen as potential for helping the analysis and repair of the damaged self of
childhood.[96] However, empathy alone is not enough to cure a defective self.
Healing and growth result from the combined impact of being empathically
understood, as well as the client interpreting the content of the understanding.[97] Here, Kohut's psychoanalytic self psychology emphasizes the importance of the investment of the analyst in the cure of the patient through
empathy, and allowing the defects of the childhood parenting to be
remedied in the new "parenting" relationship with the analyst. Kohut

further emphasizes the fact that analysis cures the problems of the formation of the self by providing a platform for the laying down of psychological structure via (1) optimal frustration and (2) in consequence of optimal frustration, via transmuting internalization.[98]

In summary, Kohut claims that the disturbances in the structures of the self are to be understood in terms of two separate, but complementary, lines of development. They are drive/biological-driven development and relational-driven development. To Kohut, the developmental goal of the child is to have a healthy cohesive structure of the self that is enhanced by the interplay between the child and the parenting environment. The cohesive self is a result of empathic responses of the mirroring and idealizing parental images of the child that are seen as self-objects. Through the empathic or accepting environment of the child, the child builds its nuclear self through adopting the structures of the care-giving environment, which is called transmuting internalization, meaning the child internalizes the structures of the parenting community. If the child does not receive the empathic approval that is needed to build the structures of the self, he/she will suffer psychologically and, hence, a fractured or fragmented sense of self ensues. According to Kohut, if the mother/mothering figure fails to respond to the child's needs empathically, as the mirroring self-object (the father or idealizing figure) can correct the fracturing or fragmentation. He also says that sometimes the non-empathic self-objects are themselves fractured due to failure of empathic responses in their own childhood development, hence, their failing their children.

Empathy is the central factor for building structure for the nuclear self. Empathy is important in the development of the self in the child. It is as important as in restoring the vicissitudes of childhood in therapy. Empathy is both a method of gathering information and a tool of the therapeutic relationship. Kohut, in highlighting empathy, is encouraging connecting with the clients in a way that classical psychotherapy did not encourage because it emphasized detachment.

KOHUT'S IMPLICATIONS FOR THE "ASIAN-INDIAN SELF"

Kohut's understanding of the development of the self has some similarities and dissimilarities with the Asian-Indian understanding of personhood. Kohut's claim that we should not see the development of human beings merely through biological drives will fit very well with the Asian-Indian understanding of the development of personhood. Kohut, therefore, brings up the importance of the role of the parenting self-objects as an important conduit towards the development of the necessary structures that will enhance the child's identity and his/her growth, with time, into an individual self. Kohut's work seemingly has the individual as its emphasis, while the traditional Asian-Indian emphasis is on the communal self, as noted in Kakar's work. The key here is to understand the differences in orientation that may exist, even among members of the same family. This is the present experience of Asian-Indian families living in the United States. Since the self of first- and second-generation immigrants is formed differently in two different cultural contexts, their worldviews, perceptions, outlooks, cultural values, cultural understanding, and cultural practices are entirely different, often opposing each other. When these two groups of people live in the same house and interact with each other, family conflict is inevitable.

Kohut discusses the curative process of therapy from a purely Western perspective that focuses on the individual, locating the individual needs and suggesting how to correct the structural deficits through the sole agency of the therapist in session with the client. This may fit well when the focus is premised on the understanding of the existence of an individual self. When dealing with communal-oriented Asian-Indians, there is need to recreate the community and locate the healing in the community. I am aware that there may be some who are embracing both (individual and community), therefore, it will be very important to hold the two in tandem. In this regard, Kohut admitted that he was not producing a dogma that should be "the" only way of conceptualizing and practicing.

I believe translating Kohut's psychological concept of empathy into the theological concept of grace is relevant to, and applicable in meeting the pastoral care/psychotherapy needs of, Asian-Indian immigrant families in the United States. As empathy is relational, grace is also relational. As empathy helps a person to "walk in another's shoes" and feel the way the other person feels, so, theologically, grace is an abstract quality and an active personal principle showing in our dealings with those who surround us. According to the New Testament, grace signifies the unmerited operation of God in the human heart, affected through the agency of the Holy Spirit. Grace is the exercise of love, kindness, mercy, favor, unconditional acceptance, and disposition to benefit or serve another. While Kohut sees the caring environment of self-objects as essential for the development of the structures of the individual self, Asian-Indian families will see the caring environment as a source of developing the child into a relational and communal self. The importance of relationality is highlighted in both, but divergent in their intended goal.

According to Kohut's self psychology, it is the self-objects that enhance fullness of the self, and this fullness is gained through transmuting internalizations. In the Asian-Indian context, the self-objects are culturally based in the community and, therefore, the failures of the primary self-objects can be overcome by the availability of communal self-objects. Kohut also subscribes to the idea that the need for self-objects is a lifelong need because of the possibility of situations that challenge the cohesion of the self. This understanding is important when dealing with Asian-Indian families in the Western world where they find their communal selves deprived of the empathy that they need to keep themselves together. This, therefore, means there is need for a model of care that can help Indian immigrants restore their communal selves. Kohut also emphasizes the importance of understanding the context before rushing to interpretation.

SUMMARY

The basic assumption of Kohut's self psychology is that the self is formed and developed in relation to other people. The self or self-concept is continually formed and reformed through ongoing interactions between self and self-objects. Kohut also emphasizes that for the formation of a healthy self, empathic understanding as well as healthy mirroring are crucial. Kohut's theory, however, is constructed on a hypothesis where only one cultural setting is present. But adding a bicultural context challenges this assumption. Living in a bicultural setting provides different cultural self-objects which mirror different values, ethoses, and priorities. This inconsistent mirroring and differently valued reinforcement can disturb the formation and growth of the self. The consequence of living in-between cultures is that bicultural setting cannot provide adequate consistency to form and nurture a strong sense of self. Therefore, the most critical symptom of living in-between cultures is the development and expression of symptoms similar to those found in Kohut's idea of the weakened self.

According to Kohut, a healthy self is characterized by the ability to tolerate loss, failure, and disappointments without breaking down. A healthy individual has the capacity to be attuned with the other, maintain relationships, and also to enjoy them. These individuals are also able to utilize their gifts and skills in order to achieve goals and ambitions, and feel fulfillment in them. However, Kohut's idea of a "healthy" self (or a "healthy" individual) is born out of his own cultural context, a Western one, which cannot be generalized and applied to other cultures. Depending on the assumptions and ontological values, every culture has different classifications of what it means to be "healthy."

Although the cultural realities may be the same in America for Indian-Americans, Chinese-Americans, and Americans of other ethnic origins, there are significant but subtle differences in their understanding of "healthy" self. For instance, first-generation Asian-Indians have their own idea of what it means to be a "healthy" self or healthy human as born in a particular cultural context of origin that they value and preserve. However, their children, the second-generation Indian immigrants, born and raised in the United States or in other Western countries, taught in American/Western public schools, have been socialized and reinforced in a Western model of healthy person, similar to that of Kohut's. However, second-generation immigrants are expected to obey their parents and pressured to adapt to parental cultural values that shaped and formed their parents' sense of self. These conflicting notions of self can cause distress and affect the formation of a coherent self.

Consequently, second-generation immigrants receive different and often conflicting messages of what "healthy" should look like. When the basic assumptions of "what a healthy self is" contradict their culture of origin and their parental culture, it is very hard for this community to form a strong and healthy sense of self and a solid identity. Therefore, one of the goals of therapy for second-generation Asian-Indian immigrants who live in-between the dominant American culture and their parental culture, is to help them understand what it means to be healthy—not as an Asian-Indian nor as an American, but as an Indian-American. I strongly believe that this new understanding of what it means to be "healthy" for them as Indian-Americans can strengthen their sense of self that is very unique and fitting to them. Further, I strongly believe that it will help both groups of this community to navigate their lives meaningfully in both cultures being aware about, acknowledging, and accepting their differences, thereby reducing the level of stress, anxiety, and family conflict. This is the end-goal of the model that I have developed using Kakar's and Kohut's theoretical components.

In the next chapter, my aim is to examine the issue of intergenerational conflict in Indian immigrant families from a pastoral theological perspective based on the theological framework of Jung Yung Lee, a Korean-American theologian, using his book, *Marginality: The Key to Multicultural*

Theology.[99] Based on Lee's theology, it is my argument that marginality and lack of empathic relationality are interconnected within the context of ethnicity and culture, resulting in intergenerational issues and cultural identity issues.

NOTES

1. Sudhir Kakar, *The Indian Psyche* (Delhi : Oxford University Press, 1996).
2. Ibid., 1.
3. Ibid., 2.
4. Ibid., 3.
5. Ibid., 5–6.
6. Ibid., 8.
7. Ibid., 9.
8. This he experienced during his wandering years in Germany while trying to find out the real meaning of life. In his personal introduction, he writes that he was in utter confusion about who he was and what he wanted to be. He could not settle down to a career or to raise a family because he needed help to unravel his tangled perception of himself and of the world. It was only after meeting Erikson that his life began to change for the better.
9. Kakar, *The Inner World.*
10. Robert B. Ewen, *An Introduction to Theories of Personality* (Hillsdale, NJ: Lawrence Erlbaum Associate Publishers.1988), 2.
11. Sudhir Kakar, *The Inner World: A Psychoanalytic Study of Childhood and Society in India* (Delhi: Oxford University Press, 1978), 140–160.
12. Ibid., 2.
13. Ibid.
14. Ibid., 52.
15. Ibid., 53.
16. Ibid.
17. Ibid., 79.
18. Ibid., 80.
19. Ibid., 80–81.
20. Kakar, Ibid,, 81.
21. Ibid., 82.
22. Gardiner Murphy, *In the Minds of Men* (New York, NY: Basic Books, 1953), 56.
23. Kakar, *The Inner World*, 88.
24. Ibid.
25. Ibid., 89.
26. Ibid.,103.

27. Ibid.
28. Ibid.,104.
29. Ibid.
30. Ibid.
31. Ibid.
32. Pinchas Noy, "A Revision of Psychoanalytic Theory of the Primary Process," *International Journal of Psychoanalysis* 50, no. 2 (November, 1969): 155–178.
33. Kakar, *The Inner World*, 108.
34. Ibid., 109.
35. Ibid., 110.
36. Brij B. Sethi, V.R. Thakore, and S.C. Gupta, "Changing Patterns of Culture and Psychiatry in India," *American Journal of Psychotherapy* 19, no. 1 (January, 1965): 445–454.
37. Kakar, *The Inner World*, 135.
38. Ibid, 6–7.
39. Ibid., 9.
40. Heinz Hartman, *Ego Psychology and the Problem of Adaptation* (New York, NY: International Universities Press, 1958), 23.
41. Kakar, *The Inner World*, 11–12.
42. Ibid., 11.
43. Kakar, *Identity and Adulthood*, xi.
44. Ibid., x.
45. Ibid., xi.
46. Kakar, *The Inner World*, 56–57.
47. Allen M. Siegel, *Heinz Kohut and the Psychology of the Self*, (New York: Routledge, 1996), 14.
48. Ibid.
49. Ibid.
50. Frank Milstead Wagon, "The Will to be Known: The Development of a Pastoral-Theological Model of the Self Based upon Deitrich Bonhoeffer and Heinz Kohut," (PhD diss., The Southern Baptist Theological Seminary, 1994), 82; Siegel, *Heinz Kohut and the Psychology of the Self*, 2.
51. Paul H. Ornstein, "The Evolution of Heinz Kohut's Psychoanalytic Psychology of the Self," in *The Search for the Self: Selected Writings of Heinz Kohut, 1950–1978*, vol. 1, ed. Paul H. Ornstein (New York: International University Press, 1978), 7.
52. Ibid., 7–9.
53. Siegel, *Heinz Kohut and the Psychology of the Self*, 44.
54. Ornstein, *The Evolution of Heinz Kohut's Psychoanalytic Psychology of the Self*, 44.
55. Ibid., 19–43.

56. Heinz Kohut, *The Restoration of the Self* (New York: International Universities Press, 1977), xiii-xiv.
57. Ibid., xx
58. Wagon, 87.
59. Michael St. Clair and Jody Wigren, *Object Relations and Self-Psychology* (Belmont, CA: Thomson Learning, 2004), 147.
60. Kohut, *The Restoration of the Self*, 2–3.
61. Heinz Kohut, *The Search for the Self*, ed. Paul H. Ornstein (Madison, WI: International Universities Press, Inc., 1978), 2, 617.
62. Kohut, *The Search for the Self*, 617–618.
63. Ibid., 618.
64. Ibid., 936–937.
65. Heinz Kohut, *Analysis of the Self* (New York: International Universities Press, 1971), 187.
66. Kohut, *The Restoration of the Self*, 310–311.
67. Ibid., 312.
68. Ibid., 311.
69. Kohut, *Analysis of the Self*, xiv.
70. Kohut, *The Restoration of the Self*, 171–219.
71. Heinz Kohut, *How Does Analysis Cure?* eds. Arnold Goldberg and Paul E. Stepansky (Chicago, IL: The University of Chicago Press), 5.
72. Siegel, 112.
73. Kohut, *The Search for the Self*, 54.
74. Kohut, *Analysis of the Self*.
75. Kohut, *The Search for the Self*, 756.
76. Kohut, *The Restoration of the Self*, 177.
77. Ibid., 178.
78. Kohut, *Analysis of the Self*, xiv.
79. Kohut, *The Restoration of the Self*, 87.
80. Ibid., 177.
81. Ibid., 216–218.
82. Kohut, *Analysis of the Self*, 50, 64.
83. Kohut, *The Search for the Self*, 205–232.
84. Kohut, *How Does Analysis Cure?* 65
85. Ibid., 82.
86. Kohut, *The Search for the Self*, 778–789.
87. Siegel, 44.
88. Kohut, *The Restoration of the Self*, 185.
89. Kohut, *Analysis of the Self*, 107.
90. Paul H. Ornestein, "Kohut the Psychoanalytic Treatment of Narcissistic Personality Disorders," in *The Search for the Self: Selected Writings of Heinz*

Kohut, 1950–1978, ed. 272. Paul H. Ornstein (New York: International University Press, 1978), 86, 89.

91. Siegel, 49.
92. Kohut, *The Restoration of the Self,* 177–179.
93. Kohut, *How Does Analysis Cure?* 83.
94. Ibid., 172–191.
95. Ibid., 83.
96. Ibid., 84.
97. Ibid., 95–96.
98. Ibid., 98–99.
99. Jung Young Lee, *Marginality: Key to Multicultural Theology* (Minneapolis, MN: Fortress Press, 1995).

CHAPTER 6

Marginality and Theology of New Marginality

INTRODUCTION

A pastoral theology for Asian-Indian immigrant families that fear intergenerational conflict and family declension that effects the development of the self must attend to the issues of marginality. Marginality is a major aspect of both first- and second-generation immigrants' experience in the United States, with each group experiencing marginality somewhat differently, like all other people of color do in every area of their lives. However, the level of marginality and the emotional pain that second-generation immigrants experience differ significantly from that of first-generation immigrants. First of all, second-generation immigrants who are born, raised, socialized, and educated in the United States, speaking the same language with the same accent, and mostly thinking and acting like their American counterparts, are often viewed as being marginal or "others" in their own land. When they return to their parental community, they are also marginalized there and regarded as a minority, as they are not considered fully Indian. It is a double marginality—marginality in mainstream American society and in the dominant immigrant (parental) community. For this very reason, the different levels of marginality experienced by those in the Indian immigrant community manifest themselves as intergenerational conflict. This requires our serious attention.

To develop a pastoral theological framework for the Indian diaspora in the United States, I am drawing primarily on the theology of Jung Young Lee, set forth in *Marginality: The Key to Multicultural Theology*. Lee is a

© The Author(s) 2017
V. Jacob, *Counseling Asian Indian Immigrant Families*,
DOI 10.1007/978-3-319-64307-6_6

prominent Korean-American theologian who writes on the nature of marginality, fashioned the "in-beyond" cultural identification model, and depicts Jesus Christ as the marginalized person *par excellence*, the one who redefines marginality. Lee is interested in how the experiences of being an immigrant, an ethnic minority person on the margins of society, affect one's way of doing theology. According to Lee, theology is autobiographical by nature, and it is only through a careful analysis of the self and one's own experiences that one's theology can be constructed. Consequently, Lee develops his theology of marginality by means of his own autobiography and redefines concepts of marginality through the perspective of Asian Americans. Lee's autobiographical insights on the marginalized Asian-American self seemed likely to prove helpful in my efforts to examine the life of Asian-Indian immigrants in general, and second-generation Asian-Indians, in particular. Lee's reviews of the cultural identification models, including his in-beyond model guided my interest in how Asian-Indians might understand their social locations in a more positive frame.

As explained in the survey, the experience of marginality is revealed in various ways such as discrimination, frustration, and cultural value conflict. Further, it culminates in manifestations of intergenerational conflicts. Sandhu, Portes, and McPhee point out that the acculturation process is a significant cause for stress as it involves the individual undergoing major changes in his/her ethnocultural orientation. The individual can experience "threats to ethno-cultural identity, feelings of powerlessness, inferiority, and alienation, as well as a sense of marginality and hostility."[1] The roots of oppression are not only in class and gender struggles, but also in racial and cultural misunderstandings in a pluralistic society. Margins are not only essential in understanding the center of any society, they are also places of "creativity" that foster hope for new interpretations of self, church, and theology.[2] The marginalized can work to exercise accountability and transformation, both for those at the margins and at the center, creating a theology of marginality that is not only a paradigm of hermeneutics, but also a key to the essence of our faith. After offering constructive criticisms of two popular cultural identification models for Asian Americans, Lee introduces an alternative model, the "in-beyond model," which emphasizes certain advantages of being Asian American correlating his new understanding of the Asian-American self to Jesus Christ, the ultimate being of marginality and the pioneer of the new marginality.

WHY A THEOLOGY OF MARGINALITY?

There are various reasons why I chose the theology of marginality. First of all, theology is derived from the experience of persons and communities and originates from the experience of an immigrant marginal and is also a theology of the minority. My investigation concerns an immigrant community that differs from other American communities, values a different culture and different way of thinking, and has unique characteristics. However, all these differences and uniquenesses are marginal in the mainstream American culture. While marginality and minority experiences are part of the outside-home experience to one group in the immigrant community (first-generation immigrants), it is both an inside and outside experience for another group of the same community (second-generation immigrants). It is also a communal experience that expresses a communal identity. "No one is isolated because we are part of others just as they are part of us. I share the experience of others just as others share my experience."[3] A theology of marginality is a theology of the living experience[4] of the immigrant community and, therefore, is very relevant to the experience of the Indian immigrant community in the United States, particularly as we seek to develop a therapeutic counseling model for them.

The discrimination, racism, and inferiority status that people experience outside the home are the sum total of marginality which creates in them a sense of shame, anger, inferiority, frustration, and guilt. When people undergo such experiences, and do not have a space in which to express their feelings and emotions in public, they bring it home and release it onto family members. While second-generation immigrants pick up Western cultural values for their survival in the wider community and bring it home, the first-generation immigrants also experience this marginalizing culture in a more complex way. However, second-generation immigrants experience marginality within their family from their parental generation and outside the family from the mainstream American culture. Therefore, marginality and cultural identity are strongly interconnected in the immigrant life experience. I believe it plays a significant role in the intergenerational conflicts that the immigrant community is experiencing. In the theology of marginality, Lee narrates a communal identity based on the harsh experiences of immigration but claims that the communal identity that is undergoing harsh experiences may be redeemed, becoming a healthy communal identity, by living "in-both" and "in-beyond."

MARGINALITY DEFINED

Marginality is both the context and the method of marginal theology.[5] To provide the method of marginal theology, Lee defines the meaning of marginality through the use of cultural and racial determinants:

> Marginality had various understandings because of the variety of determinants. Particular determinants seem to affect the intensity and significance of the marginal experience more than others. Specifically, race, gender, economic status, politics, education, occupation, and age seem to be more important determinants than others.[6]

Those determinants, being interdependent and interconnected, influence each other with their centers and margins just as in concentric ripples in water.[7] Though there are several kinds of marginality, all of them have one thing in common – they allow the individual to know what it means to be at the edges of existence. This is the experience of all Asian-Indian immigrants, in general, and second-generation immigrants in particular.

RACIAL, CULTURAL RELATION TO MARGINALITY

"Ethnicity is the most important and primary determinant that creates marginality and minority status in all areas, such as political, social, educational, economic, and other areas of the Asian immigrant lives in the United States."[8] Each one's ethnicity includes their racial origin and cultural preferences. For Lee, "as an Asian American, all other determinants are relative to but of lesser significance than my racial origin and cultural differences."[9] Manning Marable defines ethnic group as:

> a set of people who distinguish themselves socially from other groups primarily on the basis of cultural or national characteristics. However, race is a totally different dynamic and has its roots in the structures of exploitation, power and privilege. Race, further, is an artificial social construction that is deliberately imposed on various subordinated groups of people at the outset of the expansion of European capitalism into the Western hemisphere five centuries ago.[10]

However, Joe Feagin argues, "it was only in the late eighteenth century that the term race came to mean a distinct category of human beings with certain physical characteristics."[11]

In the Western world, race is often used as an ideology based on immutable physical or biological traits. These physical characteristics are often used to classify people into inferior or superior groups. Ethnicity and race are inseparable from ethnic minorities. "Though a clear distinction between ethnicity and race makes sense from the perspective of dominant group, it is not possible from the perspective of marginality. Race is inclusive of ethnicity, just as is culture. Therefore, both racial and cultural characteristics are included in the ethnicity of marginal people."[12] Racial determinants are fixed, while cultural determinants can be altered. In this context, "though, the non-white immigrants may attain a high degree of cultural assimilation (adoption of an American lifestyle), structural assimilation (equal life chances) is virtually impossible, unless the immutable independent variable (race) becomes mutable through miscegenation or cognitive mutation of the white, Anglo-Saxon, protestant (WASP)."[13] For instance, though second- or third-generation Asian-Indians may easily be acculturated (adopting an American lifestyle), they can hardly be assimilated into American society on an equal basis because of their race. Therefore, the most fundamental determinant of marginality for this immigrant community is race, while cultural prejudices also play a role. Marginality is a relative and dynamic term that includes even Caucasians who experience marginality due to gender, class, economy, religion, and sexual orientation.[14] Therefore, marginality is common ground that unites all minorities.

CONVENTIONAL DEFINITION OF MARGINALITY: IN-BETWEEN

The conventional definition of marginality is derived from the perspective of the dominant group and its primary proponent is one of the early sociologists, Robert E. Park. According to Park, marginality is a type of personality that arises out of the conflict of races and cultures.[15] The conventional definition of marginality is related to Park's adaptation of the melting pot theory. According to Park, the race-relation cycle is marked by stages of competition, conflict, and accommodation before eventual assimilation into the big melting pot. Park names these four stages of his theory as: contact (or encounter), competition (which includes conflict), accommodation (where conflict seems to disappear), and assimilation (where fusion of races takes place, as in a big melting pot).[16] In defining marginality or a marginal person, Park and Everett Stonequist borrowed insights from George Simmer and Werner Sombert and employed them to describe the individual who lives in two societies or two cultures and is a member of neither.[17]

Since the conventional definition that is derived from a dominant perspective does not seriously consider racism, it negates the marginality and marginal people. "The centralist group often regards the conventional definition of marginality as normative and, therefore, it is the general understanding of the nation's ethnic minorities."[18] Based on the conventional definition, "in-between boundaries" form a marginal condition. Consequently, the marginal are pulled toward multiple identities and deprived of a single self-image. Here I see the disintegration of the immigrant self that is fractured through the relational failure from the Kohutian perspective.

Everett Stonequist describes the marginal person as "one who is poised in psychological uncertainty between two (or more) social worlds, reflecting in his soul the discords and harmonies, repulsions and attractions of these worlds, one of which is often "dominant" over the other; within which membership is implicitly based upon birth or ancestry (race or nationality); and cohere exclusion removes the individual from a system of group relations."[19]

"To be 'in-between' two worlds means to be fully in neither, and people who are placed in these two world-boundaries often feel like non-beings. This existential nothingness caused by the perspective of two or more

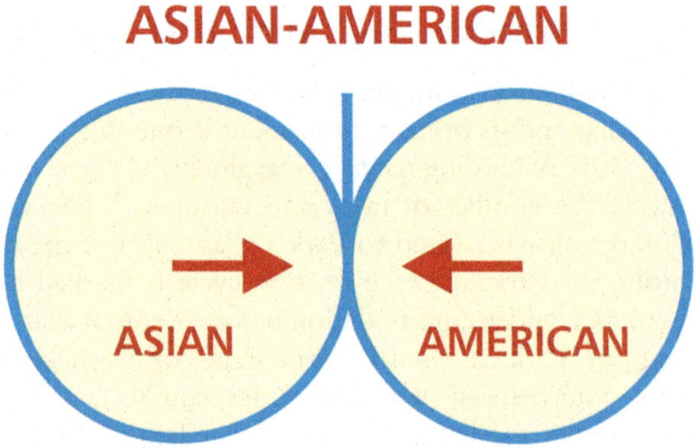

Fig. 6.1 In-between: conventional, self-negating definition of marginality defined by ethnocentric Asian and Anglo-American dominant groups (Lee, *Marginality* 57)

dominant worlds is the root of dehumanization."[20] Such a sense of non-existence can create self-alienation and unhealthy personality development. Such a self is split into two when a person is torn between two worlds. Stonequist observes, "The duality of cultures produces a duality of personality—a divided self."[21] Just as marginality arises out of two conflicting worlds, self-alienation results from two conflicting selves in a personality. Other serious effects of marginality are excessive self-consciousness and race-consciousness. "Sometimes, a marginal person can be hypersensitive about his/her racial origins and develop an inferiority complex."[22] Stonequist reports that such an experience of self-alienation has affected his every waking moment to the extent that his life has seemed meaningless and without purpose.[23]

Marginal persons, according to conventional perspective, are expected to think and say nothing. Silence and non-thinking are expressed in terms of the neither/nor way of thinking. Neither/nor thinking means the total and unconditional negation of all things. This is the reason for developing a therapeutic counseling model for Asian-Indian families, in general, and second-generation immigrants in particular.

Marginality does not have a separate existence of its own because it is always relational, for it relates worlds that oppose one another. "So marginality can be compared with a nexus where two or three worlds are interconnected. It is never closed, but open-ended, with unfolding horizons where the others come to meet and go away."[24] Therefore, the conventional definition gives us a new opportunity for a positive thought that marginality is an opportunity for creativity. With this positive outlook, marginality has been redefined in a modern way, as marginality of "in-both" worlds.

CONTEMPORANEOUS DEFINITION OF MARGINALITY: IN-BOTH

Instead of replacing the incomplete and self-negating conventional definition originating from the dominant perspective, the marginal people redefined marginality from a self-affirming and positive perspective. This new self-understanding definition of marginality, taking pride in one's ethnic roots, argues that they know how to define themselves. This self-affirming definition of marginality that emphasizes the idea of in-both, rather than in-between, and complements and balances in-between is known as a contemporaneous definition of marginality.

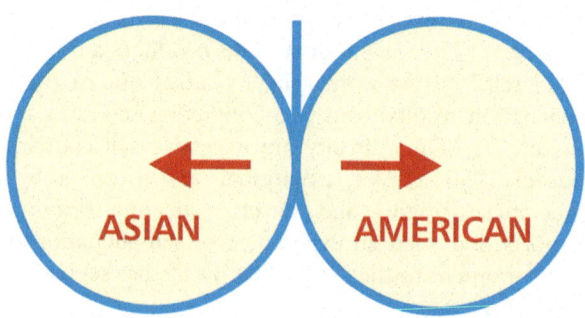

Fig. 6.2   In-both: contemporaneous definition of marginality that is self-affirming and inclusive in nature (Lee, *Marginality*, 57)

The contemporaneous definition that genuinely appreciates one's own racial and cultural heritage does not preclude an appreciation of others. This definition helps a marginal to affirm one's roots and color, without entertaining the danger of ethnocentricity. Being in-both Indians and Americans means the affirmation of Indian-ness is also the affirmation of American-ness, though that is hard to do. Lee says,

> We marginal people cannot be exclusivists. We are called to live in the margin where worlds emerge. We are, as our very nature of marginal, inclusive and open to all centers. We are pluralistic because we live in-both or in all. An exclusivist approach is unacceptable to in-both marginal people... Likewise, appreciation of our own skin color has to be accompanied by our appreciation of other skin colors as well. If we cannot appreciate the colors of other races, we cannot affirm our color. From the marginal point of view there is no sharp distinction between white skin and colored skin. Likewise, white is a color in the view of the colored people.[25]

A Holistic Definition of Marginality: In-Beyond

While the conventional definition of marginality maintains a strict, structural separation between dominant and subordinate groups, the contemporaneous self-affirming definition presupposes an emergence of the new configuration, a genuinely pluralistic society. Both these definitions are painful realities to the marginal people. For, the marginal who live in-between two worlds do not fully share the power, privilege, or resources of the dominant group. "This negative experience can be resolved only if the ethnic minorities are allowed to be assimilated into the melting pot. However, total assimilation is unrealistic and undesirable. The resurgence of ethnic consciousness and indigenous cultural values challenge the dominant paradigm of assimilation."[26]

The contemporaneous, self-affirming definition, 'in-both' acknowledges that a marginal person is living in both worlds without giving up either one. He/she is more than Asian-Indian and American because he/she is both. Therefore, "the positive, self-affirming definition of marginality is as realistic as the self-negating conventional definition and, therefore, both are acceptable as marginal people experience the negative and positive traits of marginality."[27] They are two sides of the same reality to the marginal.

Therefore, "they are in-beyond, meaning they are both in-between and in-both. Just as in-between and in-both are one in-beyond, the margin and creative core are inseparable in new marginality. The margin is the locus, a focal point, a new and creative core, where two or multiple worlds emerge."[28] Here, the new creative core, which is the margin where two or multiple worlds emerge, does not replace the old centers—the centers of centrality—because it is at the margin of marginality and they are related to each other as conventional and contemporaneous definitions of marginality together making a holistic sense of marginality. This is evident when Lee says,

> The core or new center is also the margin at the same time. However, in the new marginality, the margin is no longer the margin of the centrality, the margin defined by the dominant groups, but the new margin is the margin of marginality. In this margin of marginality, the conflict between the margin and the center disappears and reconciliation between marginality and centrality takes place.[29]

According to David Ng, "The condition of in-between and in-both must be harmonized for one to become a new marginal person who overcomes marginality without ceasing to be a marginal person."[30]

The holistic understanding of a marginal person is, therefore, a new marginal person, or a person living in-beyond. The experience of being in-between and in-both, without either being blended, coexists in the new

ASIAN-AMERICAN

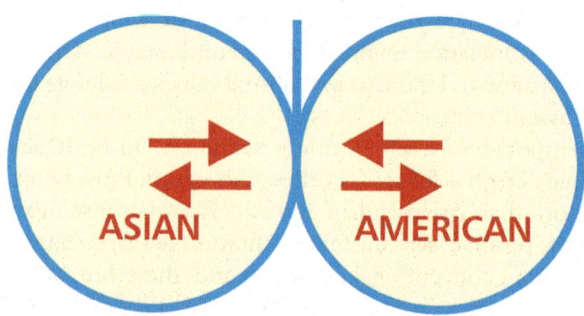

Fig. 6.3 In-beyond: new marginality: holistic definition of marginality. In-between is also In-both the interpenetration of both positive and negative experiences of marginality (Lee, *Marginality*, 57)

marginal person and the norm of the new marginality is the harmony of difference. Lee explains the in-beyond status of a marginal as follows:

> To transcend or to live in-beyond means to live in both of them without being bound by either of them. The new marginal person is a liberated person, a person who is truly free, because each is a whole person and able to be fully present in the world. Because the new marginal person is whole, he/she reconciles two opposing worlds unto the self. The new marginal person is a reconciler and a wounded healer to the two-category system... Gender, class, and religion are also other determinants of marginality.[31]

NEITHER/NOR AND BOTH/AND

The norm that validates the theology of marginality is the holistic experience of marginality itself, the experience of being in-beyond, which includes in-between and in-both simultaneously. "Therefore, marginal thinking is an inclusive, open-ended and creative link that connects multiple views, interpretations, and reinterpretations. Neither/nor thinking is a negative understanding of marginality that is influenced by the centralist perspective to indicate that in-between people are of neither this nor that world."[32] While 'neither/nor' perspective is a passive way of thinking, the 'both/and' thought process is an active form of self-expression.

In-both people are a self-directed community with a positive self-image based on their conviction about a genuinely pluralistic society. They affirm this world and that world simultaneously, and think in terms of both/and as they are in-between and in-both. "They live in and reconcile two different worlds with a blended experience of complete negation and complete affirmation. Therefore, both these experiences co-exist in a new marginal people."[33]

The both/and thought process, which is an active form of self-expression, affirms both worlds in spite of their denial. Therefore, self-assertion is the inner strength of new marginal people. "While either/or thinking excludes both/and, both/and thinking includes either/or. In in-both thinking, the two forms are complementary and form a harmonious whole, while in either/or thinking they are in conflict. Both/and thought does not eliminate opposites but complements them."[34] In this sense, "yes" is "yes" but also "no," as "no" is "no" but also "yes," because "yes" contains "no" and "no" contains "yes." For instance, typically when an Asian-Indian offers candy or something to another Asian-Indian, their initial and immediate response will be "no" before accepting it. This "no" response may be repeated twice or thrice before they accept the offer. Yet, the other keeps offering the same because they know that the "no" does not always mean "no" because it also means "yes." But when a white American (in the same context) makes an offer, if the Asian-Indian says "no" just once, it will instantly be taken away: the white American does not know an Indian's "no" also includes "yes." "Simply stated, the in-between is in-both and in-both is in-between, and these together make a new marginal in-beyond or both/and. This makes the new marginal the most inclusive, most relational form of thinking."[35]

JESUS CHRIST: THE LIBERATED MARGINAL

Incarnation theology is an immigrant theology and immigrant theology is a marginal theology. Jesus Christ is a new marginal person *par excellence*. However, the narration in Matthew Chapter 16 reveals that Peter's perspective on Jesus was from the center (though he confesses Jesus Christ as the son of the living God). When Jesus talks about the sufferings that he must undergo in Jerusalem, Peter rebukes him saying, "Lord this must not happen to you" (Matthew 16:22).[36]

Peter's thought appears to be from a human perspective of centrality that seeks the center, the position of power. Christianity in the course of time, over and over again made the same mistake of overemphasizing the power and majesty of Christ at the expense of his weakness that made him powerful and his humility that raised him to be Lord of lords. Often people emphasize the lordship of Christ over his servanthood and his resurrection over his death. "Jesus Christ is also Christ Jesus like an Asian American is Asian and American. They are inseparable that share a double identity and two facets of the same existence."[37]

INCARNATION, THE ICON OF DIVINE MARGINALIZATION

The historical background of Jesus reveals most of his marginality. John's gospel and Paul's letter to the Philippians mostly narrate the metaphysical aspect of the incarnation of Jesus Christ, while the other gospels narrate the historical background. Jesus possessed dual identity (human and divine), experienced the crisis of belonging to two worlds at the same time and, thus, offers the best model for immigrants. All descriptions, such as being conceived by an unwed woman, born far from his hometown, sheltered in a manger, visited by Eastern wise men rather than by the elite of his nation, and the flight into Egypt are the evidence of Jesus' life-long marginality. His very incarnation made him marginalized. Incarnation—leaving his heavenly abode to be born, as a human baby in this world—was an experience of marginality. His social class and economic, political and ethnic orientations made him a marginal person. He experienced loneliness and felt abandoned by his father on the cross. Therefore, God is not central to those who seek the center. Rather, God is the center to those who seek marginality, because the real center is the creative core, the margin of marginality—Jesus Christ.

According to Luke, the act of conception prior to Mary's wedding was divine, and emancipated Mary from mortal and social sanctions by the angels. Yet, she was troubled at the message of the angel (Luke 1:34). Based on the moral and ethical mores of the time, Mary realized that it was a disgrace to have a child prior to marriage. According to Matthew's gospel, Joseph, Mary's future husband, was a righteous man and, therefore, decided to dismiss Mary quietly to avoid public disgrace (Matthew 1:19). However, disgraceful, it seemed Mary's response was the symbol of true marginality. This was a divine marginalization.

The hatred he encountered from the Pharisees, the torture he suffered, the crucifixion and death as any ordinary human would, are the self-emptying process of God into a human form, was divine marginalization, the very margin of marginality. Further, Jesus came to his own people, but they also rejected him (John 1:11). Washing his disciples' feet was an act of a slave, not of a master, a non-human being at the margins. By doing so, he was entering into a neither/nor category.

However, self-emptying or humiliation, the act of taking the lowest position raised Jesus to self-fulfillment (or exaltation), the highest position.

> When he became the servant of all servants or slave of all slaves he also became the Lord of all lords. Jesus through his self-emptying process brought in the two worlds of the total negation (in-between) and total affirmation (in-both). This made Jesus Christ as the new marginal person who lives in-beyond by totally affirming the world that negated him. In this context, the incarnation of Jesus Christ can also be compared to divine immigration, in which God emigrated from a heavenly place to this world.[38]

New Marginality in the Life of Jesus

The account of Jesus in the gospel narrative reveals that the life of Jesus was a life of marginality. The flight of Jesus' human parents with Jesus to Egypt because King Herod wanted to kill Him portrays Jesus as doubly marginalized: politically by the Roman government and culturally by living in a foreign land. Later, on his return, Jesus grew up in the town of Nazareth "from where nothing good can come" (John 1:46). The act of Jesus' baptism was the symbol of his marginalization.

> When Jesus immersed into the waters of the river Jordan, Jesus was symbolically placed in-between the worlds, belonging neither to heaven nor to earth. However, baptism did not end with his immersion but ended with his rising up from the water. The act of baptism symbolizes his total affirmation that was confirmed by the vision and voice of the spirit.[39]

Jesus' affirmation and heavenly confirmation made him a new marginal person, though it did not remove his marginal status. He also became a new marginalized person in the experience of temptation.

Jesus in his public ministry, may be portrayed as a homeless man with a group of homeless people around him, though it included central-group people such as a Roman officer, a local synagogue official, a lawyer, council members, and so on. He suffered and died as a marginal person does, and was resurrected from the dead to help us live in-beyond. His disciples were marginal people—fishermen and tax collectors. In his ministry, those who were healed were marginalized—the sick, the blind, the mute, the crippled, women, widows, the paralyzed, the possessed, prostitutes, Gentiles, and the crowds of poor and the weak. All were rejected, outcast, and marginalized from the larger society. However, this marginalized community had a strong faith rooted in a strong relationship between healer and the healed.

Even after every miraculous ministry of preaching and healing, Jesus is seen lonely, homeless, rejected in his home town (Matthew 14:53–58; Mark 6:1–6) and often misunderstood by his own disciples who were more interested in centrality than marginality. Jesus, as the poorest of the poor, did not have money to pay his tax. "Even in his marginality, Jesus, as a person living in-beyond, pioneered the new marginality as a healer and reconciler."[40]

Jesus' teachings, especially the beatitudes, were given from the perspective of marginality. The majority of those who heard his message were economically, politically, and socially marginalized. He declared, "Blessed are the poor, the hungry, those who weep, and those who are hated, excluded, and cast out" (Luke 6:20–23; Matthew 5:3–7:27). "Yet he affirmed himself as the reconciler and, thus, lived in-beyond in the world, which marginalized him."[41]

Isolation and Marginality of Jesus Christ

The entry of Jesus into Jerusalem on a donkey, prior to his crucifixion, symbolizes his marginality because the horse, which the Roman rulers rode, symbolized centrality and triumph. Yet his entry into Jerusalem was a triumphal entry as he entered to conquer sin and death. This entry was the symbolic penetration of marginality into the center of centrality. Following his triumphal entry, Jesus celebrated the last supper with his disciples, which was the symbol of both death and resurrection. "Here the principle was: to live is to die and to die is to relive. Therefore, negation and affirmation, or between neither/nor and both/and, are very symbolically converged in the last supper."[42]

In the death of Jesus also this new marginality is quite clear. In Isaiah 53:3, we see that Jesus was despised and rejected by people. Peter denied Jesus thrice. After his arrest, Jesus stood isolated and alone before the council. They slapped him and spat on him. At the crucifixion, even his marginalized followers and his heavenly father rejected him. Jesus was hung in-between, belonging to neither heaven nor earth. He was completely negated. But negation and affirmation are like two sides of a coin, just as death and resurrection in Jesus are inseparable.

The cross symbolizes death and resurrection. Death symbolizes tragedy, failure, disappointment, and darkness—utter negation. Yet, death is necessary for resurrection and resurrection is possible because of death. Resurrection symbolizes hope, joy, and life renewal. It is ultimate affirmation, the fulfillment of life's hope and the divine "Yes" to humanity. It is the assertion of both/and. With resurrection, Christ transcended all marginality. He broke the bond of every cultural, racial, religious, sexual, economic, social, and regional bias that marginalized him and eventually led him to the cross. The cross that symbolizes death and resurrection was once filled and now is empty. The cross means that death presupposes resurrection and resurrection is possible only because of death. The empty cross represents triumph, joy, and hope; the cross gives us memory and hope.[43]

THE MARGIN OF MARGINALITY AND THE CREATIVE CORE

"The resurrection of Christ Jesus marks the beginning of a new age of God's reign, where all people can live in harmony and peace as children of God. Jesus, through his resurrection became a new center or a creative core. The resurrection of Christ brought the scattered disciples together, back to Jerusalem and eventually, a new marginal community of believers was formed, and its head was Christ Jesus himself (1 Corinthians 12:12–26). The creative core is where the son, spirit, and father are present. At this core, God reigns with genuine pluralism."[44] It is true that though one may not be absolutely free from marginality in this world, it is possible to live in-beyond because of this creative core. For this very reason, immigrant marginal can live in both worlds and transcends their negation and achieve affirmation as shown in Fig. 6.4.

The creative core invites reconciliation between two different or opposite worlds. Here is where the potentiality of the immigrant community is found, especially the potentiality of the second-generation immigrants. Being between these two margins, an individual reconciles each and lives in-beyond the two. He/she is at the creative core. In Christ, every marginal determinant is nullified and each can overcome his/her marginality. "The creative core, Christ Jesus, includes all things. It is the authentic center where God reigns over the world. To recognize this creative core, one must put his/her center in God, who is the margin of marginality."[46]

GOD'S MARGINALITY IN THE CREATION ACCOUNT

The creation account in the book of Genesis explains that God created everything in its own kind; in difference. Variety and plurality for God's self is both different and plural in trinity.

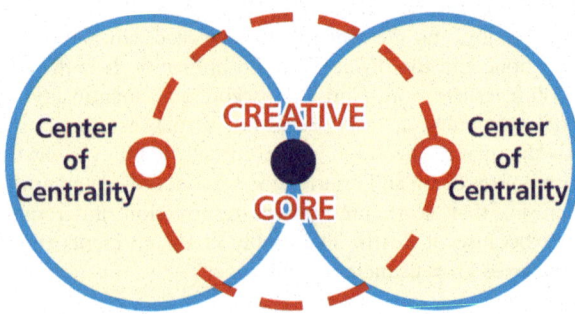

Fig. 6.4 Creative core: the creative core represents 'in-both' and 'both/and' thinking (Lee, *Marginality*, 98)

This creative core is a new transforming center that marginalizes the center of centrality and brings the marginal towards the creative core. The new core does not dominate rather it harmonizes margins with coexistence because it is dynamic, creative, and transforming. Here the former marginality is overcome by a new marginality, a creative core and everyone can move toward the real center, where marginality is overcome by marginality. "In this way, countless cores of new marginalities are formed because Christ Jesus is present in each core."[45]

While difference and plurality are fundamental principles of creativity, and are interdependent variables in the creative process, centralists deny differences and they exclude others from their right to existence, freedom, and to have their own space to make their own history and civilization. The repudiation of difference relinquishes equality and creativity. "God is the creative core of marginality, marginality and creativity are interconnected. To be marginal means to be creative and to be creative means to be at the margin. Margins are both in-between and in-both. If there were no difference or plurality, there would be neither marginality nor creativity. Race and ethnic differences are the creative designs of God's marginal people."[47]

Based on God's creation principle, sameness and oneness cannot be creative and therefore indifference is the denial of God's creativity. However, sameness and singularity are the norm of the centralist approach. It negates God's creative order by negating the existence of difference. When dominant groups make a normative frame and assume that anything that does not fit into that normative frame is abnormal, the life of ethnic minorities and immigrants is interpreted as abnormal and pathological. Here, they deny racial and ethnic plurality and make the harmonious coexistence of ethnic minorities impossible. Difference cannot peacefully coexist when sameness dominates, especially when they insist on homogeneity—expecting others to think and act as they do.[48] This approach insists the dominant norm to be the norm for the ethnic minorities. This single norm subjugates and marginalizes minorities whose norms are pluralistic.

Like white supremacists, many ethnocentrists value singularity over difference and diversity. For them, their ethnicity becomes a centralist norm, which marginalizes those of different ethnic and cultural orientations within in the same ethnicity. (For instance, first-generation Asian-Indians can be ethnocentrists in nature to the second-generation immigrants.) By elevating a single ethnic group as an ultimate value, unity is stressed through uniformity. The more people are marginalized by centralists the more they become close to original marginality. That is why those who are poor and marginalized are closer to the reign of God.[49]

TOWER OF BABEL AND EXODUS: SYMBOLS OF EMIGRATION

The tower of Babel in the book of Genesis is portrayed as a rebellion against God's original intent of decentralization. The intention with the tower of Babel was to move from God's plan of decentralization to human plan of centralization. But God's salvation begins by scattering or decentralizing humankind. The history of the people of Israel begins with the scattering of people—the removal of Abraham, Sarah, and their family from their homeland to a strange land (Genesis 12:1–9). God's call for them to leave their homeland of Ur and go to a strange land made Abraham and family marginalized people. Abraham is seen as the first successful immigrant. He built bridges with foreign communities and became father of three major world religions. Wherever he went, his strategy was to build an altar and build a bridge to connect with God and different cultures. In this way, he overcame cultural differences, generational differences, and faith differences. Biblical stories like the Tower of Babel, the displacement of patriarchs such as Abraham, Isaac, Jacob, Joseph, David, Paul, and many more, the exodus, the different captivities of Israel and Judah, the flight of Jesus to Egypt, the life and work of apostles and so on all narrate that immigration or sojourning in a strange land is the initial step in becoming a marginal person.

Immigration is the most vivid and profound symbol of marginality for Asian-Indians in the United States, just as it is for every other ethnic immigrant. As immigrants completely detach from their country that protected and nurtured them, immigrants also are estranged from the centrality that previously protected them. Rather than the suffering and alienation Abraham and his family endured in a strange land, faith and blessings are the focus of the biblical authors. Abraham and family were in-between the two worlds. "If Abraham's and Sarah's lives symbolized Israel's faith, that faith demands scattering to strange places and a marginal existence. In this process of immigration, God's call was the first act, Abraham's response in faith is the second act, and God's blessing is the third act.[50]".

Further, the descendants of Abraham lived in Egypt for more than 400 years and became like permanent Egyptian residents or citizens. The land was filled with them (Exodus 1:7). Yet they had Hebrew roots and so were in the margins, again like our present second, third or fourth-generation Asian-Indian immigrants in the United States who, no doubt, identify themselves as Americans. However, "Exodus shifts the human marginalization into divine marginalization that helped the people of Israel to live in-both."[51]

Moses is another new marginal person. Born to the Levi tribe and then growing up in Pharaoh's palace as an Egyptian prince, he was a man in-between two worlds. His natural parents were Hebrews and his foster parents were Egyptians. By education and growth he was an Egyptian but by birth and traits he was a Hebrew. Therefore, he was neither/nor and both/and, in-between and in-both.

God's call is closely related to the discovery of one's identity as a marginal person. Ultimately, Moses intensely identified himself as a Hebrew and defended his people when he saw their suffering and mistreatment by Egyptian rulers (Exodus 2:11–12, 14). "The public demonstration of his Hebrew identity marked the beginning of God's call to Moses to become a marginal person."[52] From centrality, he moved to marginality, where he encountered God and responded to God.

The life of wandering in the wilderness for 40 years was an experience of in-between and neither/nor in the land of Egypt and in the Promised Land. Several times the Hebrews wanted to return to Egypt as the pain of marginality was far more severe than the pain of oppression. It was a choice for them to depend on human centrality or to place their dependence on God. However, in the course of time, they wanted to be in the center of centrality rather than on the margin of marginality. According to Joachim Jeremias, "the people of Israel under the kingship were bound by the political, economic, and social situation, rather than by the covenant. The kingdom of David represented the center of centrality."[53] Many, though not all, prophets of God warned against the centralization of Hebrew power

(1 Kings 22:6, 8). Finally, God decentralized them and repentance occurred with decentralization. In this respect, the kingdom of David represents, the tower (or city) of Babel and the Babylonian captivity represents the scattering of people.[54]

MARGINALITY: THE MARK OF TRUE DISCIPLESHIP

The gospel of Luke Chapter 4, Verse 18 is known as the "Nazareth Manifesto." Here, Jesus announces his mission from the perspective of marginality, "preaching good news to the poor, freedom for the prisoners, sight to the blind, liberation to the oppressed." Jesus began, continued, and completed his ministry from this perspective. His act of choosing disciples reflects his perspective on choosing the marginal people of God. For instance, the rich young ruler portrayed in Luke 18:18–30 represents the central-group; he could not become God's marginal person as he was not willing to give up the centralist position inherent in his wealth (Matthew 19:16–30; Mark 10:17–31). This reveals that "marginality is a precondition for entering the new marginality one experiences when he/she becomes a disciple of Jesus Christ. It may not be possible for the centralists to become new marginal people unless they become marginalized first."[55]

All the disciples, including Paul, were marginal people. Though Cornelius and Nicodemus, representing the dominant groups, came to Jesus, they did not become disciples of Christ, like the others, because they could not give up their centrality. However, when Paul gave up his centralized position and accepted the marginalized status, he became a new marginalized person and creative as God's person. "The affirmation and acceptance of marginal status is very important for becoming the new marginalized of God and, hence, creative people."[56]

MARGINALITY AND CREATIVE POTENTIALITY

The church, as the dynamic community of new marginal people, is the servant of the world, who saves the world from centralist domination. According to Lee,

> Centrality is based on hierarchical value, while marginality is based on egalitarian principle. Centrality is interested in dominance, while marginality is interested in service. Centrality views control while marginality seeks

cooperation... Because of this same polarity, margin is not the new center rather it is only a creative core.[57]

True reconciliation includes liberation and, therefore, liberation is impossible without reconciliation. Therefore, the goal of marginal people is a reconciliation and liberation, meaning harmonious coexistence of all people in the genuinely pluralistic society. Based on the marginal experience of Asian-Indian immigrant families, in general, and the needs of the second-generation Asian-Indian immigrants, in particular, I would summarize this section by quoting Don S. Browning, who defines "practical theology as the reflective process which the church pursues in its effort to articulate the theological grounds of practical living in a variety of areas such as youth, work, sexuality, marriage, aging and death."[58] His compelling model is called practical reason with an outer envelope and an inner core, in which he integrates theory and practice in an ongoing process of action and reflection.

Standing in the gap to bridge the widening gulf between generation, culture, and worldview are important features of counseling Indian immigrants. I think the metaphor of pilgrim, traveler, or wanderer may not be very comfortable and relevant to the emerging immigrant generations, although it might have been for their parents. For emerging immigrant generations, it is not as much a geographical dislocation as a cultural displacement. Diaspora theology is more aptly suited for the second generations, which deals with the complexities of the multiple cultural influences, multicultural identities, and global network of communities. Cultural uprootedness can be a positive force for greater openness to an intercultural community of God that pursues an identity beyond ethnocultural realities.

In the revised critical correlation approach, Elaine Graham, Heather Walton, and Frankie Ward observe that Tracy attempts to mediate between cultural concerns and theological truth claims. Tracy argues that in the process of hearing the claims of modern culture in all its urgency and complexity, Christian theology itself must be prepared to undergo revision.[59] Conversely, when faith is considered an important dimension of the context itself, the particular religious beliefs, theological assumptions, religious rituals and symbols must find their way into the therapeutic context. To make theology meaningful and life stress-free, the traditional theology and dogmas also need to be revised based on the context.

The traditional understanding of the Indian church was that an individual who is born in a Christian family/community "behaves" in a certain manner and "belongs" to the community around him/her, which determines his/her religious orientation. Whether one personally "believes" in Christ or not, he/she remains as a part of the church and community by virtue of his/her birth. However, theologically, an individual first becomes a Christian by "believing" in Jesus Christ and then he/she joins a faith community and finds his/her "belonging." Then they begin to imitate others around them, based on what is being taught at church, which determines his/her "behaving."

In the former, the starting point is behavior, but in the latter it is belief. However, in both cases, belonging plays a central role. Here, the church and theology need to transcend tradition and ideologies to the extent that the immigrant community can live meaningfully. Implementing a code of behavior should undergo radical revision to make Christian theology applicable to believing and belonging to this community.[60]

THE AUTHENTIC CHURCH: THE COMMUNITY OF NEW MARGINALITY

The concept of church can be divided into two parts: the practicing church and the ideal church. What I refer to in this section is the authentic church as the ideal church. Rather than critiquing the practicing church, I would like to narrate briefly my vision of an authentic church. If at all I critique, I can only critique the Asian-Indian Pentecostal Churches,[61] of which I was a member from birth and in which I served as a pastor for more than 23 years, both in India and in the United States. So, my knowledge about the church is personal and limited. However, based on my personal experience I have a vision of an ideal church.

An authentic church is the community of God's marginalized people, and Jesus Christ is the highest norm of this new marginalized community. In other words, "the church is a community of new marginal people, who are conscious of the presence of Jesus Christ as the margin of marginality, where the genuine fellowship of brotherhood and sisterhood is experienced and the original order of creation is restored."[62] Those who occupy the center of centrality distance themselves from the margin and unconsciously avoid the presence of Christ.

The success of the ministry of the church should be judged by the marginal values of Jesus Christ—love, humility, and service—rather than the centralist values of personal power, wealth, and glory. An authentic church should be centered on the life and events of Jesus Christ:

> The church at the center of centrality must die so that the genuine community of marginality will resurrect from its corpse. Just as resurrection is not possible without death, there is no resurrection of a new church without the death of the old church. . . . The church as a Christian community must in-between the world now and the world that is to come. Both worlds, are however, one and inseparable, so it exists in-between and in-both at once.[63]

Jesus Christ as Spirit, who transcends temporal and spatial limitations, must become the locus of our church and the basis of our existence as a community of marginal people. The love that loves one another as Jesus loved us (John 15:12), the love that bears all things, believes all things, hopes all things, and endures all things (1 Corinthians 13:7), must be the character of the community of new marginal people. Such love makes the church a genuine community of marginality possible.

The new marginal community's theology should be developed from contexts of its distinctive understanding of the Christian faith. It requires an ongoing dialogue of plurality of faith expressions and understanding. The church as a living community of marginal people must relate to other communities. A common tendency of minority communities, like that of Asian-Indians, is to become closed so as to gain a temporary, false emotional security to combat alienation and marginality from the dominant group.

In Asian-Indian churches, schisms and division are common. Most Asian-Indian Pentecostal Church services have a time of testimony[64] (also called praise report). Quite often, the dominant group uses the time to gratify their emotional needs. These dominant people in the ethnic community are marginalized by the mainstream American society on the basis of race, gender, and social/economic status. Due to limited freedom, language, and law, dominant people in the ethnic community also cannot express feelings of marginality to the mainstream American society. Therefore, they use the church's time of testimony to mask their frustrations and shame, using the pulpit to show off their ability, eloquence, and greatness to others.

Many male Asian-Indian immigrants are well educated and many held professional, technical, and managerial positions in India and Middle-East prior to their emigration to the United States. They were the source of good income for the family, spending it without anyone's restrictions. But in the

United States, many of those same men are simply the family babysitters and cooks while their wives are working. Due to this role change, many husbands feel inferior to their wives. Even those men who work are discriminated against because of their skin color and accent. These frustrated men often find the church/religious/cultural centers to be the only place for recognition. Receiving recognition is important, but its desire is often germinated in an inferiority complex and is a means for proving that they are at the center of centrality.

The more Asian-Indians are marginalized, the more they seek public recognition in their ethnic congregations. They pay a lot of money for power, position, and recognition. Many ministers often exploit such weakness to gain financial profit. People who give more money are given more chances to use the pulpit to achieve public recognition. Their names always appear in the sermons and bulletins. The church, thus, profits by stressing the centralist values that attract marginalized people. The function of the church should not be to exploit its members' weaknesses but to help them realize that the power they seek actually marginalizes them.

Second-generation Asian-Indian ministers born, raised, and socialized in the United States, and aware of their new marginality, should be encouraged to minister to the people. The so called "youth pastors," who directly landed in the United States from India without being aware of the identity issues of Asian-Indian youngsters in the United States and are not trained in the American social and cultural contexts, have to be replaced by these second-generation Asian-Indian ministers who can identify with the youth and growing adults. Most of the first-generation Asian-Indians are not sufficiently familiar with PowerPoint presentations, note-taking, and so on in worship. Even praise and worship itself is a community activity that is led by the pastor. While all these Westernized and globalized forms of worship are brought into the Sunday service, effective methods and strategies for meeting the spiritual needs of growing young adults are often not contemplated or carried out.

Most first-generation immigrants insist that their children, who are born and raised in the United States, whose primary language of communication even at home is English, should join them in their Sunday services conducted in an Indian vernacular. In most Asian-Indian churches, first-generation immigrants are the dominant group, the center of the centrality. Even those who do not know how to communicate in English insert English vocabulary during their conversations and testimonies to impress others. However, those people often vehemently oppose the church's plan to offer a separate English service for their children. Here, second-generation immigrants are marginalized. These situations have to be changed.

In many Asian-Indian Pentecostal Churches, pastors are not theologically trained and there is no proper church administration. Anybody who has money, power, and ability to speak can become a pastor. Often pastors are the paid workers of the church and, therefore, trained pastors have no freedom to reform the church based on the needs of the congregation. If trained pastors do not "dance to the music of the church committee/council," they will be transferred or terminated. The dominant group in the church does not hesitate even to destroy the social reputation and image of such pastors. Some pastors, with no consultation and dialogue with the church members, do whatever they want. They claim they behave as they do because the Holy Spirit told them to talk and act in such a way. Several second-generation respondents told me in public that they are fed up with such dramas in their parents' churches and, therefore, are not interested in attending.

The mission of the church, according to the Apostle Paul, is to proclaim, admonish, and teach every man and woman in all wisdom to present them mature in Christ (Colossians 1:28–29). In other words, the church is to help the people to reconcile and live as a new marginal community in-between and 'in-both.' Reconciliation is not possible without justice. A church without justice cannot become a community of reconciliation. Therefore, dismantling centralist ideology is essential for transformation.

The attraction to centralist inclinations fails to make the church a community of new marginal people. "Those who are unaware of their marginality cling to the norm of centrality and are victimized by it. As Jesus Christ is the symbol of the margin of marginality, marginal people are Christian in principle."[65]

Today, many Asian-Indian ethnic minority churches are influenced deeply by the dominant ideology and fail to see their marginality. When marginal people do not see themselves, as marginal people, not only do they fail to be other-directed, they are also misdirected. The Asian-Indian church can help Asian-Indians discover their identity only when it discovers its own and shifts its norm from a centralist to a marginal perspective. People are the church and, therefore, personal discovery is the church's discovery of identity as marginal people of God. Transition from tradition to transformation is hard. It will face a lot of resistance because the false idea of centrality gives them a false sense of safety and security.

CHURCH: AN INTERCULTURAL COMMUNITY

To experience community is to "know the joy of belonging, the delight at being known and loved, the opportunity for giving and growing, and the safety of finding a new home."[66] Community for me is a point of commonality, not of residence. A meaningful community is a meaningful relationship that enriches people to discover their passions and purpose in life. According to Kohut, the human self is shaped and developed in relation to other people. He emphasizes the need for human relatedness in the development of self to be mirrored and to idealize. For Kohut the external objects are the real people and the internal objects are mental representations of people or things that exist within the self. Therefore, the human self is a relational self.[67]

Asian-Indian Christianity and churches are intricately interconnected with culture and faith. Mostly they practice a culturalized Christianity, invariably propagating Indian culture in the name of God. Most first generations, in the name of culture and tradition, try to recreate their childhood family, community, and faith memories, without realizing that it does not give their children the same sense of connection or meaning. Often this is done unconsciously and is evident across linguistic, ethnic, doctrinal, and denominational lines. The church is unconsciously expected to be a socialization vehicle to nurture the next generation in the culture, but not necessarily biblical faith. Sometimes behaving the Indian way takes precedence over the Christian or biblical way. Sometimes Asian-Indian Christianity is reinforced with unflinching zeal in the name of tradition, in order to preserve it from adulteration by American Christianity.[68]

I believe that the Asian-Indian churches in the United States, as a community, must engage with the realities of their host culture. The ethnic church leadership must take all necessary measures for critical contextualization and relevancy of ministry to the emerging generation. The ethnocentric nature of the Indian churches requires a transformation like that of Peter in the book of Acts, Chapter 10, whose perception was characteristic of the people of his time when Christianity was centered on Jewish ethnicity. The ethnocentricity of the Indian church should be its strength for making it an intercultural community of growth, support, and development.

The church as a community—both dominant white American churches and the dominant first-generation Indian churches—must focus on ministry to second-generation immigrants. When second-generations, in particular, suffer neglect from both ends, the church and pastoral caregivers, as a community, must be sufficiently capable to engage the theological issues in the present situation to make it relevant for the emerging generation and respond to the challenges of a postmodern culture.

Church history reveals that the church has always been the same but always changing. The issue of relevancy calls for a flexibility regarding expressions of faith and beliefs. First-generations must be willing to change or incorporate newer ways of doing church, instead of keeping Sunday morning reminiscent of the faith they grew up with back in India. Seeing the turbulence of our times and the uncertainties of the future, they resort to living in the idealized past. They are trapped in a time capsule thinking that things back home are the same as when they left, decades ago. It is time for the first-generation Indian churches to take a non-judgmental approach, avoiding "right/wrong" and "do/don't" language. For the benefits of the emerging generations, the question concerning issues should be "Is this the best way to do this?" instead of "Is this the right thing to do?" Moreover, the church as a community in a consumer culture that seems to focus on self-fulfillment should reveal the self-giving love to its members and be less judgmental.

Pastoral caregivers and clinicians from the Western culture must be aware of and not be influenced by the popular/centralist beliefs of the American society into which the second-generation Asian-Indians are assimilating, absorbing Western culture and seeking to fit into it without appreciating their ethnic roots. Similarly, ethnic pastoral counselors should also be aware of the sameness and differences of the second-generation immigrants so that they may not be treated as one of the counselor's kind and expected to fit right into their home culture. Pastoral counselors and theologians must reinterpret their practices and traditions in order to give a new understanding for the new generation in the new cultural context. Rediscovering some of the traditions for original meaning and giving them a fresh life by articulating its relevancy in contemporary language is also required of the pastoral care-givers. It is equally important to redeem traditions and create new traditions relevant to the immigrant generations. It is time to distinguish traditions for the sake of traditions from traditions for the purpose of building a sustaining community.

Since second generations do not have a fixed boundary between sacred and secular, the theology for this emerging generation needs to be a theology that bridges the gap and sees all religious experiences as human experience. It must be a community-oriented theology with sufficient individual freedom that is shaped and conditioned by the context in which it is rooted. Here again, the action and reflection should be the praxis for understanding this immigrant theology. Thus, it should be a holistic, relational, and culturally sensitive theology.

A THEOLOGY OF NEW MARGINAL COMMUNITY

Jesus Christ is the self-emptied God who pioneered a new marginal people. His followers are the new marginal people of God. The phrase "children of God" is often used to describe the familial relationship with God. "Because we are children of God through Jesus Christ, we are also joined him in the family of divine Trinity."[69] Liberation from marginality does not mean that we are free from marginality, nor does it mean that we are to be at the center that dominates the margin. Rather, liberation from marginality means transferring one form of marginality to another form of marginality that is, moving from the human centrality to the new marginality of divine presence in the world.

Therefore, the envisioned new marginal community is a group of people that affirms human worth, provides a sense of belonging, and helps people connect with spiritual resources and other life-sustaining aid. It is a community of new marginality. The aim of this theology of community of new marginality is human wholeness or shalom, relationality, and community. This is theology of an intercultural community that helps its members to interpret and reinterpret the realities and traditions until the subjects discover the true self. It is a theology with fewer judgments and one that ascribes higher value to individual differences and cultural diversity. In other words, it is not uniformity but unity in diversity that is the focus of the theology of the community of new marginality. This theology enables the community to be mutual and reciprocal. This is a community in which people are less judgmental and more open, interactive, and supportive. The theology of the community seriously considers the need for belonging and makes its gatherings informal, less structured, fellowship-driven, and non-hierarchical.

The theology of the community of new marginality is rooted in the conviction that wisdom does not belong to only one group, generation, race, ideology, or faith. Emmanuel Lartey calls it a polylingual, polyphonic, and polyperspectival community.[70] It should be a community that connects the multiplicity of cultural self. In this communal theology, many voices are spoken, listened to, and respected for meaningful and effective living. This theology considers all religious experience as human experience.[71] Action and reflection need to be the praxis to understand theology. There needs to be an integration of both male and female aspects of spirituality in this community since every human experience is relational, holistic, and culturally shaped.

A THEOLOGY OF OPENNESS

Marginal theology is a theology of openness. According to Jürgen Moltmann, the crisis of the present-day churches is a double crisis – the crisis of relevancy and crisis of identity. These two crises are complementary. The more theology and church attempt to become relevant to the problems of the present day, the more deeply they are drawn into a crisis of their own identity. The more they attempt to assert their identity in traditional dogmas, rights, and moral notions, the more irrelevant and unbelievable they become.[72]

Most second-generation immigrants are uncomfortable in Indian churches where they cannot speak or understand the language of worship. Openness allows us to understand the mystery of God by understanding each other and the needs and cultural heritages of others. Human beings are the creations of God in various cultures with deep and hidden meanings. Openness is not a process of approving or confirming the preconceived ideas. Rather, it is the willingness to enter, exit, and re-enter into the differences and sameness of others and oneself. The theology of openness creates meaning-making through healthy and meaningful relationships, taking a not-knowing approach. The centralist approach of value judgment and prejudice has no place in the theology of openness.

Tolerance is one of the major components in the theology of openness. Religious truth should be seen in the context of relationship. Unconditional love and acceptance are the basis of the theology of openness. Here, truth is not understood in an absolute sense, but in a relational sense. It is derived from an understanding that divine truths are mysteries that cannot be understood at any one time, or completely at any given stage. Nalini Arles argues that theology of openness is less dogmatic and more pragmatic, less authoritarian and more participatory.[73] Such a theology should provide growth, change, and development to the people. Briefly stated, whatever came from the center would eventually return to the center because of the margin. Marginality is defined only in relation to centrality because there is no center without the margin as there is no margin without the center. They are mutually relative, interdependent, and coexistent.[74]

Therefore, when we mention center we should also acknowledge margin and vice versa. When one is overemphasized, the other is ignored. Therefore affirming the one without ignoring the other is the actual openness.

NOTES

1. D.S. Sandhu, P.R. Portes, and S.A. McPhee, "Assessing Cultural Adaptation: Psychometric Properties of the Cultural Adaptation Pain Scale," *Journal of Multicultural Counseling and Development*, 24, no. 1 (January 25, 1996):15–25, at 22.
2. Jung Young Lee, *Marginality: The Key to Multicultural Theology* (Minneapolis, MN: Fortress Press), 1.
3. Ibid., 3.
4. Ibid., 2.
5. Ibid., 32.
6. Ibid., 33.
7. Lee uses the image of a pond in a park near his town to define center and marginality, illustrating many ripples created by fish, or a stone thrown or leaves falling into it. He beautifully explains that these ripples created through various means have many centers and margins.
8. Lee, *Marginality*, 33.
9. Ibid.
10. Manning Marable, "The Rhetoric of Racial Harmony: Finding Substance in Culture and Ethnicity," *Sojourners* 19, no. 7 (August–September, 1990): 16.
11. Joe R. Feagin, *Racial and Ethnic Relations* (New York: Prentice Hall, 1978), 6.
12. Lee, *Marginality*, 34.
13. Ibid., 35.
14. Ibid.
15. Robert E. Park, *Introduction to Everett V. Stonequist's The Marginal Man: A Study in Personality and Cultural Conflict* (New York: Russell and Russell, 1961), xvii.
16. Robert E. Park, "Our Racial Frontier on the Pacific," *Survey Graphic* 56, no. 3 (May, 1926): 196.
17. Stanford M. Lyman, *The Asian in North America* (Santa Barbara, CA: ABC Clio Inc., 1977), 12.
18. Lee, *Marginality*, 42.
19. Everett V. Stonequist, *The Marginal Man: A Study in Personality and Cultural Conflicts* (New York: Russell and Russell, 1961), 43.
20. Stonequist, *The Marginal Man*, 45.
21. Ibid., 217.

22. Lee, *Marginality*, 46.
23. Stonequist, *The Marginal Man*, 148.
24. Lee, *Marginality*, 47.
25. Ibid., 50–51.
26. Ibid., 56.
27. The common assumption is that the second-generation Asian Americans reject their ethnic roots and strive for full assimilation in the dominant American culture and that is why they are in the state of being in-between. This assumption further holds that the third-generation Americans seek their roots in ethnicity, which is often called, "the law of third-generation return." However, this assumption is no longer true because the second-generations experience both worlds simultaneously. Even some of the third-generation immigrants with whom I shared my views agreed that they, too, experience discrimination and rejection as the first- or second-generations experience, though the intensity of these experiences may vary from person to person or from generation to generation.
28. Lee, *Marginality*, 59–60.
29. Ibid., 60–61.
30. David Ng, "Sojourners Bearing Gifts: Pacific Asian American Christian Education," in *Ethnicity in the Education of the Church*, ed. Charles R. Foster (New York, NY: Scarit Press, 1987), 14.
31. Ibid., 57.
32. Ibid., 66.
33. Ibid., 67.
34. Ibid., 69.
35. Ibid.
36. Unless otherwise noted, all scriptural citations are from the New Revised Standard Version of the Bible (Oxford: Oxford University Press, 1991).
37. Ng, "Sojourners," 78.
38. Ibid., 83.
39. Ibid., 84.
40. Ibid.
41. Ibid., 86.
42. Ibid., 89.
43. Ibid., 95.
44. Ibid., 96.
45. Ibid.
46. Ibid., 99.
47. Ibid., 106.
48. It is a monoculturalist assumption that "What is good for us must be good for you." While this is the attitude of the dominant whites in the United States to the Asian Indians (like all other ethnic minorities), the dominant

Asian-Indian parental community shows the same attitude to the second-generation marginal, minority groups as well.

49. Ng, "Sojourners," 109.
50. Ibid., 111.
51. Ibid., 112.
52. Ibid., 113.
53. Jehoachim Jeremias, *Jerusalem in the Time of Jesus* (Philadelphia, PA: Fortress Press, 1981), 74–76, 95–97.
54. Lee, *Marginality*, 117.
55. Ibid.
56. Ibid., 118.
57. Ibid., 151.
58. Don S. Browning, *A Fundamental Practical Theology* (Minneapolis, MN: Fortress Press, 1991), 10.
59. Elaine Graham, Heather Walton, and Frankie Ward, *Theological Reflection: Methods* (London, UK: SCM Press, 2005), 159.
60. Sam George, *Coconut Generation: Ministry to the Americanized Asian-Indians* (Niles, IL: Mall Publishing Co., 2006), 107–108.
61. Indian Pentecostal Church here does not mean the IPC denomination, rather the Pentecostal churches in India.
62. Lee, *Marginality*, 123.
63. Ibid., 130.
64. In every Indian Pentecostal Church, irrespective of denomination, a particular amount of time (between 30 and 45 minutes) is devoted to testimony in Sunday services. Testimony is actually is meant to share in public what great things people received from the Lord throughout a week and what great things they attempted for the Lord. However, this time is often used to boast, compete with one another, and indirectly accuse each other. Hence, the time becomes a major source of fights and schisms in the church.
65. Lee, *Marginality*, 143.
66. John Ortberg, *Every Day is Normal Till You Get to Know Them* (Grand Rapids: Zondervan, 2003), 40.
67. Refer to Chap. 5 and footnote 60 for more information.
68. George, *Coconut Generation*, 106.
69. Lee, *Marginality*, 101.
70. Emmanuel Y. Lartey, *Pastoral Theology in an Intercultural World* (Cleveland, OH: Pilgrim Press, 2006), 124.
71. Lartey, *In Living Color: An Intercultural Approach to Pastoral Care and Counseling* (London: Jessica Kingsley, 2003), 33.
72. Jürgen Moltmann, *The Crucified God* (New York: Harper & Raw, 2006), 7.

73. Nalini Arles, "Spirituality and Culture in the Practice of Pastoral Care and Counseling," in *Spirituality and Culture in the Practice of Pastoral Care and Counseling: Voices from Different Contexts*, eds. John Foskett and Emmanuel Lartey (Fairwater, UK: Cardiff Academic Press, 1998), 89.

74. Ibid.

CHAPTER 7

Cohesive Self and New Marginality: A Mutual Critical Correlation

INTRODUCTION

The purpose of this chapter is to present a mutually critical correlation which brings into conversation Lee's theology of new marginality (in-beyond), Kohut's psychology of the self, and Kakar's concept of communal identity. Kakar's view of the self in relation to community is generally in agreement with notions of the self in Lee's understanding of marginality. However, Lee's presentation of the self in a new marginal community is Christ-conscious, whereas Kakar's view is focused on Hindu mythology, though ultimately connected with God. I correlate some of the concepts of Kohut and Lee, such as the understanding of the self, the vicissitudes of the self, and the cure for the disintegration of the self in the development of a model of pastoral care for Asian-Indian immigrant families in the United States. The theological method of mutual critical correlation that is used in this chapter includes a way of analyzing data through an integrative perspective that allows the fields of theology, psychology, and culture to be in mutual dialogue.

Selected themes that have a bearing on the development of a pastoral psychotherapeutic method for intervention with Asian-Indian persons and families are highlighted in this chapter. Particularly important are the concepts of in-between, in-both, and in-beyond from Lee's theology, which help illuminate and solidify concepts that are fundamental to the understanding of the Asian-Indian cultural situation in the United States.

© The Author(s) 2017
V. Jacob, *Counseling Asian Indian Immigrant Families,*
DOI 10.1007/978-3-319-64307-6_7

A number of concepts from Kohut are also helpful in understanding the impact of primary relationships on the psychological dynamic, both in human development and in the healing of wounds from conflicts encountered in life. The intent of this chapter is to develop an approach that focuses on developing material that will meet the spiritual/emotional care needs of the Asian-Indian individuals and families living in the United States, and in similar cultural environments, who are feeling immobilized due to a sense of loss of identity resulting from cultural clashes, marginality, and intergenerational conflicts.

In developing a method of intervention with Asian-Indian immigrant persons and families in the United States, my major focus from the Indian perspective is rooted in family and community. Development of a healthy self, or new marginal person, and individual and family functionality are from the Western perspective. These concepts are well-connected with interdependency or collective identity, also referred to as relationality. This is important because marginal experience, cultural value differences, fear of family declension, and intergenerational conflicts disconnect or disintegrate one another. Such experiences often lead to lack or absence of empathy, grace, love, and caring.

Understanding Kohut's and Lee's Positions on the Self

According to Kohut, the self develops through two parallel lines of development that he terms the bipolar self.[1] For Kohut, this means that the development of the self on the one pole occurs through drives, as hypothesized by Freud, while the other pole of the development of the nuclear self is constituted by the relationships of care givers to the developing child, that is to his or her self-objects. For Kohut, self is "a psychic configuration – the self – that has become a center of initiative, a unit that tries to follow its own course."[2] Kohut sees the self and the development of the self from an individualistic perspective, as well as from the process of establishing one's sense of initiative.

The disintegration of the self, according to Kohut, is caused by the failures of the developing child's environment. The environment of the developing child is comprised of its caretakers/self-objects, in general, with the mother typically the main care giver. The disintegration of the self is caused by unempathic responses to the child's narcissistic needs that form the core of the child's development into a cohesive nuclear self. Kohut speaks of the fragmentation of the self, due to unempathic responses from the mirroring and idealizing self-objects in the child's life. Discussing the fact of disintegration of the self, Kohut says,

> Subsequent to an Oedipal phase that is marred by the failure of the parents to respond healthily to their child, a defect in the child's self is set up. Instead of the further development of a firmly cohesive self, able to feel the glow of healthy pleasure in its affectionate and phase-appropriate sexual functioning and able to employ self-confident assertiveness in the pursuit of goals, we find throughout life a continuing propensity to experience the fragments of love (sexual fantasies) rather than love and fragments of assertiveness (hostile fantasies) to respond to these experiences of childhood– with anxiety.[3]

In writing about development of the cohesive self, Kohut puts great emphasis on the primary caregivers for the child. Still, he suggests that failures may be caused by the parents' own history of childhood failures in forming a cohesive self. Here therapists can help the clients to understand their parents' empathic failures. Kohut notes,

> First and most important: the self-psychologically informed psychoanalyst blames no one, neither the patient nor his parents. He identifies causal sequences; he shows the patient that his feelings and reactions are explained by his experiences in early life, and he points out that, ultimately, his parents are not to blame since they were what they were because of the backgrounds that determined their own personalities. . . .[4]

Though Kohut does not blame the primary caregivers, it is the case that he sees the causes of the disintegration of the self are placed in relationship to primary caregivers. This relationship issue can either be the primary caregivers' own issues or they might be inherited from the parents. In other words, the cause of the disintegration of the self happens either because of relational difficulties with primary caregivers, who can be the parents of a child, or it can be a result of relational issues that lie or lay between the child's parents and their parents. Ultimately, Kohut describes different ways in which humanity's experience of disintegration of the self happens. It is either in the drives or in the realm of needs of the nuclear self.

While Kohut deals with the subject of the self from the perspective of self-psychology, Lee deals with self from the perspective of theological anthropology. His understanding of the self hinges upon relationality or in-both/in-beyond as the proper understanding of what it means for human beings to be created in the image of God. His goal is to develop a social or communal understanding of the concept of the "new marginality" as a response to the dissipation of the self in modernity. Relationality and empathy are required when everything is the same, but even more so when everything is different and yet relational. In this regard, Lee says,

> Difference and plurality are essential aspects of creativity. They are mutually dependent and constitute interdependent variables in the creative process. The interdependent relationship seems to be a key to understanding dynamism and creativity in the Old Testament. This plurality is the condition of marginality. If everything is the same and singular, marginality is not possible.[5]

It is clear that Lee's understanding of the self is communally based. He calls for the rightful context of reconceptualization of the self as occurring in and through the community. He argues that the modern understanding of the self is focused on the center of centrality, the craving for a single or normative form that oppresses and marginalizes the minority whose norms are pluralistic. The imposition of sameness over difference and singularity over plurality are the centralist ideology of dominance.[6] Lee further indicates that change and growth of self are possible as marginal can transcend from neither/nor (in-between) to both/and (in-both and in-beyond). Self, in Lee's understanding, is multidimensional with multiple connotations in relation to both sociological anthropology and theological anthropology.

A true understanding of the self in Lee's theology is the new marginality, which is structural and relationally oriented. He posits that the structural understanding of the self is always the center of centrality that emphasizes the ideology of singularity and sameness while denying the existence of plurality and differences. However, this structural self is able to transform and transcend. As the marginal self (in-between) is transcended or transformed it becomes a new marginal (in-both and in-beyond), conforming to the margin of marginality (Jesus Christ).[7]

The relational understanding of the self presupposes a harmonious relationship between oneself, others, and God. One cannot understand himself/herself unless he/she understands others who are in them. They are included in them, and the reverse is true. This unity presupposes difference in plurality. The relational self is also connected with the Godhead as found in the high priestly prayer of Jesus, found in the gospel of John (17:21).[8]

This understanding visualizes that the disintegrated human self is able to reflect, or mirror, God in a way that the human being obediently reflects the will of God, revealed by their life and action. The emphasis here is on the relationship between human and human, and also between human and God. The authentic church is a community of new marginal people, where the genuine fellowship of brotherhood/sisterhood is experienced, where original order of creation is restored, and where people reflect the nature of God.[9] It is an internal transformation that is externally expressed as the awareness of marginality begins from below and moves upward, that is, it moves from the margin to the center.

When people accept their marginality and understand its power, they can resist moving towards the centralist ideology, knowing that God is with them at their margin.[10] We can further understand self as the marginality in-between and in-both in the context of the community, as well as in relationship with God as its fullness found in Jesus Christ, the new marginal person *par excellence*.[11] Therefore, a true understanding of self is also communal and relational.

Concerning the disintegration of the self, Lee would agree with Kohut that the disintegration of the modern self is due to the empathic failures of the caring environment of the marginal. His argument is that the true understanding of self must begin from self-awareness and move toward the community, culminating in Jesus Christ, the margin of marginality. In other words, the disintegrated self should be aware of its centralist (unempathic) nature and move toward the experience of healing. To explain it in a different way, the self in the in-between situation should move to in-both and further culminates into in-beyond experience that makes a creative core which, includes all kinds of differences as in the creative order of God.[12] He clearly and categorically declares that his intention is to foster the renewal of the Christian communally constituted soul out of the ashes of the centered self.[13]

Concisely, while Kohut understands the disintegration of the self as a result of empathic failures in early childhood, which is basically due to the failures of the parenting figures in helping the child develop a nuclear and cohesive self, Lee from the marginal perspective understands disintegration of the self as a result of empathic failures of the centralists who dominate the marginal with their dominant ideology and discriminatory attitude.

EMPATHY

Empathy is central to Kohut's self psychology because it defines his theoretical approach to psychotherapy. He calls it a "vicarious introspection" and the capacity to think and feel oneself into the inner life of another person.[14] He believes that it is only through empathy that we are able to understand the other person's world as we use introspection, or allow ourselves to feel what the other person feels to the extent of "putting ourselves in their shoes," so to speak. Therefore, empathy is the core of his therapeutic model, both as a research tool and as a healing tool. It is empathy that helps the therapist to connect with the world of the counselee to the extent of understanding their archaic needs and wounds. For Kohut, empathy is also a God-given gift that is available to everyone, only that some need to keep working on it more than others.[15]

The therapeutic power of empathy is the therapist's ability to help mend the fractured or disintegrated self by positive regard, or healthy responses. Through empathy, the counselee will be able to complete whatever developmental stage was not fully completed. Through the empathic response of the therapist, the counselee is able to develop a cohesive nuclear self in the therapeutic relationship. The therapy allows the counselee to heal their fractured self through transmuting internalization (taking in the groundedness of the therapist into the core of oneself). For Kohut, empathy is the mode by which and through which the development of the self is formed and repaired. It is through its ability to create a supportive environment conducive to the growth of persons of all ages who are seeking to be cohesive, healthy selves.

Lee does not use the term empathy in his writing, but uses terms such as reconciliation and compassion as the acts of God that allow persons to be fully who they are.[16] Reconciliation, acceptance and inclusivism are the terms that Lee mostly uses to indicate empathy. It is a metaphor for a very deep level of relating that takes place in the community of God. While Kohut emphasizes a cohesive individual self, Lee's focus is a new marginal community that is implied in the community of God.

Incarnational theology is an immigrant theology. The act of incarnation, God's grace through the coming of Christ, has opened the door for to all to enter into relationship with God and to live in beyond, even in the midst of marginality. Christ is the new marginal through his incarnation, and church is the community of God's marginal people. Hence, our true identity calls us to share our common identity with others in the community. This community of new marginality with its true identity reflects genuine brotherhood/sisterhood, accepting the differences and plurality as the creative order of God. Hence, Lee views empathy at a higher level. For him, empathy is not only a human quality that connects people with each other, but also connects them with God.

Lee presents the entire Bible from the perspective of emigration and marginality. Further, he sees such immigrant communities as bridge-builders between cultures, other communities, and God. Ultimately, Jesus Christ is narrated as the new marginal and his church as the new marginal community. In the following section, I explore further the role and importance of relationships in understanding the self, comparing it to Heinz Kohut's conceptualization of empathy and self.

RELATIONSHIPS

One of Lee's major concerns is the development of a genuine and inclusive relationship that accepts differences. This genuine and inclusive relationship is the true self, which is also a communal or collective self. He claims that identity can only be understood in terms of being in genuine relationships, which is the true marginality. His starting point is Jesus Christ, the image of the invisible God who migrated from one realm to another realm and became the new marginal, a relational self. Lee views all of scripture from the perspective of migration, marginality, and relational self. He posits that the creative core, or new marginality, invites reconciliation as a new marginal person is a reconciler of two or more different or opposite worlds. Being in-between two margins, the new marginal reconciles each and lives in-beyond the two.[17]

Lee sees humanity's relationship to God as the only way humanity can realize its true identity. He sees marginalization, domination, and racial discrimination, which do not accept God's creative order of plurality, as alienation from God. Harmonious coexistence of the ethnic minorities is not possible when dominant groups deny racial and ethnic differences. Difference cannot coexist when sameness dominates and insists on homogeneity.[18]

According to Lee, the coming of Christ is an act through which God seeks to restore the relationship with humanity that was broken by humanity's propensity toward self-centeredness. The resurrection of Christ Jesus marks the beginning of a new age as it offers the reign of God, where all people can live in harmony and peace as children of God.[19] The significance of relationships for Lee is that he values the community as the source of one's identity.[20] This relationship recognizes the importance of the community as the doorway to a true understanding of our true identity or communal self.

For Kohut, the healing power of relationships is in the therapist's ability to use empathic attunement. The empathic therapist helps the client to heal the childhood wounds of unempathic responses by the parenting figures. Relationships are important for Kohut, as they are for Lee. While Kohut sees the importance of relationships in the formation and healing of the self, Lee views relationships as the way we should understand our identity as intricately intertwined with God and community. While Lee holds that our relationships make our identity a shared identity, Kohut posits that relationships help us form our own individual identities. Lee emphasizes that the inclusive relationships of the new marginal community have a healing status, while Kohut emphasizes the significance of therapeutic relationship. Their views share similarities, but also have differences.

SIMILARITIES AND DIFFERENCES IN LEE'S AND KOHUT'S VIEWS OF THE SELF

Both Lee and Kohut highlight the importance of relationships that help form human identity and the way in which these relationships impact a persons' self-understanding. Though Lee and Kohut differ in how they see "self" from two different disciplines, they agree that the fragmentation or disintegration of self is to be remedied or resolved in relationships. Kohut focuses on the individual and how relationships help or hinder the development of the self in his estimation of the psychology of the self. Lee views it through the lens of marginality and theological anthropology focused on the communal self and how this understanding of the self is based on the creative order of plurality.

Kohut sees the disintegration of the self as a failure in the caring relationship of the child's parental figures that may be caused by deficits in the parents, or their own childhood empathic failures. This view presents the self as being affected by its relationship to parental figures. However, Lee seems to blame disorders of the self on the dominant group holding a centralist approach that disapproves of difference and plurality, which is the creative order of God.

The dominant group is unempathic to marginal minority persons. As a result, marginal people have to create an empathic community and relationship in relation to Jesus Christ, the new marginal person and become his new marginal people. Lee views self as more communal than individualistic and found in relationship with others and God. Kohut sees relationships as self-objects, objects that help the individual to grow and develop as true selves. Kohut's presentation of the self in self psychology follows a developmental approach similar to Freud and Erikson, but he provides his own unique and distinctive approach. Lee, on the other hand, presents a self that is understood from a theological-anthropological perspective.

Clearly, both Kohut and Lee are dealing with the disintegration of the self and the need for healing in two different ways, namely psychological and theological. They differ only in their understanding of the nature of healing. Lee conceptualizes the disintegration of the self as the loss of relationship with others and God, and sees restoration or healing as enhanced through union with Christ and community. Kohut, however, sees disintegration in terms of psychological damage that needs to be resolved in a psychotherapeutic relationship. Kohut sees empathy through the action of the therapist as the key to the healing of the psychological vicissitudes. Empathy and grace are both concepts that entail the emptying of love for the sake of the other born out of a deep understanding of the condition of the other through kenotic action. For this purpose, centralists and marginals should move toward the creative core where God is the center, accepting all differences and restoring God's creative order of plurality.

From his research and observation, Kohut claims that the child is full of initiative, strives psychologically to be in relationship with significant parental figures, and seeks out significant others in the process of seeking to be a self. However, the child is affected either positively or negatively, depending on the parental figures' reaction to it. This is the theme of relationship that is carried out in therapy because Kohut sees the success of the therapy in the therapist's ability for empathy.

Both Kohut and Lee provide very important material for working with those migrating to the United States/Western cultural worlds from different ethnic and cultural backgrounds. Their different perspectives on personhood are very helpful in understanding persons who seek therapy. The importance of empathy and the availability of grace to everyone are important in dealing with the loss suffered by the persons and families that come for counseling. Therefore, my intention for the purpose of developing a model for Asian-Indian immigrants in the multiple cultural spaces of the United States is to look further at the implications of the information previously discussed from both Kohut and Lee.

IMPLICATIONS FOR DEVELOPING A MODEL FOR ASIAN-INDIAN IMMIGRANTS IN THE WESTERN CULTURAL WORLDS

To this point, I have explored the correlation between the psychological theory of Kohut and theological method of Lee selected for developing a model of counseling with Asian-Indian immigrant persons and families who fear the "death or declension of family"[21] and are undergoing intergenerational family conflict due to clashing cultural values and cultural identity issues. Kohut's theory of the self in an individualistic perspective and nuclear family context may seem inapplicable and not relevant to work with the Asian-Indian immigrant persons and families in therapy. On the other hand, Lee presents a theological view of marginality that emphasizes self-in-community that appears to be more applicable to the therapeutic needs of Asian-Indians, as discussed in Chap. 2. However, it must be noted that the experience of migrating to the United States or other Western cultural worlds cannot be homogenized to the extent that one theory fits all, because for instance, Asian-Indian families living in the multiple cultural spaces of the United States comprise both Indians and Americans.

Concepts from Kohut's and Lee's theories have promises as well as limitations for understanding Asian-Indian persons and families living in the United States or in any other Western cultural world. The cultural backgrounds of these persons make it necessary only to borrow those aspects of the theories that are consistent with the communal orientation brought from the Indian culture. Because of cultural and identity issues, there may be instances where one of the concepts may be applied in therapy, while in other cases both must be applied. This will depend on the structure of the family, persons, and the impact of globalization.

Based on my therapeutic experience with Asian-Indian immigrant families, there are a number of factors that help assess the need of each theoretical component in different cases—cultural generation (whether first or second), the level of acculturation among family members, parental communities' environment of upbringing, and the impact of migration on them. Lee's conceptualization of marginality in three different ways (in-between, in-both, and in-beyond) and relationality with oneself, others, and God is easily applied in the Asian-Indian cultural context. However, his understanding of community seems limited to the ecclesial community, whereas the Asian-Indian understanding of community consists of different castes, classes, religions, languages and cultures. However, the church as the new marginal community and Christ as the new marginal person as its center, is inclusive of all differences in castes, classes, religions, languages, and cultures. It is important to be in relationships with others and in relationship with God.

I am sure that almost all Asian-Indians will resonate with the Kohutian understanding of the importance of a child's primary relationships with its caregivers (parents, grandparents, and other family members) for a healthy development of the self, as the collective effort of raising a child is a very important concept among Asian-Indians. I am also sure that no Asian-Indian will disagree with Kohut in his theoretical elaboration on empathy and its importance as a vehicle through which healthy relationships are developed. However, there can be disagreement regarding Kohut's understanding of the normal development of a child leading to independent self rather than an interdependent self. This is due to the Indian under-standing that the self is not an individualistic self but rather a communal self, as discussed in Chaps. 2 and 3.

Though the Indian community is close-knit, due to the influences and impacts of globalization, along with the influence of the dominant individ-ualistic culture of the United States, community support is often lacking when a person finds himself/herself in crisis. Moreover, many people often use the crisis of another as opportunities to gossip and spread the details of that personal experience throughout the community. It is in these situations that the therapist may need to be willing to journey with the Asian-Indian immigrant families in order to identify the issues that make their life mean-ingless and dysfunctional.

Lee consciously divides the understanding of church into two: the prac-ticing church and the ideal/authentic church. But the churches where immigrant families find themselves are all-too-often practicing churches, which are informed by the centralist approach, controlled by the rich, dominated by traditions, dogmas, and "groupism." Therefore, even for many immigrant Christian families, it becomes a great challenge to find the relational ecclesial community, the community of acceptance and relationality they so desperately need.

Lee speaks to the importance of understanding the self from a point of marginality that is developed of in-between, in-both, and in-beyond perspec-tives. He also presents Jesus Christ, the people of Israel, Moses, the disciples of Jesus, and many other biblical characters and figures as the immigrants who experienced marginality only to become successful bridge-builders and reconcilers. He posits this as a comprehensive understanding of the self and the self's relationship with God and others. Therefore, the implication of this in the development of a liberative pastoral care model for use with Asian-Indian persons and families calls for a deliberate and informed understanding of the history of the persons who are coming for care. As discussed in Chap. 2, Asian-Indians (whether first- or second-generation) have a history that warrants an intentional engagement that will bring forth some level of cultural and historical sensitivity.

Kohut speaks of the need to be able to employ empathic introspection for the sake of helping the client. Understanding the history of brokenness and experiences of subjugation and oppression that caused multiple identities will help bring forth informed methods of care that are sensitive to the needs of those seeking care. A meaningful and appropriate care can be provided only when the therapist understands the history of the brokenness and disintegration. Lee also emphasizes the importance of knowing the history of the marginalized immigrant in terms of their ethnic, racial, and cultural heritage, and brokenness.

While the concepts of these Western and Asian writers may be useful for the development of a model of care for Asian-Indian immigrants in the United States facing intergenerational conflicts and declension of family, they must be examined for their applicability to and relevance for the persons and families seeking care. The cultural experience and context of Asian-Indians should determine the usefulness of these concepts. Since concepts and methods have the power to determine and influence outcomes, Asian-Indian and Indian-American cultural norms of being, life, and health must be given an important place in the development, application, and evaluation of offered methods of care.

Two questions that are seriously considered in the development of the pastoral care model for Asian-Indian immigrant families in the United States or any other Western cultural world are:

- What are the theoretical concepts from Kohut concerning human development and methods of counseling that are culturally relevant to the care needs of Asian-Indian families and persons?
- How does marginality affect Asian-Indian immigrants in ways (such as conflicting values and level of acculturation) apart from the cultural identity issues?

It is very clear that any relationship that does not affirm and accept the other is disintegrating the self. Any relationship that does not affirm or reinforce the identity in the community is not healing. This is what is happening in the marginality experience. However, the therapist as a healer, in the place of Christ, offers a holy and healing space with a renewed relationship to facilitate healing and health. Since relationship is the basic cause for the disintegration of the self or identity, it is by a renewed relationship that healing and cohesiveness are attained. Therefore, for me, the in-between, in-both, and in-beyond experiences of marginality are similar to Kohut's disintegrated self, which is formed through relational failure, the healthy self, which is formed through therapeutic relationship, and the cohesive self which is developed and attained through repairing the relational experience and restoring the relationship for further relationship with oneself, others, and God.

NOTES

1. Heinz Kohut, *The Restoration of the Self* (New York: International Universities Press, 1977) 56.
2. Ibid., 245.
3. Heinz Kohut, *How Does Analysis Cure?* (Chicago: University of Chicago Press, 184), 24–25.
4. Ibid., 25.
5. Lee, *Marginality*, 105.
6. Ibid., 108.
7. Ibid., 101.
8. Ibid., 105.
9. Ibid., 121.
10. Ibid., 145–146.
11. Ibid., 78.
12. Ibid., 108.
13. Ibid., 121
14. Kohut, *How Does Analysis Cure?* 82.
15. Ibid., 83.
16. Lee, 75.
17. Ibid., 99.
18. Ibid., 107.
19. Ibid., 96.
20. Ibid.
21. See Chap. 1, footnote 10 for the definition of "death/declension of family."

CHAPTER 8

The Praxis–Reflection–Action Model: An Interdisciplinary Approach to Pastoral Care and Psychotherapy

INTRODUCTION

Based on the historical perspective of understanding the pastoral care needs of Asian-Indians as discussed in Chaps. 2 and 3, along with the empirical data analyzed and interpreted in Chap. 4, this chapter proposes a pastoral psychotherapeutic model for Asian-Indian families living in the United States and other Western worlds which share similar cultures. The development is premised upon the following questions:

- What are the care needs of Asian-Indian immigrant families dealing with alienation resulting from immigrating to the United States, and other similar cultural settings as informed by an understanding of their cultural reality?
- Based on their care needs, what kind of a counseling model is required for doing appropriate and effective pastoral counseling with Asian-Indian immigrant families in the United States, taking seriously their cultural heritage and the ensuing cultural clash between multiple cultural generations?
- What, if anything, do various resources premised on a Western perspective of identity development have to offer in the construction of an interdisciplinary approach of pastoral care and counseling with Asian-Indian immigrants considering the difference in culture and the two notions of self—the individualistic self (Western) versus collective identity—which Asian-Indian immigrants navigate?

© The Author(s) 2017
V. Jacob, *Counseling Asian Indian Immigrant Families*,
DOI 10.1007/978-3-319-64307-6_8

To recapture the context of this research and to refresh readers' memories, the issue that prompted the development of this model is briefly restated here. Next, the reflection method of Whitehead and Whitehead, the liberative model of Lartey, and the family systems theory of Murray Bowen are examined for their applicability to a pastoral counseling model for the Asian-Indian families in United States. Finally, I present my five-stage counseling model and examine two case studies through the lens of this model to illustrate how it effectively addresses the care needs of Asian-Indian immigrant families in the United States and other Western countries.

RESTATEMENT OF THE PROBLEM

Traditionally, Indian families have been greatly influenced by a patriarchal, joint family system, with mothers, fathers, grandparents and others playing significant roles in socializing young children into culturally expected behaviors. Asian-Indian parenting typically practices authoritarian parenting styles,[1] emphasizes academic achievement,[2] and familial bond and solidarity (i.e., importance of family and respect for elders).[3] Because of the history of caste system in the Asian-Indian culture, marriage within the same community and religion is encouraged.[4] Dating and premarital sexual relations are generally considered unacceptable.[5] These values and beliefs are often acquired implicitly rather than explicitly through a culturally determined learning process.[6]

Like other immigrant parents, Asian-Indian immigrants continue to emphasize specific values and goals for their second-generation children—values that were instilled in them during their own upbringing in India (e.g. pride in cultural heritage, familial interdependence). However, as a result of immigration and acculturation, Asian-Indians experience a sense of displacement when their perspectives and the parameters of their original environment no longer function within the new environment.[7] Living in a culturally incongruent community, first-generation parents perceive themselves as having sole responsibility for imparting cultural values to their children, which results in restrictive behaviors placed on children by their parents.[8] Within this context, actively reproducing traditional culture and establishing a cultural identity in their children become important parenting goals for these immigrants.[9] For first-generation immigrants, their culture, cultural values, and cultural identity are very true and real. However, for the second-generation immigrants, their parental culture is foreign to them. When the parental generation unconsciously or consciously demands that their children behave as they behave and adhere to parental cultural values, beliefs, and practices, this becomes intolerable for the second-generation immigrants. At the same time, when the second-generation children acquire certain values of the host culture and bring them home, the parental community finds this very offensive. This practice of living in the midst of opposing cultural values—Indian versus American—creates significant intergenerational stress, conflicts, and individual/family dysfunction among the members of multiple cultural generations living together in one home. The research detailed in this book is an investigation of the mental health needs of first- and second-generation Asian-Indian immigrants living under the same roof.

When Asian-Indians seek counseling/therapy for their culturally formed or conditioned issues, they need a method of care that is sensitive to their cultural milieu. My counseling experience with Asian-Indian families has revealed to me that, though there are several books that discuss the cultural and psychological needs of Asian-Indian immigrant families, there is almost no material that speaks to the counseling model needed for Asian-Indian immigrant families in the United States. The Asian-Indian immigrant community is very complex, consisting of two main groups: the parental generation (the dominant group whose personhood is formed in communal culture and collective identity) and the second-generation group (whose personhood is formed partly in the communal culture and collective identity of their parents' culture but also in the individualistic culture of the dominant American society). Both groups are influenced by the communal culture and collective identity. Therefore, even when therapy is offered to second- or third-generation Asian-Indian immigrants, the therapist should understand that these people's experiences cannot be isolated from their parental cultural experience. For this very reason, I claim that using Western theories exclusively, without translating them into the immigrant cultural world to fit the needs of immigrant families, will do more harm than good for the counselees.

INTERDISCIPLINARY APPROACH OF PASTORAL CARE AND PSYCHOTHERAPY

The pastoral care and psychotherapeutic model I propose here is a praxis–reflection–action model, which combines elements of the family systems theory of Murray Bowen, the formulation of the correlation method due to

Whitehead and Whitehead, and the liberative pastoral praxis of Emmanuel Lartey. For each of these three resources the starting point is human experience. I call my model a praxis–reflection–action model because it is based, primarily, on Lartey's definition of the term praxis: "to convey the sense of constant interactions between action and reflection."[10] Though the correlation method of Whitehead and Whitehead and Lartey's liberative pastoral praxis are pastoral theological methods, both approaches are premised on the counselee's experiences. Though family systems theory originates in the North American cultural context and the term "family" is understood in the Western context, there is ample room to apply this theory in the extended Indian family. "The family remains with us wherever we go... and unresolved emotional reactivity to our parents is the most important unfinished business of our lives."[11] One of the major focuses of pastoral care and counseling is the liberation of counselees from the experiences that bind or impede their experiencing of wholeness. In this regard, Lartey's method of identifying pastoral praxis as liberative is quite relevant.

Process theology has played an important role in the development of liberative theories and practices of pastoral care.[12] Process theology, which was developed primarily by Alfred North Whitehead in *Process and Reality*, asserts that God is involved in the lives of people trying to bring about a perfect society that is not yet realized but is in the process of becoming, because to have a perfect society was the original intent of God.[13] Pastoral care and counseling/psychotherapy has adopted process notions of becoming and the ongoing creative and redemptive activity of God in creation. A process approach to pastoral care and counseling/psychotherapy also calls for dialogue between experience and theological convictions. Process theology is compatible with a revised correlational theological method that calls for a dynamic relationship between theology and human experience. In a revised correlational approach, questions and answers come from both spheres.

In the following section, I briefly present Murray Bowen's family systems theory, which is used in the development of my praxis–reflection–action model. I then discuss the contributions of Whitehead and Whitehead and those of Lartey for the development of my model. Those approaches capture some of the issues that family systems theory does not address, particularly the role of other traditions. After presenting these three sources, I briefly examine some specific concepts from Winnicott's object relation theory and the narrative therapy approach of Clandinin and Connelly that are helpful in developing my model.

THE FAMILY AS A SYSTEM

Family systems theory is an important component of my model of pastoral counseling because it shifts the focus from the individual to the patterns of relationships and considers family as the network of relationships. The perspective of family systems theory is congenial to the family focus and communal identity of Asian-Indian immigrants. Family systems theory de-emphasizes the notion that our conflicts and anxieties are due primarily to the intrapsychic instinctive drives and our unconscious personalities. Rather, it suggests that our individual problems have more to do with our relational networks, the influence of the makeup of other's personalities, where we stand within the relational systems, and how we function within that position. It understands the symptom-bearer to be only the identified patient, rather than the cause of the problem. The problem is seen as symptomatic of something askew in the family itself.[14]

The concept of homeostasis is very helpful in looking at problems existing among the Indian immigrants in United States. Family systems theory is a useful lens through which the therapist may see his/her own life and the way in which that life interfaces with the life of the family or groups. In addition, upon seeing the layered landscape of family and community, the therapist may better understand his/her role as a facilitator of health and healing.

In family systems thinking, all parts of the systems are interdependent forces influencing one another. Each part of the system is connected to, or can have its own effect upon, every other part. Each component, therefore, rather than having its own identity or input, operates as a part of a larger whole. The components do not function according to their "nature" but according to their "position" in the network. According the family systems approach, it is the structure that becomes the unit of study.[15] To take one part out of the whole and analyze its nature will give misleading results, first, because each part will function differently outside the system and second, because even its functioning inside the system will be different depending on where it is placed in relation to the others.[16]

Human relationship systems are so inextricably connected that the functioning of any member can best be understood in terms of the presence of the others. Therefore, the "sick" part does not have to be removed or corrected if other components in the system can be made to function differently or their relationships with one another changed. The possibilities of change are maximized when we concentrate on modifying our own way of functioning and our own input into the family/system.

According to Bowen, the cause of an individual's problems can be understood only by viewing the role of the family as an emotional unit. The family system perspective holds that individuals are best understood through assessing the interactions within an entire family. Symptoms are often viewed as an expression of a dysfunction within a family; these dysfunctional patterns are thought to be passed on across several generations.[17] According to Corey, this approach is grounded in the assumption that a client's problematic behavior may (1) be a function or purpose for the family, (2) be a function of the family's inability to operate productively, especially during developmental transitions, or (3) be a symptom of dysfunctional patterns handed down across generations.[18]

Bowen's family systems approach holds that the client is connected to living systems and that change in one part of the unit reverberates throughout other parts. Therefore, a treatment approach is required that comprehensively addresses the other family members and the larger context, as well as an "identified" client. Because a family is an interactional unit, it has its own set of unique traits. It is not possible to assess an individual's concerns accurately without observing the interaction of other family members, as well as the broader context in which the person and the family live. To focus primarily on studying the internal dynamics of an individual without adequately considering interpersonal dynamics yields an incomplete picture.[19] Further, the family is viewed as a functioning unit and, therefore, the family provides a primary context for understanding how individuals function in relation to others and how they behave. Actions by any individual family member will influence all the others in the family, and their reactions will have reciprocal effect on the individual. Therefore, a therapist needs to view all behavior, including the symptoms expressed by the individual, within the context of family and society.[20] "By working with the whole family system or even community system, the therapist has a chance to observe how the individual acts within and serves the system's needs, how the system influences and is influenced by the individual and what intervention might lead to changes that help the couple, family, or larger system as well as the individual expressing pain."[21]

From the systemic perspective, an individual may carry a symptom for the entire family. Further, an individual's level of functioning is a manifestation of the way in which the family is functioning. According to Bowen, human relationships are driven by two counterbalancing life forces: individuality and togetherness. Each one needs companionship and a degree of independence.[22] Bowen identifies eight key concepts as being central to his theory: differentiation of the self, triangulation, the nuclear family emotional system, the family projection process, emotional cut off, the multigenerational transmission process, sibling position, and societal regression. Though Bowen identifies eight key concepts being central to his theory, I primarily employ his concept of differentiation in developing my model for pastoral counseling.

DIFFERENTIATION OF THE SELF

A central concept in Bowen's theory is differentiation of the self, which involves both the psychological separation of the intellect and emotion as well as independence of self from others. Therefore, it is both an intrapsychic and interpersonal concept. Differentiation of the self means the capacity of a family member to define his/her own life's goals and values apart from the surrounding togetherness and having the ability to say "I" when others are demanding one say "you" and "we." It includes the capacity to maintain a (relatively) non-anxious presence in the midst of anxious systems.

At the same time, this concept is entirely different from autonomy and narcissism. Differentiation means the capacity to be "I" while remaining connected. It is the maintaining of self-differentiation while remaining part of the family that optimizes the opportunities for fundamental change. Differentiation of the self is the capacity to think and reflect, not to respond automatically to emotional pressures, whether internal or external.[23] Differentiated individuals are able to choose between being guided by their feelings or by their thoughts. Undifferentiated people have difficulty in separating themselves from others and tend to fuse with dominant emotional patterns in the family. These people will have a low degree of autonomy, they react emotionally, and they are unable to take a clear position on issues. Similar to psychoanalytic theory, the process of individuation involves a differentiation whereby individuals acquire a sense of self-identity. This differentiation from the family of origin allows one to accept personal responsibility for one's thoughts, feelings, perceptions, and actions.[24]

When this concept of the differentiation of the self is compared with the communal cultural nature of interdependence in the Asian-Indian community, there is a possibility of misunderstanding interdependence as dependence. Interdependence is not absolute dependence—having no ability to think and act or being unable to be guided by one's own feelings and thoughts. Interdependence is the ability to mutually depend on each other. Therefore, interdependence cannot be equated with emotional dependence or "un-differentiation" of the self.

It has already been noted that Bowen's multigenerational family systems theory ascribes importance to the whole family and that it is a relevant tool in developing a psychotherapeutic or counseling model for addressing the intergenerational family issues of Asian-Indian immigrant families in the United States. The approach focuses on changing the individuals within the context of the system. It contends that problems that are manifest in one's current family will not significantly change until relationship patterns in one's family of origin are understood and directly challenged. Any action involves various steps and stages. "It is necessary to decide the course of action of all the circumstances involved. It is important to anticipate consequences and effects of the proposed action."[25] Action requires a planned strategy and program of action that have evaluative and reflective phases. To that end, I have chosen the action–reflection method of Whitehead and Whitehead.

WHITEHEAD AND WHITEHEAD: CORRELATION/ ACTION–REFLECTION METHOD

In developing my model of praxis–reflection–action for pastoral counseling or psychotherapy, I utilize the term developed by Whitehead and Whitehead and draw on their development of a method for ministerial reflection leading to ministerial action. Whitehead and Whitehead suggest that ministry should be practical. It should also be reflective. In other words, the ministry of pastoral care and psychotherapy should be a praxis–reflection–action model. According to Whitehead and Whitehead,

> Christian ministry today requires a method of reflection that is at once theological and practical. As theological, it must attend confidently and competently to the resources of Scripture and the historical tradition. As practical, it must be more than theoretically sound; it must be able to assist a wide range of ministers in their efforts to reflect and act in complex pastoral contexts. The method must be sufficiently clear and concrete that it can actually be used by persons and groups in the church. And it must be focused on action.[26]

This statement makes it clear that the authors intend a method of reflection for ministry. Though the term "Christian ministry" involves a lot more than pastoral care and psychotherapy, here I use it related to the ministry of pastoral care and counseling/psychotherapy. The Whiteheads are concerned with the practical applicability of theological reflection to the contemporary issues that arise from people's experiences. The method of reflection presented is a correlational method that is conversational in nature. It respects the value of whatever comes from various sources without privileging one over the other.

In its actual sense, the authors are presenting a model and a method of doing theological reflection in ministry which is very practical. Pastoral care, psychotherapy and counseling, like theological reflection, should not end in mere theoretical formulation. It should lead to practical application or action that brings transformation in thought processes and patterns. With regards to this model, the Whiteheads have identified the Christian tradition, personal experience, and culture as the sources of information that are relevant to decision-making in contemporary ministry. The authors make it clear that "faithful and effective pastoral activity depends on the ability of Christians and, in a special way, Christian ministers, to recognize and use the religiously significant insights available in these three sources."[27] With regards to this method, they suggest a "three-step process, which includes attending, assertion, and pastoral response, through which this information is clarified, coordinated, and allowed to shape pastoral action."[28]

As previously mentioned, the model they discuss is one that is conversational in nature, as is pastoral care and counseling. According to the Whiteheads, "theological reflection in ministry instigates a conversation among three sources of religiously relevant information: the experience of the community of faith, the Christian tradition, and the resources of culture."[29] The practices of pastoral care and counseling instigate a very similar conversation. The tradition brings to the conversation how God has been active in the history of the community. Since it is the truth of that particular community, it also allows other truths to be present. It recognizes and accommodates the plurality of interpretations and, hence, tolerates diversity.[30] The authors also emphasize befriending the tradition in such a way that one develops a familiarity that includes both an appreciative awareness of tradition and a comfort with its diversity and contradictions.[31]

The praxis–reflection–action (PRA) method starts in experience because it is ignited by a pastoral challenge. According to the Whiteheads, the key ingredient in this experience is the existence of self-awareness. This awareness encourages an engagement with tradition that is conversational in nature. The community is reminded of its religious past but advised that it is not supposed to cling to what has been received; instead the community must have the courage to penetrate this ongoing experience anew and have the ability to apply its new awareness in contemporary life.

Culture deals with the attitudes, values, and biases that constitute the social milieu in which we live.[32] Pastoral caregivers need to carefully attend to the presence of cultural influences because, though often invisible, they are pervasive, very powerful, and influential. Culture speaks in many voices and pastoral caregivers need to be able to recognize those cultural voices. Culture does not merely entail the given or the past. It also influences the present, current life context of the community.

What makes the PRA model so dynamic is its inclusion of and reflection on tradition, personal/community experience, and resources of culture as important elements in pastoral decision-making. Therapists who employ the PRA model and engage in the therapeutic relationship with second-generation Asian-Indians in particular are aware that the roots of their Indian ethnicity, the routes of their migration, shoots of their American education, and fruits of their destiny are all closely tied together. It is easy to deny or ignore some of the factors that constitute an irrefutable part of them. When therapists turn a blind eye to some of these multiple aspects, something within them dies and for the rest, life seems incomplete. Therapists who deal with this community using this model also include the framework of ADDRESSING (Age and generational influences, Developmental and acquired Disabilities, Religion and spiritual orientation, Ethnicity, Socio-economic status, Sexual orientation, Indigenous heritage, National origin and Gender).[33] Though Whitehead and Whitehead emphasize only the Christian tradition, it is my contention that any experience evolved from any tradition should be in conversation with culture and reflection. The reflection model offers a way to structure our conversation, paying attention to three sources of information—cultural setting, religious heritage, and experience.[34] This method of reflection suggests a process of pursuing communal discernment by moving from listening/attending, to assertion, and, finally, to practical pastoral response.

By attending, we seek out, or gather, information on a particular pastoral concern that is available in personal experience, tradition, and cultural resources. It is a process of collecting facts. One of the major conscious choices of the pastoral caregiver is, at this point, to suspend premature judgment. An active and empathic listening to the meaning, feeling, and content of the story, not only the dominant/elite group but also of the whole community, is required in this part. It also entails an honest exploration of the information available from the sources of tradition, experience, and culture.

During the assertion stage, we bring to bear the contribution of these sources in an assertive relationship of challenge and confirmation. This is based on the assumption that God is revealed in all three sources and that the religious/spiritual information available in each source is partial.[35] What is very important is that in this reflection model is the conviction that "our faithful efforts to both recover and overcome our religious past are facilitated by placing the tradition's insights on a pastoral concern in assertive dialogue with the community's experience and with cultural information."[36] This statement highlights the need of mutual respect for the insights drawn from a community's experience/cultural information and the interpretations of those insights born from all the sources previously discussed. The Whiteheads use two metaphors: conversation and crucible,[37] which are very important at the stage of assertion.

In conversation, the different voices that we have heard in the attending stage are now allowed to speak to one another. In the crucible, diverse information is poured into a single container, where insights and convictions are allowed to interact with one another.[38] Assertiveness, while acknowledging one's own needs and convictions, also respects the needs and convictions of others. This reflection model provides tremendous space for embracing diversity.

Pastoral response is the third and final stage of this method. Here, insight gained is translated into action. This stage is initiated by focusing on the best insights gained in the assertion stage. The goal of reflection is to reach a pastoral decision on pastoral challenges arising from the context of the community. It is against this context that the authors argue that theological reflection in ministry fails when pastoral decisions ignore the communities in which they will be implemented. Thus, consensus building, which is the ability to move from honored diversity to shared action, becomes an important skill of pastoral reflection.[39]

The PRA model is applicable to the practice of pastoral psychotherapy and counseling with people living in a multicultural context. Though this model may be criticized for valuing scripture as more important, in my understanding, tradition, culture, and experience are presented as conversational partners with equal voice and status. Further, the method of reading and interpretation of the scripture I envisage in the PRA model is not a traditional, conservative and colonial one, rather a re-reading and reinterpretation of the scripture.

Whitehead and Whitehead emphasize the mutuality of the community. They have placed theological reflection at the center of the community in which all voices should be heard, and where the art of listening is required. This makes this model relevant to the Asian-Indian's worldview in which everything is placed at the center of the community. This model also allows the engagement of the cultural context, thereby broadening the horizon of the different texts at play. As mentioned earlier in this chapter, I will extend Whitehead and Whitehead's method beyond the Christian context on which they focus and consciously include the Asian-Indian tradition, which also includes other religious traditions. I do this in order to meet my people in their true context.

According to Whitehead and Whitehead, the assertive interaction of tradition, experience, and culture generates insight.[40] This claim is based on the assumption that God is revealed in all three sources (tradition, experience, and culture), and that the religious/spiritual information available in each source is partial. This stage further leads to a pastoral response in which insight gained is translated into action.[41] The reflection itself is to reach a pastoral decision on pastoral challenges arising from the context of the community.

LIBERATION AS PASTORAL PRAXIS

The third resource I utilize in the development of my PRA model of pastoral counseling and psychotherapy is Emmanuel Lartey's concept of liberation as pastoral praxis. Lartey emphasizes the cultural diversity that is inherent in the Asia-Indian families living in the United States, other Western cultural worlds as well as in India. He makes it clear that using an intercultural approach captures complexities so as to avoid the dominant culture defining "normality" for others.[42]

Understanding the Asian-Indians who come to the United States from various religious, cultural, and language backgrounds is a complex task. When such families expand into multiple cultural generations in the United States, they become even more complex, making it difficult to understand the differences that may be inherent, even within the same family. Here, Lartey argues for the term intercultural in preference to cross-cultural or transcultural because it attempts to capture the complex nature of the interaction between people who have been influenced by different cultures, social contexts and origins, and who themselves are often enigmatic composites of various strands of ethnicity, race, geography, culture, and socio-economic setting.[43]

Lartey further explains that the way an intercultural approach seeks to counter such developments and to enhance interaction is by giving many voices from different backgrounds a chance to express their views on the subject under review in their own terms. It does not then rush to analyze or systematize them into overarching theories that can explain and fit everything neatly into place. Instead, the intercultural approach ponders the glorious variety and chaotic mystery of human experience for clues to a more adequate response to the exigencies of human life.[44]

Lartey also explains that liberation theology makes its priority the experience of the oppressed, the poor, or marginalized. Theology comes second because "the theologian begins from a position of being immersed in the experiences of poverty, marginalization and oppression."[45] It is quite true that the starting point of any serious pastoral theological method should be grounded in people's experiences. The very act of the incarnation of Jesus Christ shows that God is quite serious identifying with and experiencing the human condition as people seeking liberation. Further, Lartey makes it clear that liberation theology can help in bringing about change if it considers the psychological bondage of the people, as well as bringing about a new hermeneutic that privileges the stories of the people and their experiences and interpretation of biblical stories according to their stories. He advocates for a strong and mutual interconnectedness of the hermeneutical task in relation to pastoral concerns for healing and growth.[46]

While Lartey discusses the pedagogical cycle for liberative pastoral praxis and the cycle of social therapy, he identifies five phases that he has "adopted in facilitating learning within a group of people from different countries and cultures, of different ages, men and women, lay and ordained, of different Christian backgrounds, as well as other traditions, with varying degrees of commitment to and challenges of their various heritages who all want to learn how to be reflective practitioners of pastoral care in one form or another."[47] He states that the normal starting point is with concrete experience. The learning practitioners are in a placement where they are involved with people who bring their real life experiences. This is important in order to ground the theoretical discussion in the lived experience of living people rather than in some generalized facts and figures.[48]

The second phase, situational analysis, "is an attempt to combine the social analytical mediation of Latin American liberation theology with the religiocultural analysis of African and Asian liberation theology."[49] The psychosocial analysis, or "social perspective taking," that pastoral caregivers and counselors use is also discussed here. At this stage, the emphasis is on bringing into play an analysis that is multiperspectival by using only selected perspectives from different disciplines to help give a clear understanding of the situation and avoiding the rigors of an interdisciplinary approach. Experts from other disciplines are also invited to comment on the situation in an effort to foster collective seeing.

In the third phase, faith perspectives are brought in to question, both the concrete experience and situational analysis. At this point, according to Lartey, the following questions should be raised: (1) What questions arise from my faith concerning what I have experienced and the analysis of it? And (2) How have thinkers in my faith tradition approached the issues raised?[50] This is the stage where all participants need to look into their faith tradition for some recorded views to which to relate their ideas.

The fourth stage is a critical analysis of the traditions of faith. The question in this phase is "How adequate is my tradition's formulation in responding to the concrete experience encountered?"[51] In the fifth stage the group explores the response options that are available in the light of the whole cycle. They then return to test this in their practice with the real experiences of the persons in context.

Lartey's intercultural stage approach is very relevant and applicable in developing a counseling model for the Asian-Indian immigrant families living in the multiple cultural spaces of the United States. However, I am concerned about his emphasis on written sources at the third stage when dealing with people from traditionally oral cultures. At that stage, Lartey strongly suggests that written sources are necessary in order to relate one's own ideas to other recorded views on the subject. In my perception, we may be creating other issues when we value, primarily, the written records. I feel this is particularly true for Asian-Indians because, in the Asian-Indian cultural context, most cultural beliefs, practices, and values are handed down from generation to generation not in written form, but in oral form and through practice. Therefore, when we deal with immigrant families, it is sometimes difficult to find recorded views on the subject, or in some cases, even if we find them, the recorded views on the subject may have been generalized so much that they do not speak to the specifics or particularity of the current problem. In some cases, recorded views are influenced greatly by Euro-Western views that may have overlooked a persons' cultural–religious heritage. Further, sometimes written words blur the meaning or miss it due to the unavailability of transportable or corresponding meanings between languages and cultures.

ADDITIONAL CONTRIBUTORS TO THE PRA MODEL OF PASTORAL COUNSELING

In addition to the three main sources previously discussed, there are the two other Western theories, which I found helpful to translate and apply to the PRA model of psychotherapy and counseling . In each case, I draw specific concepts from these two larger theories because they benefit the development of my model. I draw on D.W. Winnicott's object relation theory, which strongly emphasizes that life happens in "potential space" between inner psychic reality and external reality, and on a narrative therapy approach, specifically the "three-dimensional narrative inquiry space" of Clandinin and Connelly, which focuses on temporality—personal, social, and place.[52]

Winnicott contends that when we speak of persons we speak of them along with the summation of their cultural experience. In his book, though Winnicott focuses his studies specifically on children, I believe his findings on the impact of culture are applicable to all ages. He finds that life is really experienced not in intra-psychic dynamics but in "potential space," somewhere between inner psychic reality and external reality.[53] Winnicott developed this concept by focusing on the developmental stage of the baby where separation–individuation is taking place and a basis is formed upon which the child experiences life.[54] Though his concept of empathy is a prerequisite for developing a healthy self, autonomy[55] is not an applicable concept when dealing with Asian-Indians as their characterization of a healthy self is not independence but interdependence. Winnicott's argument that "those who care for children of all ages must be ready to put each in touch with appropriate elements of the cultural heritage and then look into potential space"[56] is highly relevant in the therapeutic context of the Asian-Indian immigrants. Further, it is that very aspect of potential space which I am proposing is the key to helping the Asian-Indian immigrants in the United States.

The narrative approach of Clandinin and Connelly argues that experience happens narratively and, hence, it should be understood from a narrative perspective. This information is helpful in providing a road map narratively engaging with Asian-Indians in the United States and in similar cultural environments as they deal with cultural clashes that occur as they transition into a new cultural environment. The three-dimensional narrative inquiry space of Clandinin and Connelly that focuses on temporality, personal, and social place is most relevant in development of my model. This is one theory that acknowledges the importance of context and continuity. It allows that the past and the future are present in the present.[57] It also highlights the importance of making sure the voices of research "texts" are allowed to speak for themselves and not drowned out by the voice of the researcher.

According to the narrative counseling approach, "life is complicated, so we find ways to explain it." These explanations, the stories we tell ourselves, organize our experience and shape our behavior. The stories we tell ourselves are powerful because they determine what we notice and remember, and, therefore how we face the future. The narrative approach focuses on expanding clients' thinking so as to allow them to consider alternative ways of looking at themselves and their problems. For Nichols, "stories do not mirror life, they shape it."[58] Instead of having a problem or facing a problem narrative, therapists encourage clients to think of themselves as struggling against their problems. Neither the client nor the family is the problem. The problem is the problem, because narrative therapists externalize the problem. Narrative therapy is not interested in the family's impact on the problem but rather the problem's impact on the family.

THE PRAXIS–REFLECTION–ACTION (PRA) MODEL

Based on the resources previously discussed, the next step is to develop my five-stage PRA model where actual care, psychotherapy and counseling can be made possible. These are both distinct and interconnected to reflection stages.

Praxis Stage

Praxis is the process by which a theory, lesson, or skill is enacted, practiced, embodied, or realized. Praxis may also refer to the act of engaging, applying, exercising, realizing, or practicing ideas. The end goal of knowledge gained through praxis is action. Praxis as the manner in which we are engaged with people's experience/stories has its own insight or understanding prior to any explicit formulation of that understanding. According to Lartey, "the term praxis is used to convey the sense of constant interaction between action and reflection."[59] Therefore, this is the first stage where the practitioner of pastoral counseling and psychotherapy plunges himself/herself into the crisis situation in order to fully understand the presenting problem for individuals, couples, families, extended families, and small groups that seek some resolution to their problem. A pastoral caregiver at this stage listens to the meaning, feeling, and content of the person's/group's story and values their experience and culture to help them cope with the problem and facilitate healing.

Analytic Reflection Stage

This is the second stage, the point at which the practitioner of pastoral care draws on the multiperspectival approach from a variety of behavioral and social sciences for the purpose of assessing the human dynamics at work in the crisis situation. To achieve a thorough assessment, intrapsychic, interpersonal, psychological approaches, developmental theories, family systems theories, intercultural and cross-cultural theories and contextual and indigenous theories are applied.

Spiritual Assessment Stage

In this third stage, the pastoral care practitioner examines the beliefs and convictions that operate in the persons and families caught up in the crisis situation. This step informs the therapist as to how his/her client spiritually and theologically understands their problems and how they view their problems from the perspective of spirituality and faith system. In all crisis situations, there are some kinds of spiritual, religious, and theological convictions at work. Be they explicit or implicit doctrine, the convictions and beliefs need to be identified.

In a recent study conducted by faculty from the department of psychiatry at McLean Hospital, Harvard Medical School concludes that, "belief in God, but not religious affiliation, was associated with better treatment outcomes. With respect to depression, this relationship was mediated by belief in the credibility of treatment and expectations for treatment gains."[60] Therefore, it is important to determine the spiritual/theological elements that promote meaning and hope for clients, even in the midst of crises.

Dialogical Stage

This is the fourth stage of the PRA model. In this stage, the behavioral and social sciences disciplines from the second stage enter into dialogue with the spiritual convictions and beliefs identified in stage three. The purpose of the dialogical stage is to recognize how the behavioral and social sciences multilevel assessments can provide a holistic assessment of the problem. This holistic assessment leads to identifiable findings concerning the nature of the problem that can be used in the final stage of the model, the intervention or action stage. The key for the dialogical stage is to recognize and draw on the similarities between the disciplines using the principle of similarity in structure. Thus, the therapist draws on the reflection approach and invites dialogue between the different disciplines. However, therapists should be aware that similarity does not mean the disciplines are identical, rather that they are only philosophically similar, as all life is interrelated.

Action/Strategic Intervention Stage

This stage begins when the assessment and dialogue phases end, where there is an articulated summary statement of the presenting problem and an understanding of the behavioral and social sciences/theological dynamics that are at work. Based on the expanded understanding of the existing issue, the counselee returns to act towards his/her healing and growth. The key for this stage is applying the various elements of pastoral care—healing, sustaining, guiding, reconciling and empowering. Ultimately, this leads (or should lead) to the healing and growth of all.

THE SIGNIFICANCE OF THE MODEL

First let me say that I do not claim my PRA model to be *the* model of counseling and psychotherapy for the Asian-Indian immigrant individuals and families living in the United States or in similar cultural environments. It is only an attempt at a model that points to the possibility of a holistic approach that can bring health, healing, and wholeness to Asian-Indian immigrant families living in the multiple cultural spaces of the United States and in similar cultural environments.

Though there is extensive literature that discusses Asian-Indian immigrant issues and cultural conflicts, so far there is little or no research, literature, or a clinical tool that deal with a psychotherapeutic or counseling model for the Asian-Indian immigrants dealing with intergenerational conflicts and declension of family. Therefore, this model hopes to provide a resource for counseling Asian-Indian immigrant persons and families facing cultural value conflicts, intergenerational conflicts, lack of individual and family functionality, and the declension of family, not only in the United States, but any Western culture similar to that of the United States.

This research is a contribution to the field of intercultural pastoral care and counseling for individuals and families from communal-oriented cultures. It also challenges the boundaries of individual-centered therapy to a certain extent. It is interdisciplinary and intercultural in nature, a combination of resources from Western, Asian, and African psychoanalysts and theologians. While the concepts of self psychology, narrative approach, object relation theory, family systems approach, and correlation method are derived in the Western cultural context, the marginality theology of Lee and Kakar's development of the self in the Indian context are Asian and Asian-Indian. Further, liberative pastoral praxis is the resource of an African pastoral theologian, Lartey.

Another significance of this model is its awareness of uninformed application of the dominant culture's monocultural concepts, which may lead to misdiagnosis and non-therapeutic treatment when it does not seriously consider the cultural components of the counselee from another cultural context, especially people from non-Western cultures. Therefore, the PRA model developed in this book is an interdisciplinary, intercultural, and holistic approach that is meant primarily for those seeking professional counseling and psychotherapy from the family-oriented cultural community perspective and whose self is a communal self.

Finally, since Asian-Indian immigrant families consist of first- and second-generation immigrants whose cultural identities and values are different, I have combined Western writers, Indian thinkers, and Asian and African theologians adequately to make the proposed pastoral care and counseling model relevant to those whose identities are developed in the Asian-Indian culture, and whose identities are also formed and developed in the mainstream, white American culture.

For the purpose of this book, I present these stages in a linear form, though in the delivery of pastoral care, psychotherapy and counseling, the use of stages may not necessarily be chronological and linear. Rather, they can be cyclical and/or spiral as life for Asian-Indians is understood to be intricately intertwined.

NOTES

1. S. Jambunathan and K. P. Counselman, "Parenting Attitudes of Asian Indian Mothers Living in the United States and in India," *Early Child Development and Care* 172, no. 6 (2002): 659.

2. N. Tiwari, A. G. Inman, and D. S. Sandhu, "South Asian Americans: Culture, Concerns and Therapeutic Concerns," in *Culturally Diverse Mental Health: The Challenges of Research and Resistance*, eds. J. Mio and G. Iwamasa (New York: Brunner-Routledge, 2003), 191–209.

3. S Jambunathan, D. C. Burts, and S. Pierce, "Comparisons of Parenting Attitudes among Five Ethnic Groups in the United States," *Journal of Comparative Family Studies* 31, no. 4 (2000): 398.

4. S. Parthanikanti, "East Indian American Families," in *Working with Asian Americans: A Guide for Clinicians*, ed. E. Lee (New York: Guilford Press, 1997), 84.

5. V. Dhruvarajan, "Ethnic Cultural Retention and Transmission among First-generation Hindu Asian Indians in a Canadian City," *Journal of Comparative Family Studies* 24, no. 1 (Spring, 1993): 65.

6. Terry Arendell, *Contemporary Parenting: Challenges and Issue* (Thousand Oaks, CA: Sage, 1997), 16.

7. R. Hedge, "Translated Enactments: The Relational Configuration of Asian Indian Immigrant Experiences," in *Readings in Cultural Contexts*, eds. J. Martin, T. Nakayama, and L. Flores (Mountain View, CA: Mayfields, 1998), 318.

8. G. R. Sodowsky and J.C. Carey, "Relationship between Acculturation Related Demographics and Cultural Attitudes of an Asian Indian Immigrant Group," *Journal of Multicultural Counseling and Development* 16, no. 3 (July, 1998): 121.

9. Dhruvarajan, "Ethnic Cultural Retention and Transmission among First-Generation Hindu Asian Indians in a Canadian City," 65.

10. Emmanuel Y. Lartey, *In Living Color: An Intercultural Approach to Pastoral Care and Counseling* (London: Jessica Kingsley, 2003), 122.

11. Michael P. Nichols, *Family Therapy: Concepts and Methods* (Boston, MA: Pearson, 2006), 115.

12. See Jackson, Gordon E. *Pastoral Care and Process Theology* (Washington, DC: University Press of America, 1981).

13. Alfred North Whitehead, *Process and Reality* (New York: Free Press, 1978), 342–351.

14. Gerald Corey, *Theory and Practice of Counseling and Psychotherapy*, 5th ed. (Pacific Grove, CA: Brooks/Cole Publishing Company, 1996), 367.

15. Ibid., 368.

16. Ibid., 368.

17. Nichols, *Family Therapy*, 115.

18. Corey, *Theory and Practice of Counseling and Psychotherapy*, 367.

19. Ibid., 368–369.

20. Ibid., 375–376.

21. Ibid., 367.

22. Nichols, *Family Therapy*, 117.
23. M. E. Kerr and M. Bowen, *Family Evaluation* (New York: Norton, 1988), 72.
24. Corey, *Theory and Practice of Counseling and Psychotherapy*, 374.
25. Lartey, *In Living Color*, 122.
26. James D. Whitehead and Evelyn Eaton Whitehead, *Method in Ministry: Theological Reflection and Christian Ministry*, rev. ed. (Lanham, MD: Sheed & Ward, 1999), x.
27. Ibid., ix.
28. Ibid.
29. Ibid., 6.
30. Ibid., 7–8.
31. Ibid., 9.
32. Ibid., 11.
33. M.G. Constantine and D. W. Sue (ed.), *Strategies for Building Multicultural Competence in Mental Health and Educational Setting* (New York: John Wiley & Sons Inc. 2005) 22.
34. James D. Whitehead and Evelyn Eaton Whitehead, *Method in Ministry*, 13.
35. Ibid., 15.
36. Ibid.
37. Ibid.
38. Ibid.
39. Ibid., 17.
40. Whitehead and Whitehead, *Method in Ministry*, 27.
41. Ibid., 23.
42. Lartey, *In Living Color*, 32.
43. Ibid., 12.
44. Ibid., 32.
45. Ibid., 115.
46. Ibid., 128–130.
47. Ibid., 130.
48. Ibid., 131.
49. Ibid., 132.
50. Ibid., 133.
51. Ibid.
52. Jean Clandinin and Michael Connelly, *Narrative Inquiry: Experience and Story in Qualitative Research*, (San Francisco, CA: Jossey-Bass, 2000), 50.
53. Donald W. Winnicott, *Playing and Reality* (New York: Routledge, 2005), 133.
54. Ibid.
55. Ibid., 146.
56. Ibid., 148.

57. Clandinin and Connelly, *Narrative Inquiry,* 50.
58. Nichols, *Family Therapy,* 337–38.
59. Lartey, *In Living Color,* 122.
60. David H. Rosmarin, et al., "A Test of Faith in God and Treatment: The Relationship of Belief in God to Psychiatric Treatment Outcomes," *Journal of Affective Disorders* 146, no. 3 (April, 2012): 445.

CHAPTER 9

Application of Praxis-Reflection-Action Model of Pastoral Counseling

In this chapter, I present two case studies through the lens of the PRA model to demonstrate its applicability to the care of Asian-Indian immigrants experiencing family conflict arising from intergenerational and intercultural conflict.[1]

CASE STUDY 1 DEVIN:[2] DEALING WITH INTERGENERATIONAL AND CULTURAL CONFLICT

Praxis Stage

In this stage, the goal is to collect as much information as possible from the individual and/or family concerning their care needs. The major tools used in this stage are active listening to the feeling, meaning, and content of the presenting problem and its source, and empathic understanding to the person. Further, considerable attention is paid to the counselees as they narrate their stories so that the therapist knows how the counselees understand their problem and their lived experience.

Devin is a 22- year-old-second-generation Asian-Indian, single, currently enrolled in undergraduate school, majoring in computer science. Though Devin did not have much respect for Asian-Indians in general, some of his best friends who know me from church introduced me as a "different Asian-Indian who can understand others" and encouraged him to consult with me. Thus, Devin gave me a call and made an appointment to see me, but changed his mind and canceled the appointment the next day. Later he called again, made an appointment, and came to see me. I believe he came to me with the expectation that I would be able to understand him based on his friends' remarks about me.

Devin presented himself in the counseling/therapy room with a little reluctance, but eventually relaxed and kept a smile on his face. However, as I began to actively listen to the meaning, feeling, and content of his story, I recognized that Devin's smile and his deeper emotions did not match. His smile masked his resentment and anger towards his father and, to a great extent, towards himself.

Devin's primary reason for seeking counseling was to find direction for his life. He did not really know what he wanted to do upon graduation. He also wanted guidance for handling relational problems. According to Devin, he often "felt helpless, lonely, and depressed." In his school, most of the students were Caucasians and African Americans, with a minority of Asian-Indian students recently arrived from India, who usually spoke their vernacular and socialized among themselves. Though they welcomed Devin in their group and he tried to interact with them, Devin often felt that he could not get as close to them as he was with his American friends. Not only did Devin find it difficult to speak the vernacular his Asian-Indian friends spoke, he also realized that they spoke a different kind of English from him, with a different accent. In addition to the language barrier, Devin also felt a cultural difference. Though Devin was warmly welcomed in their small world, he felt he was merely a guest at their gatherings.

Devin associated more closely with his Western friends because he could speak the same language with the same accent. Yet though Devin stated that he had good relationships with his Western friends, he also often felt that he did not have a close friend among them. Devin spent a lot of time with his Western friends, claiming they were easy going and people it was not that difficult to get along with. With a sense of pride, he told me that he had no issues or confrontations with his friends. Even though Devin enjoyed being around his friends, at times he felt a void within himself, which he found difficult to articulate. He simply knew that he felt lonely even when he was in the midst of his friends.

I invited Devin to explain further the stories and experiences, which led him to those feelings. After a long pause and several attempts, Devin blurted out, "I don't know who I really am. I don't like myself when I am around people. I don't know what is wrong with me." I realized that these questions of self and self-identity had haunted Devin for a long time. Devin described to me a couple of situations in which his Western friends encouraged him to stand up for himself as a man with a 'backbone.' Such situations really embarrassed and startled Devin. Though he rationally accepted their encouragement, realizing that they had a genuine concern for him, emotionally he felt that he was weak and unstable. Following that experience, Devin began to often question himself and worried about how he was perceived by others and who he really was. He began to ask some fundamental questions that disrupted his inner image of himself.

Our therapeutic relationship was growing and during several sessions we kept talking about Devin's relationship with his friends. Devin had a circle of friends with whom he socialized. In one of our sessions he admitted that he felt more comfortable when he spent time with his female friends. When I asked him to describe the nature of his relationship with his friends, Devin said "Definitely I am not a leader but only a follower." Devin says he is cool, easy-going, with no enemies and with no close pal. With a long sigh Devin said, "I wish I had a close friend, whether male or female." I sensed his longing for an intimate relationship with someone who would understand and accept him for who he is. In that session, he finally made a cry for help, "When I don't know who I am, how can others understand me?"

Devin's Childhood

Devin's father, Daniel, went to Kuwait when he was 25 years old. There, he started working as a software engineer and remained in that position for about three years. While he was in Kuwait, he got a chance to come to the United States on a work visa. After securing a job in the United States, Daniel went back to India to visit his family. At that time, his family proposed his marriage to Daisy. She had earned her bachelor of nursing degree and was working as a registered nurse in one of the high-tech hospitals in India. After their wedding and a 45-day vacation, when Daniel was about to leave India to return to the United States, he learned that Daisy was pregnant. Daniel left Daisy in India with her parents and returned to the United States. After a year and a half, Daisy received the necessary legal clearance to come to the United States. However, Devin could not go with his mother, but was left behind with his maternal grandparents. He only remembers the love and care his grandparents gave him.

Devin was brought to the United States when he was two years old. After coming to the United States, Devin remembers both his parents going to work in the morning and leaving him in a small apartment with a nanny who spent her time watching television and not caring properly for him. As he was growing up, he learned to operate the television and change channels, spending most of his time alone before and after school, even though there was a caregiver at home in the absence of his parents. He had a lot of toys to play with, but even when the parents returned home from work, he was not given adequate care and attention due to his parents' stress and tiredness. Though Devin's father did take him to different places, he does not remember much about interaction with him. He remembers his father always sitting at a computer when he was at home.

Devin remembers that after some time, there were constant argument and fights between his parents. Meanwhile, his paternal grandparents, with whom Devin had no emotional connection, were brought to the United States on a tourist visa. While his parents were sleeping in two different bedrooms, Devin was forced to sleep with his grandparents. Devin remembers that at that time he was not emotionally connected with anyone in the family. Even when everyone was at home, Devin was in his own world of video games, toys, and television.

Devin's Family Relationship

Devin claims that he was closer to his nanny and maternal grandparents than to his parents. His memory of his father is that he was authoritarian, demanding, and always expecting much from him. His father forced him to do everything, using encouragement or discouragement. In other words, Devin's father either said "do this," or "do not do this."

Devin was always expected to maintain good grades in his studies, behave like a model child, not to bring shame upon the family, and to save his family's face in the community. According to Devin, his father was a man who could never be satisfied. He recollected and described several occasions when his father became very angry and burst out about something Devin did or did not do. His father scolded him whenever he did not meet his father's expectations, either in school or at home. Whenever Devin tried to clarify or defend his stance, he was scolded even more for talking back and being disrespectful to his parents. In such situations, Devin would go to his nanny who, he thought, understood him better than did his parents.

Devin's paternal grandparents returned to India following the expiration of their visas. At the same time, Devin's nanny stopped coming to the family's home for a while. Devin felt that he was completely alone and a sense of abandonment began to envelop him all the time. After a few weeks, another nanny was hired for Devin.

In the midst of these transitions, Devin began school. He did not much like school. In his first-grade class, he remembers that no one would be friends with him and that he played alone. He began to realize that he looked different from the other students. Though some students were friendly, most of them were mean. He remembers that he was called ugly names by some of his mean classmates.

As years went by, Devin was able to make more friends, and in middle school he adapted well and had several friends. One of his major concerns was observing his friends in order to understand their behavior so he could imitate them and fit into their group. Devin did not want to draw any attention to himself that would highlight his difference. Academically, he performed well, but was always insecure because he felt his performance was not good enough. Nonetheless, he always tried to secure good grades to gain his father's acceptance.

By high school, Devin had more friends. He socialized more and put more effort in to fitting in with his circle of friends, trying very hard to behave as they did. At the same time his relationship with his father hit rock-bottom. His father, who did not like Devin's friends, began yelling at him. In those situations, Devin told himself, "I don't have to listen to you and you cannot control me." He wanted nothing to do with his father. Out of rebellion, he continued to stay out with his friends most of the time, which fueled his father's anger. During the counseling session, Devin said, "Maybe that might be the only way of controlling my life and showing my father that he cannot control me."

Devin was accepted to a good college. He lived at home and commuted to campus. During his college years, there was intense tension between Devin and his father. The conflicts stemmed mostly from Devin's low grades and his staying out late. After every argument with his father, Devin would leave the house and return home very late in order to avoid confrontation with his father. Even in those circumstances, Devin tried to listen to his father's advice and respect him, leading Devin to expect his father to respect him and not yell at him when he decided to do something other than whatever his father suggested. Devin compared his father to those of his Western friends, whose parents seemed to respect and support their children's choices. Though Devin tried to listen to his father and always obey his wishes, he felt he was never good enough. He tried his best to make his father proud, but felt he could never live up to expectations, even when he completely complied with his father's decisions. Devin resented his father and was angry with himself for not being able stand up to his father and make his own decisions.

Even now Devin has a split relationship with his father. His mother is completely detached from everyone, though she lives in the same house. When she is working, she leaves home early. When she is at home she is on the telephone talking with someone. Whenever Devin approached his mother wanting to share his struggle with her, she would scold him and avoid him saying, "You and your father are friends, go and settle it with him. I don't want to know about it." While Devin desired his father's acceptance and approval, he also expected his father to respect his choices and decisions. Even in counseling sessions, it was evident that Devin was striving to receive his father's acceptance while at the same time carrying great resentment toward him.

Daisy, Devin's mother, is in her early 50s and still works as a registered nurse. She now realizes that she experienced culture shock when she left her village in India and was thrust into the American culture. She was raised and educated in the same village where she was born. Daisy grew up in a family with meager financial resources. Thus, as a child, she did not have many luxuries. The first time she travelled outside her village was for work. Before completing her probationary period as a nurse, her marriage was proposed and conducted. After her wedding, Daisy did not work.

According to Daisy, soon after she arrived in America, her husband forced her to wear clothes, which she was not used to wearing, and to attend parties where men and women drank and danced. She was told her English was not good and was always reminded that she needed to improve her English. Devin also corrected Daisy's English. Her husband's constant criticism gradually developed into defensive argument, causing Daisy to develop a sense of low self-esteem. Daniel's criticism also contributed to her feelings of inferiority. She contends she was criticized for anything and everything she did. Thus, she began to withdraw from Daniel and the entire family. Moreover, her in-laws supported Daniel and blamed Daisy for all the family's problems. She was expected to be modern and act like others. This forced her to distance and disengage from everybody at home, because this was more pressure than she could bear. Her thinking was that God gave her a chance to come to the United States and that the privilege of being here was not for self-boasting, partying, and celebrations.

Devin's father subtly forced his wife and children to do things to improve their life in the United States. He said, "When everyone is looking at us, we should maintain our dignity and prestige in the society. We cannot act here like those who are living in the village." In a sense, it is true. Asian-Indians are a close-knit community and teach their children to watch their actions because others are always watching them. This was the cultural value Daniel expected his wife and children to observe. Daniel wanted his children to be smart, his wife to be modern, speak good English, and maintain a desirable social image in the community. Though his intention was good, there was no empathy in his action towards his wife and children.

In the midst of all this, Debie, Devin's younger sister, acted with complete indifference and flat affect, spending her time reading and writing without joining anyone in any activity. During the family counseling session, she cried loudly, covering her face with her palms. She did not like to hear or share the "dirty things" going on in her family. She said, "I don't want to live with them in the house, but I live there because I don't want to bring shame on them."

THE ANALYTIC REFLECTION STAGE

At this stage, the tools of behavioral and social sciences are employed to assess and analyze the experience from the previous stage. Theories from family systems, cultural and contextual thinking, Kohut's self psychology, and other theoretical concepts that help understand human dynamics at work are applied to gain insights and assess the situation for an integrated understanding.

Most of the time, Devin was quiet and gentle, considerate, selfless, and always yielding to others. Though his appearance did not indicate it, Devin was restless, with low self-esteem. Further, he was angry with himself. He felt that he was unable to stand up for himself and that he could not speak out and articulate what he wanted in any given situation. When Devin went out with his friends to eat, he felt that what the others ordered was good for him, too. However, in very rare situations, when Devin disagreed, he could not stand firm regarding his thoughts and desires. While Devin saw this inability as a problem, his friends began to mock at him, saying he was not independent enough.

Devin's upbringing in two different and opposing cultures has been a major reason for his inadequate sense of self/his low self-esteem. Kohut broadly defines self as the center of initiative and a recipient of awareness and experience. However, simultaneous awareness and experience of two contradicting cultural elements negatively affect oneself and the growth of self. Self-objects and responses to the self are necessary components for the formation of the self. The underdeveloped self merges with self-objects, whose responses are used in the formation and growth of a sense of self.

Devin's self-objects, whose response would affect the development of Devin's self, have been the two cultures in his life: Asian-Indian and dominant American. As Kohut theorized, a non-responsive self-object can lead one to feel helpless and empty with low self-esteem. Devin's self-objects, however, were not non-responsive but responded in culturally particular ways which often misaligned with Devin's distinctive way of being.

In his early years when he was brought up only in the Asian-Indian cultural context (by his first-generation Asian-Indian parents), his self-object, Asian-Indian traditional cultural values, provided the responses that affirmed his self. However, enrolling in the Western education system, his self-object, the Asian-Indian culture, could no longer provide responses that were accepting and upholding his self. Devin's thought patterns and values became distant from the Asian-Indian cultural values and practices of his parents.

Though Devin was very cautious and obeyed his parents most of the time, if he tried to defend his stance on a matter, his self-assertiveness was interpreted, (particularly by his father), as rebellion, disobedience, and disrespect (talking back and impudence). Traditional Indian culture very particularly insists on children's obedience and commitment to the parents. Children are supposed to obey their parents' words as final in all circumstances. With such a mindset, Devin's parents felt upset at his perceived lack of respect for them. They began to question his views on obedience, submission, and duty as a male child in the family. Quite often, Devin's parents began to compare him with his other sibling, yelling at him questions such as, "Why are you always talking back? Why are you so rebellious?" "Why can't you be obedient and submissive like your sibling?" Devin's behavior did not conform to that of a submissive son. Devin's grandparents and parents were always very critical of him. In the course of time, he became absorbed in his sense of self as an "unfit" son and an inadequate person.

Relationally, Devin was viewed differently by those from the Western culture. His behavior was perceived as different because he could not completely abandon his Asian-Indian cultural values, which were deeply embedded in his unconscious. Devin neither critiqued nor challenged others because he felt it was "bad." Devin's teachers and classmates branded him a "mild" person and "invisible." For the most part, no one reacted to or resisted Devin because it was known that he could not stand up for himself.

Though Devin was externally quiet, internally he was very disturbed. Several of his friends told him that if he did not stand up for himself, nobody would do it for him, and that if he does not claim his rights, nobody will give them to him. Though Devin intellectually understood these admonitions, he could not apply them in his real life because of his fear of rejection, disrespecting his parents, and being regarded as too selfish. As Devin was living in the peripheries of two dominant cultures, he could not develop personal qualities that were desirable in either culture. Rather, he was stuck in the middle of the two cultures, trying to accommodate himself to the best in each culture. Acceptance was not possible.

Kohut describes normal narcissism as psychological health. Normal narcissism develops as a result of being accepted and affirmed by self-objects. However, Devin did not receive consistent mirroring that affirmed his "self." Instead, he received criticism and negative affirmation because his actions were neither consistent nor acceptable in either culture. He did not receive mirroring of acceptance and delight. Rather, was reminded that his behavior was not acceptable for the people in either culture. As a result, he was also unable to develop a healthy narcissism, self as a love object. This deficiency would not allow him to later develop into a secure sense of self.

Kohut also contends that the core self develops through the responsiveness of self-objects. The core self is made up of two parts: the grandiose self and the idealized parental image, both of which need empathic responsiveness from self-objects. The grandiose self is established by self-objects approving the child's grandiose self. The idealized parental image is established by the self-object (parents), permitting the child to idealize it (the parents). In Devin's case, he was not really allowed to develop either part of the bipolar self that would become his core self.

Like many other cultures, Asian-Indian culture is very patriarchal, and children's status is always below their parents. The role of the child is to respect and obey parents. Hence, unless the child is exercising the virtues and values of the traditional culture, such as obedience, compliance, maintaining harmony, academic excellence, and saving the face of the family, their grandiose self is not permitted to flourish. The idealized parental image is contradictory to the grandiose self in which it is implied that someone else, often the parent, is perfect. In this case, the child experiences a sense that "you are perfect and I am a part of you." This feeling also has to be received empathically by self-objects. If not, the experience will lead to fragmentation of the self.

Like many other second-generation immigrants, Devin's idealized parental image was not fulfilled. First of all, Devin was not proud of his parents. Rather, he was embarrassed by them for various reasons. His mother did not speak fluent English and even when she did speak, it was with heavy accent. He did not like to introduce his parents to his friends because they could not agree on anything and argued over everything. Because of their inadequate language and inferior social status, Devin lost respect for his parents. Thus, he began to disobey his parents and question their authority. Moreover, Devin did not receive any logical explanation as to why he should obey his parents' decisions. Therefore, he began to be resentful and frequently angry at his parents, particularly his father for his unreasonable orders. Because of cultural differences, Devin could not idealize his father.

On the other hand, Devin's father did not want Devin to idealize him. This was due to Daniel's own sense of inadequacy, inferiority, shame, and guilt. Daniel encouraged Devin not to become like him, but to study more and to work for money and prestige. So Devin's father over-pressured his son regarding his education. That contributed to Devin's negative sense of self. Unrealistic expectations and excessive pressure from parents are two of the major issues with which second-generation Indian immigrants in the United States must contend.

DSM-IV and V are other tools that are helpful for further analysis of the situation. Based on DSM-IV, symptoms of acculturation problem (V62.4, Z60.3), parent–child relational problem (V61.9)/parent relationship distress (V61.29, Z62.898), adjustment disorder with mixed disturbance of emotions and conduct (309.4), and problems related to neglect are evident in the case of Devin and his family. According to its definition, "this category can be used when the focus of clinical attention is a problem involving adjustment to a different culture (e.g., following immigration)." Daniel had already achieved an enormous level of acculturation as he was exposed to foreign cultures when working with Americans in Kuwait and then migrating to the United States before bringing other members of the family to the United States (while Daisy was still in the traditional Asian-Indian culture in India). And because Devin and his sister, Debie, were raised, socialized, and educated in mainstream American culture, their level of acculturation was entirely different from that of the others in the family. This is evident from the differing thought-patterns of Devin and his father.

Along with acculturation issues, Devin's situation also involved relational issues due to the multiple cultural generations involved. As is the case in most Asian-Indian families, Devin's family structure is very hierarchical. His father is a typical domineering father, demanding obedience from his children. His father's voice of command was the ultimate authority. Devin's relationship with his father was strained because his father demanded obedience from Devin, always. This is Daniel's understanding of how a dutiful son behaves.

Devin's father chose Devin's clothes, even his college major without inquiring of Devin about his interests. Devin's resentment towards his father grew with each demand for complete obedience and to live according to his father's cultural values and standards.

Devin's choice of friends was another issue that escalated the tension between him and his father. Daniel did not accept Devin's associating with certain of his friends. According to Daniel, Devin's friends had to be from well-educated families, and should be well-mannered and smart. Devin's and Daniel's relationship was aggravated further during Devin's senior year of high school when Devin chose friends unacceptable to his father. Devin felt that his father was a racist because he tried to keep Devin away from his friends from other cultures. Devin never disclosed his relationship with his female friends to his father.

Enormous conflicts erupted whenever Devin missed his curfew. Daniel would yell at Devin, saying that Devin was ruining his future, wasting his time, and that he would be only be a professional janitor. Though Devin realized that his friends were somewhat of a negative influence on him, he continued to socialize with them as a passive–aggressive way to rebel against his father's authority.

Devin also carried a lot of guilt and shame in relation to the way he performed his role as a son, for yelling at an authority figure, for overstepping his bounds, and for bringing shame to his father. Devin felt that he was a failure as a son, and this sense of failure was very heavy while he was in the presence of his father. He never felt at home with Asian-Indian cultural practices, which also created guilt for him.

A cultural and intercultural assessment of this case can be very revealing. Asian-Indian cultural values take priority over regard for one's own feeling. Parents fulfill their obligation to their children— both in terms of traditional and modern culture—by providing financial security and meeting material, physical, and educational needs until their children get married, sometimes even beyond. In return, children are expected to fulfill their obligation to bring honor to the family by obeying and respecting the parents in all choices and decisions they make for the betterment of their children. Therefore, when a son who is supposed to maintain the honor of the family by continuing the family values and traditions becomes unable or unwilling to fulfill his role, it is unrealistic to expect empathy from parents who are predisposed to become critical and frustrated. In such situations, rather than receiving the empathy needed for the growth of a healthy self, these youngsters often receive words of criticism, dissatisfaction, anger, and rarely cursing from their parents.

Devin's pattern of blaming and his inability to make decisions had transferred to relationships with his Western friends. However, his Western friends considered those behaviors as a sign of his immaturity. They suggested he swallow his pride and admit a wrongdoing of his inability to exercise good judgment. Their comments, intended to encourage him to stand up for himself, made Devin all the more inadequate. Without realizing that the immature behaviors were inherited from his home Asian-Indian culture, Devin continued to question his own maturity. It is interesting that certain behaviors encouraged in one culture are seen as weak and inadequate in another.

Whenever Devin was with his Western friends, he always played a passive role. He did not make any decisions regarding where to go, what to eat, or what to do because he did not want to make wrong decisions. He was fine with whatever decisions his friends made, even when his friends considered it strange that he did not express an opinion. His friends perceived it as strange that someone would not voice their own desires, assert influence, or stand up for himself. They regarded that behavior as weak, wishy-washy and spineless, and encouraged Devin to say what he wanted to eat instead of accepting what others ordered for him.

No matter how Devin tried to be a part of each culture, he was not well received in either. Further, his experience of being marked as "different," combined with feelings of shame, led him to confusion of identity. Having a self that was not fully formed or anchored in either culture caused Devin to act in ways that were seen as atypical or indifferent by both cultures, making him feel in-between, rather than in-both, cultures. Devin's in-between status in two cultures made him feel powerless, lonely, and inadequate. Caught in-between two opposing cultures, being an outsider in both and belonging to neither deprived him of opportunities to form a strong and healthy cohesive self.

Devin was an outsider in the dominant immigrant world of his father and considered an outsider by the dominant Western culture which rendered him powerless and voiceless in navigating his own future. He was also helpless to explain his own position to his father because he feared his father's reprimanding behavior: he would certainly interpret Devin's attempt to explain his position as talking back and disrespect. So Devin decided to suppress his own thoughts, feelings, and choices and endure the sense of powerless. This was absolutely against the principles and cultural values that he learned in Western schools and from the United States culture.

Fueled by the sense of inequality, injustice, and powerlessness Devin experienced in his relationship with his father, he built a wall around himself, rejecting his father, and the culture and community his father represented. At the same time, this act of rejection also developed a sense of shame and unworthiness in Devin because he felt that he was not good enough to assimilate in that culture.

While Devin and his father have issues of control and blame between them, their relationship as father and son is also strained. Both Devin and his father operate from different understandings and orientations of self. Daniel's understanding of self is formed by his Asian-Indian allocentric, patriarchal, family-oriented culture. Therefore, his self is a self in community. However, Devin has a different understanding of self and finds it difficult to relate with his father's cultural self, values, and practices. Devin is living with the simultaneous tension of accepting and resisting. Devin's actions are not grounded in self-orientation or in his own thinking. Therefore, his relationships lack intimacy and transparency. Finally, father and mother are disengaged, parents and children are distanced, and the whole family is dysfunctional.

The relationship between Devin and Daniel can be described as fused. Out of the allocentric, family cultural understanding of the role and responsibility of a father, Daniel sees Devin as an extension of himself. He feels responsible for Devin making good choices. Therefore, in many areas, he made choices for Devin and demanded Devin carry out the decisions made for him. As many Asian-Indian parents do, Daniel also thought it was not a social life but an academic life that was more important for his son at this stage. Further, Daniel may have thought that his son did not have adequate ability to critically think and analyze life situations as he does.

Based on his ethnic cultural understanding, Daniel was making numerous choices for Devin. Whenever Daniel's decision did not work, Devin readily blamed his father. As long as Daniel was making choices Devin continued to blame others without seeing his responsibility for his actions.

Devin's wish was to major in fine arts at an out-of-state university. But his father decided he would study computer engineering at a nearby university in his hometown and asked him to commute from home. It was at that point that Devin began to spend time with his friends, attracted by commonality, watching movies, smoking and drinking, doing everything but studying. Devin's grades dropped, which became a huge issue between Devin and his father. In heated arguments, Devin yelled at his father that everything was his fault because he chose a college and major for Devin, neither of which Devin would have chosen for himself. Thus, Devin continued to believe that his father's refusal to let him choose his desired major and school led him to all his failures.

THE SPIRITUAL ASSESSMENT STAGE

The purpose of this stage is to examine the beliefs and spiritual convictions that are involved or at work in the given issue. Religious, spiritual, and theological convictions play an important role in understanding and resolving problems. While taking Christian theology seriously, we also should pay due respect and give consideration to people's spirituality and cultural theology, as well. The aspect of interconnectedness, family values, and respect for parents are at the center of the Asian-Indian worldview.

As most Indian Christians do, Daisy approached her priest to talk about her struggle. But neither her priest nor any parishioners responded to her positively, so she stopped going to church. In her understanding, church is a community that acts in love at the time of crisis. Daisy also believes that the privilege God gave her should not be abused or be a source of false pride. Her lifestyle is simple and influenced by her cultural upbringing. She often quotes verses from the Bible to prove that God is siding with those who are humble and meek, though her definition of humility and meekness were not very clear. According to Lee, "the church is a community of new marginal people, where the genuine fellowship of brotherhood/sisterhood is experienced and where the original order of creation is restored."[3] Lee further adds that "the church as Christian community must be in-between the world now and the world that is to come. Both worlds, however, are one and inseparable, so the Christian community exists 'in-between and in-both' at once."[4] Devin's family, as an immigrant community, was living in-between, but not in-both or in-beyond.

Daisy also believes that an evil spirit is operating in the entire family. In this context, it is very important to understand the cultural theology and traditional religious belief of good, evil, and spirit. The problem in this family also invites us to probe into their beliefs and understandings about evil spirits. That exploration is very important to bring an integrated picture of the issue from their perspective through the lens of theological, practical, and traditional good sense. When each one sees the complete picture of what is happening in the individual and in the family life, using these resources will help family members to verbalize the issues and engage in fruitful dialogue.

THE DIALOGICAL STAGE

In this stage, the insights gathered from the analytic reflection stage and theological assessment are brought together in a dialogue that leads to a holistic assessment of the problem. The major element lacking in this issue is just empathy. Empathy is a psychological term, primarily from Kohut, that entails the need for positive relationship that stimulates and sustains persons. Grace can be considered and described as its corresponding theological counterpart, a way of showing unconditional love. This is the greatest need in the case of Devin's family, as family members, especially Daniel and Devin, need to reach a deeper level of understanding and connection with each other for the sake of reducing the anxiety level. Empathy invites people to care for one another, for each one's wellbeing and wholeness, and to stand together as a family.

Here the family, especially the father as the head of the family, should come forward to express his empathy or grace toward his son. Devin should be given the grace to explain his stance and why he has acted as he has. Again, Daniel, as the father, should show compassion and grace as the father-figure in the story of the prodigal son showed compassion and mercy to his son.

The same mercy and empathy is needed for Daisy, as well. Instead of waiting for Daisy to pick up life in a new culture, she was being pushed to make the transition at a quicker pace than suited her. Identity is negatively affected as a result of living in-between cultures; when there is no awareness of words for defining the self, one can only accept definitions already made. Being told who one is, where one belongs, and why one belongs in that space, restricts the boundaries of one's thoughts, including imagined possibilities of the self. It places one in a static space. More importantly, being confined to a space with boundaries, one loses the potentiality of having one's future unfold on one's life journey. Thus, one's life remains pressed, compacted, and unable to open out in numerous potential directions and multiple ways. This is simply because in that space the multiplicity and potentiality of the selves cannot be realized. This is what happened in Daisy's life. She needs grace to see the situation in a wider perspective and to forgive to her husband.

Daniel might be working to prevent the disintegration of the family as family is a large part of his identity. Yet, Daniel needs to open up and communicate with the family so that his wife and children will understand his intentions and, perhaps, may feel valued and respected.

While Devin is the identified patient, the entire family has an issue that needs to be addressed. It is important to keep in mind that while Daniel and Debie represent the dominant American culture, Daniel is the representation of a more accultured person into the dominant American culture. Meanwhile, Daisy represents the traditional Asian-Indian culture. This has happened because of the different cultural generations and different times of immigration for Daniel and Daisy. In some instances, recent arrivals do find it difficult to feel connected to a church that is not communal in the same way they had experienced back home.

In conclusion, this is a case study about a problem of four persons in a three-cultural generational family, whose members came to the United States at different times. Their migration broadly involves two different major cultural generations and two different major cultures, the dominant American culture and traditional Asian-Indian culture.

Action/Strategic Intervention Stage

The strategic goal in this case was to work with the family to enable family members to find a way to resolve their problem relationally and to foster empathy for one another. This was especially important for the dominant person, the father, Daniel. Further, those in the in-between space needed empowerment. The goal was chosen based on the goals of pastoral care: healing, sustaining, guiding, reconciling, and empowering.

The primary step towards this goal was to foster reconciliation. On the whole, the family had a lot of disconnections and breakdowns in communication, especially between Daniel and Devin, and between Debie and Daisy. After several individual sessions with Devin, I invited Daniel to get a broader understanding of the picture and had a few sessions with him. Then, with Daniel's permission and knowledge, I invited Daisy into the therapy session. (Debie did not join the individual sessions but joined the family sessions.) Then I invited Devin and Daniel, who are the two powerful representatives in the family. Within the family, primarily they represent the clashing cultural generations, the power dynamics, as well as the communication breakdowns, other than that between Debie and Daisy.

As I provided them a safe space and non-anxious pastoral and healing presence, and guided them with active and empathic listening, they began to pour out feelings, views, intentions, and emotions that they had not shared for several years, even though they were living in the same house. As their communication progressed they began to see and understand their problem from a broader perspective. Using empathy and grace as the therapeutic tools, I also guided Daniel, Devin, and Daisy to talk about what it would look like to be in the others' shoes, wherein Daniel realized that he was judging his son and over-pressuring him without realizing his son's cultural understanding, emotional world, and peer pressure. Daniel also realized that he was expecting too much of Daisy in terms of her understanding American life the way he did in Kuwait and when he came to the United States. He also realized that though his intentions were good, he was trying to control the entire family without empathizing with them in their emotional struggles. Devin also realized that the intentions of his father were different from what he had assumed. His father's confession made him realize his true heart. Daisy was very angry but realized that she was fighting her feelings of powerlessness and grieving the loss of the supportive family and community that she enjoyed in India.

Debie realized that rather than finding ways and possibilities of connecting and relating, she was withdrawing into her own inner personal space. She also realized that in her inner personal space, she was able to control who came in and out of the space, who was an insider and who was an outsider. She allowed only a few people to come into her personal space. She also realized that she was reducing the space for others but enlarging it through her own ideas and fantasies. Thus, she was disconnected from family, though she pretended that she is normally connected with everyone.

From these family sessions, the entire family realized and agreed that the problem was a family problem and it was affecting the functionality of all members in their family. They agreed that they were all dealing with the same feeling but differently. They also agreed that they need to move on toward family functionality. That will require each of them to encourage one another with patience and grace, understanding each one's abilities and weaknesses.

In the final meeting, I asked Daniel and Daisy if they have any close family friends in whom they trust and who they would be comfortable bringing into therapy. Thus, they brought a couple with whom Daniel and Daisy used to share their burdens. Fortunately, the couple's son and daughter were also close to Devin and Debie. I consciously grabbed this chance to re-create a communal gathering that will provide support and strength here, as in the case of an Indian extended family.

CASE STUDY 2: MEENA:[5] CULTURAL CLASH, INTERGENERATIONAL CONFLICT, AND EMOTIONAL PROBLEMS

Praxis Stage

Meena is a 21-year-old, second-generation Asian-Indian, studying nursing. Though it is only a short distance from her parents' home to her school, Meena is sharing an apartment with her friends "for the convenience of her studies." One day Meena's roommates contacted her parents to inform them of a particular incident that had happened in Meena's life. According to her roommates, one night Meena walked out of her room, in the middle of sleeping, and did a back flip in the living room in front of her roommates. Following this incident, Meena's parents brought her back home and sent her to a psychiatrist for further evaluation. According to Meena, this back-flip incident happened when she was not taking the medication prescribed for bipolar disorder because she felt okay. (She was diagnosed bipolar when she was 19 years old, almost two years ago).

Though Meena started therapy with a Western therapist, her parents were not happy with that relationship. After she was brought back home, Meena was brought to me for therapy because her parents had got to know me while I was volunteering as an associate pastor for pastoral care and counseling in their church. At the same time, Meena was also seeing a female psychiatrist who strongly recommended therapy for her. Meena came to me for therapy every Wednesday evening on her way home from school. She was very regular and punctual in her routine.

In her initial appearance, Meena seemed to be very happy. She was alert and talkative. She always presented herself in expensive clothes, handbags, shoes, sun-glasses, watches, matching earrings, and make-up. She sometimes moved from topic to topic, talking at a fast pace. She was interested in talking more about others than about herself. Several times I had difficulty bringing Meena back and refocusing the conversation to her.

Our initial session was about her family, hometown, the school in which she studied, and everything she hated, including some of her friends. Meena felt that most Asian-Indians were weird and strange. She said she was frustrated because she could not complete her school simply because of her crazy friends. Meena felt that she was acting like a mother to one of them, constantly telling her what to do next because it was thought that she was not good at making decisions. Meena informed me she was in therapy for a year and said, "Therapy was more help to me than my friends were, and I am able to make better choices than before."

In the following session Meena talked about her struggles and the difficulty of having no boyfriend and feeling unlovable. Our therapy began to progress as her trust and our therapeutic relationship developed. Thus, Meena began to bring up experiences that revealed her real lifestyle was more ostentatious and that her life was progressively less controlled. Alcohol consumption was an issue for Meena. Several times she drove while under the influence of alcohol, though she was aware of, and suffered, the consequences of that decision.

When I probed further about the behavior, she was very cavalier about it, saying "Well, everyone does it." When she was in the school, she drank alcohol and skipped classes. As a result of this behavior, Meena was dismissed from her school. She also smoked and used drugs. She was still drinking when she went out with her friends.

Meena had several boyfriends because she felt she wanted to be loved. She also said she did not want to be alone and without a boyfriend, because she felt abandoned without someone to love her. During this session, she also talked about a "wonderful guy" whom she met at a social gathering. She engaged in unprotected sex with this new boyfriend, as well as with several other male friends. Meena's parents are frustrated with Meena's wild behavior, and conflicts with her parents have occurred regarding her boyfriends, drinking, going out, partying, and other behaviors that bring shame after shame upon the family.

Shopping sprees are another behavior of Meena's that causes conflict with her parents. She feels good when she realizes that people notice her. She wore expensive clothes, jewelry, shoes, and bags to get the attention of others. She charged up several credit cards and her parents paid off most of them. She also reported that she had a couple of panic attacks and continued to experience them. She could not be still when alone, so she kept herself busy with cleaning, laundry, or watching television.

Meena's Childhood

Meena's father, Mathew, was a civil contractor in India prior to his marriage. He grew up in a wealthy family. The Mathew–Mercy marriage was arranged and conducted by both families and relatives according to their custom, tradition, and religious rites. Since Mercy's parents had filed a petition of migration for Mercy, she left for the United States after two years of her marriage. She was four months pregnant with Meena when she left India. Meena was primarily cared for by her grandparents until her family moved to Georgia. Thereafter, they hired a nanny for Meena. The sense of abandonment by her mother was still noticeably present 20 years later when she came for therapy with me.

Meena is the only child of her parents. Her mother, Mercy, now in her early fifties, migrated to the United States when she was 27 years old and pregnant. Meena's father, Mathew, joined Mercy after 20 months, when Meena was almost one year old. Since Mercy did not pass the registered nurse exam, she took up work as a certified nursing assistant. She worked in two different nursing homes to meet the family's needs and pay the bills. She worked 12-hour shifts five or six days a week.

Mathew was hired in a grocery store a few months after he arrived. So, both parents were mostly absent from Meena and she hardly remembered them during the day. Meena was raised by her maternal grandparents during the early years while Mercy and Mathew were at work. One of Meena's childhood memories was her parents bringing her some clothes and toys. Meena does not remember requesting anything from her parents because her parents always gave her everything she needed even before she asked for it.

Meena said she cried a lot during the initial week of her schooling because she did not like to go to school. She used to play alone with toy kitchen sets at school. Other students would take away her toys and would not be friends with her. In such situations, all that Meena could do was cry softly. Meena recalled that she was a very shy girl and did not know how to defend herself. In those days, her teachers gave a lot of attention to teaching her "proper" English. She did not have many friends in the school because she could not speak English like other students and she did not understand them. Even now she remembers the pain of being different at school. Even though Meena felt a distance from her classmates, she adjusted relatively well to the Western school system.

At the beginning of middle school, Meena's parents moved the family to Georgia for better employment prospects. They continued to be away from home (and Meena) most of the time. To make matters worse, Meena's grandmother, who was her primary caregiver, could not move to Georgia with Meena and her parents. With a tearful and broken voice Meena told me, "I was always alone." She was always by herself, locked in a huge house, watching television until her mother returned home after dark. Though her mother used to call her to check on her every now and then, Meena felt very lonely and was scared being all alone. Meena remembers well the loneliness she felt coming home from school to an empty house, especially during her middle school years.

In the absence of Meena's grandmother, her parents hired a nanny. The nanny, who could not speak English very well, would open the front door for Meena. But Meena had to change her clothes, eat the food that was prepared for her, then stay alone in her room until her parents returned from work. Meena learned to turn on the television and change the channels, which later helped her escape from her sense of fear and loneliness.

When Meena was 13 her nanny stopped working for the family. Meena then had no choice but to sit all alone. As she grew up, she felt neglected and began to be angry when she realized the possible dangers of being alone. One of the major problems Meena presented in therapy was her resentment and anger towards her mother for neglecting her.

This lonely life at home continued until Meena was in tenth grade. During that time, Meena began to insist that her mother buy her dresses that exposed her body parts, but her mother strongly resisted the request. Meena then began buying herself the "sexy" dresses she wanted. As Meena continued dressing in ways which her parents disapproved of, they began yelling at her, and Meena would yell back. Her mother would begin yelling at Meena in English and end up shouting in Malayalam. Meena deliberately used foul words and ugly names to express her anger and frustrations. Finally, when Meena became very violent, her mother would break down and cry, thus ending the fight for the day.

When Meena was able to afford a car and drive, she began to spend time with her friends at their houses. In those situations, Meena was exposed to drugs. Gradually she began to smoke, drink, take drugs, and became sexually active, and because of these behaviors, her grades began to fall. This caused further damage to her relationship with her parents, especially with her mother. When Meena was dismissed from school in her senior high year due to misconduct, her parents decided she was unmanageable. Thus,

Meena gained the upper hand in the ongoing power struggle. Her mother could no longer control Meena's behavior with "bribes," and she feared that Meena's wild behavior would bring shame upon family and they would lose face in public.

Initially, Meena's mother felt guilt, shame, and regret about her daughter's rebellious behavior. Later she accepted it remarking, "I did whatever I could in the given situation." Now the mother's plan is to complete Meena's education somehow, get her a job, and get her married to someone so that she can have a life of her own. Even now it is Meena's mother who supports Meena, paying her tuition, books, car payment, insurance, therapy, and pocket money. Meena's mother is essentially fulfilling her role like every other Asian-Indian that financially supports their children until their marriage. In this context, Meena is controlling her mother and exploiting her mother's sense of guilt, knowing that her mother will accept her demands at least until she completes her studies. In other words, Meena manipulates her mother and threatens to quit school if at any time her mother tries to advise her about her school, friends or behaviors. Meena knows that when she threatens to quit school, her mother will yield to her demands. Therefore, Meena uses "quitting school" as a tool to manipulate her mother and ensure her demands are met.

According to Meena, her parents were very strict and demanding of her, academically. Meena and her parents went through the most difficult time when Meena was in high school, but becoming very frustrated, soon left her alone. With a strange look on her face, Meena told me, "My parents gave up on me." Meena believes that her relationship with her parents is good since they decided to leave her alone. Though she used to be open to her mother, Meena now hides things from her, such as drug use, boyfriends, and sexual activity. Even now, when Meena is at home, she is alone, as her mother works throughout the day.

Meena does not have a cordial relationship with her father since he beat her for talking back to him. That caused great trouble for the family, including community involvement. However, Meena believes that her father knows everything going on with her as her mother discusses everything about Meena with her father.

THE ANALYTIC REFLECTION STAGE

I use Diagnostic and Statistical Manuel of Mental Disorders, fourth and fifth editions (DSM-IV and V) as one of the tools to asses a person in the analytic reflection stage, and based on this tool, bipolar 1 disorder, most recent episode hypomanic (269.40/296.41; F31.11) is a part of Meena's story. This prompted me to look into the possibility of following issues such as adjustment disorder with mixed disturbance of emotions and conduct (309.4)/oppositional defiant disorder (313.81, F91.3), acculturation problem (V62.4, Z60.3), parent–child relational problem (V61.9)/parent relationship distress (V61.29, Z62.898), and problems related to neglect. The cultural adjustment problem for Meena and her family is very visible in her story. However, intergenerational conflicts and relational issues are also present and require attention.

Infants and toddlers discover their self in relationships when the self is growing in the context of nurturing self-objects. In Meena's case, it is evident that she did not receive adequate nurturing from her-self objects. Meena's mother, who served as her self-object, disappeared one morning and, thus, discontinued her role as Meena's self-object. Although Meena's grandmother served as the primary caregiver for Meena in the absence of her mother until Meena was 10 years old, it all changed suddenly when Meena's parents moved to Georgia and a nanny took over as her primary caregiver.

Therefore, Meena's grandmother could no longer fill the role of self-object for her and so her sense of abandonment and loss of self-objects obstructed her growth of self.

When a child does not get mirrored, disallowing integration with her growing self, certain inappropriate behaviors are inevitable. Driving under influence of alcohol and sexual promiscuity/engaging in dangerous sexual behaviors might have been the ways in which Meena's fragile self found expression. She was arrested a couple of times for driving under the influence, her license was revoked more than once for not paying the fine on time, and finally she was arrested for driving without a license.

Shopping sprees were another example of inappropriate behavior Meena used as her other self-defense mechanism. Meena maxed out three credit cards, buying expensive clothes, shoes, bags, colognes, etc. She also used her mother's credit card to make about $2000-worth of purchases. These expensive purchases became her idealized self, making her feel more powerful when wearing and carrying expensive clothing and accessories.

Meena was mirrored inappropriately by both cultures. Interestingly, the optimal frustration that would strengthen her self was also absent in her. Her parents worked hard, holding second jobs, in order to provide everything for her, even at the expense of feeding Meena's fantasy. In therapy, it was realized that this particular relational pattern had lost its possibility of strengthening Meena's fragmented self.

As time went on and Meena grew up, the dominance in relationships shifted. The mother–daughter roles reversed in such a way that her mother began to provide everything to Meena to appease her and try to bring under her mother's control. Meena was carrying a sense of rejection and abandonment since her parents always left her alone. She is still not sure whether or not her parents love her. In therapy, Meena visited and revisited that experience several times, always with pain. Meena is angry with her parents for leaving her alone at home at a young age. She is frightened about it even now. This fear and anger have forced Meena to develop a doubt about the genuineness of her mother's love towards her, which in turn led her to doubt her own self-worth. Consequently, she started struggling with low-self-esteem.

Meena's life of living in-between cultures has also brought emotional conflicts, loneliness, and individual dysfunctionality. To satisfy her loneliness, Meena acted in ways that made her feel loved and accepted in company of other people. Meena grew up in a hierarchical family. Though her father was present and was one of the decision-makers, Meena did not have much interaction with him, though her father was aware about everything that was going on with her. His authority came to Meena through her mother, as Meena had a closer relationship with her mother and it was her mother who represented the hierarchical authority in her growing-up.

Meena's mother advised her every day about what she was supposed to do. Along with authority and advice, Meena's mother also loved her, lavishing her with all sorts of toys, clothes, and almost everything Meena wanted. However, this luxury was conditional and came with the agreement that she would earn good grades and behave properly. For new clothes, shoes and bags, Meena was supposed to obey her mother because her mother was the dominant figure and most influential of her parents.

Meena's parents were the self-object representing Asian-Indian culture, but Meena did not feel supported or loved. Rather, she felt neglected. Her grandparents also representing the traditional Indian cultural self-object, mirrored back a faulty, deficient self, one that Meena internalized. After a few years when Meena visited India, her paternal grandmother asked her,

"If all my grandchildren speak to me in Malayalam why can't you also do the same? My five-year-old Jennifer speaks better Malayalam than you do. Why are you talking back to your mother? You should be more respectful to your mother. You are a girl and so you should learn how to cook, clean and serve." Meena, in those days quite often felt that she was being judged according to the typical traditional Mallu[6] culture. Nothing she did was satisfactory in her grandmother's eyes. Indian culture as a self-object was never empathic, supportive, encouraging, or nurturing for Meena. Rather it was critical and judgmental because Meena was not being Indian enough. Meena's self was formed while living in two cultures, mirrored back as a self that was deficient, bad, and inadequate. Self-object as the Asian-Indian culture for Meena was either non-responsive (as her parents) or critical. Therefore, it could not support the growth of narcissism that would eventually lead to a healthy sense of self. Meena was left with a fragmented and lonely self.

However, Meena felt more accepted and less judged in Western culture, even though she felt invisible in it. She paid more attention to Western culture as it affirmed her fragile self and began to idealize it as her self-object. She sought more attention, love, and relationship with males. She began to know that she was attractive and she used her beauty to get attentions from boys. Getting attention from others helped her to feel better and forget her sense of abandonment and loneliness. She began to go to bars with boys of her own age and taste liquor, engage in unprotected sex, drive when intoxicated, and skip class because she was hung over from late-night partying. She sought positive mirroring, albeit sexual, from her continuous flow of boyfriends. Meena often went out with her friends to avoid being alone and to avoid her childhood memories. According to Meena, the memory of her child abandonment made her anxious. As long as she was using the external stimuli to hide or cover her internal wounds, she was simply bandaging her hurt without any real healing.

The relationship between Meena and her mother can also be fused. A fused relationship cannot be the same as an intimate and connected relationship. Rather, in a fused relationship, both parties are acting in certain ways to make them feel secure. For instance, if Meena drops out of school, it will bring shame on the family and her mother's parenting skills will be questioned. So to avoid that shame, Meena's mother bribes Meena with the promise of things she wants. Meena, being aware of this, manipulates her mother's vulnerabilities to be sure she satisfies Meena's demands. Here, excessive energy, not intimacy, is used to control one other.

Meena always prefers Western friends, yet reports that girls are immature and not good for socializing. This reveals that Meena does not have an engaging relationship with other girls.

THE SPIRITUAL ASSESSMENT STAGE

The major spiritual issue I see in Meena's case is the lack of love in a theological sense, an unconditional love. Meena's parents were busy making money and meeting the material needs of their daughter. Though both Mathew and Mercy were traditionally Christians, they did not find time to have family prayers or to go to church on Sundays. The disunity in the family also caused a spiritual void that further resulted in dysfunctionality and illness. Meena's family was not strongly connected with any community. Most Asian-Indians believe that our connection with family and community is also a factor in determining our connection with God.

Another influence of the Asian-Indian worldview is *karma*. Mercy believes that what she is experiencing with Meena is her karma, or fate. Though *karma* is considered a Hindu philosophical teaching, it has a modified influence on almost all Asian-Indians from any faith background. Mercy believes that Meena's bipolar disorder is the result of Mercy's wrong actions. Also, Mercy believes that if Meena gives up all her bad behaviors, God will heal her. Mercy has a typical, bargaining relationship with Meena and God. Here this family's concept of faith healing and good works is clearly evident. This is another common worldview of Asian-Indians. Mercy also believes that "God abandoned her" when she was only focused on money and future "without caring for the God of the future." When I invited her to talk more about this, she said, "I did not set apart time for my daughter's and my spiritual life. We don't have family prayer nor regular Sunday Service."

The theological concepts of guilt, forgiveness, and reconciliation should be explored at various levels. Reconciliation and new meanings in life are needed between Meena and her father, who do not communicate with each other. The harmonious relationship is lost in the family. To restore the harmonious relationship of the family and alleviate the guilt, the concept of God's grace is to be introduced to the family. The need for respect and unconditional positive regard also should be recognized by each member of the family. Forgiveness should take place between Meena and Mercy as well. There is also a need for exploring the family's spiritual life so as determine their experiences and resources for dealing with spiritual matters.

The idea of being loveable and unlovable in Meena's life should be redefined in relation to God's unconditional, unchanging, and unfailing love. In the same way, the sense of abandonment and the meaning of God's care and immutable presence should be redefined for Meena. Kohut's concept of empathy and the theological term of grace are both very much needed by each member in the family. Empathy must be first of all generated in Meena's parents so that Meena will mirror it, perhaps developing a more healthy self.

THE DIALOGICAL STAGE

An appropriate care approach to the problems of Meena and her family would be a holistic approach that integrates the spiritual and the sciences. It is already assessed that bipolar 1 disorder, most recent episode hypomanic, is a part of Meena's story (DSM-IV 269.40/DSM-V 296.41; F31.11). This also forces me to look into the possibility of following issues such as adjustment disorder with mixed disturbance of emotions and conduct (309.4), oppositional defiant disorder (313.81, F91.3), acculturation problem (V62.4, Z60.3), parent–child relational problem (V61.9), parent relationship distress (V61.29, Z62.898), and problems related to neglect.

Another area which requires immediate attention in the story of Meena, is living in-between cultures or cultural dominance. Meena's case indicates that living in-between the Asian-Indian immigrant culture and mainstream Western culture did not provide an adequate environment for her self to form and grow. Rather than having one culture as a self-object to mirror back her sense of self, Meena had multiple self-objects competing for her attention. They did mirror back to her not the self they represented but the expectation from each culture.

Analysis of the reasons for the misalignments in Meena's behaviors makes it clear that it is not only the others' expectation that deformed her growth of self, but, because Meena was positioned on the lower rung of the patriarchal hierarchy, she did not have much power to exercise. Obedience was her duty. Without power in relationships, people may experience injustice and, as a result, bitterness and anger that can lead to depression.

The children within the system, with the same internalized values of the parents, often rationalize and accept their role as obedient children. However, Meena was exposed to the Western cultural values of equality and exercising power so that she began to claim her authority. How could Meena develop and grow a positive and healthy self when there is no safe space in which to express or verbalize her anger, bitterness, and desire to retaliate against her family? What could Meena do with all the negative energy pent up inside her? How can her self flourish in a helpless environment? What is the condition of the emotional and psychological health of Meena's parents? These theoretical questions demand immediate attention for the healing and radical development of a deformed and underdeveloped self.

Another aspect of Meena's story that invites attention is the relational difficulty between parents and children stemming from cultural expectations, alienation, and misunderstandings. Meena and her parents, especially Meena and her mother, experienced relational difficulty. Meena's parents worked long hours in order to meet all her material needs. Though they sacrificed many of their privileges, especially her mother, for the sake of their daughter, they could not provide the love and care in the way that Meena wanted and needed. Some of the cultural expectations regarding talking back, clothing choices, boyfriend relationship, drug use, and premarital sex also played major roles in the area of relationship issues, intergenerational conflict, and individual and family dysfunction. None of the things that Meena's parents offered her was good enough to heal her emotional/childhood wounds created by the sense of abandonment, feeling unloved, and being left alone. This further developed Meena's anxiety and resentment towards her parents.

Meena looked for acceptance in relationships outside her home. She targeted love and acceptance from boys. Though it is normal at her age, in Meena's case, it was a reaction from the perceived sense of rejection by her parents, which stemmed from cultural misunderstandings. Meena's behavior resulted from her need for acceptance and approval. Though she succeeded in her effort to gain acceptance and approval from others, her behavioral pattern served to mask her low self-esteem rather than moving her toward growth and empowerment. Meena also began to hate her parental community, projecting and transferring her frustration onto her interpersonal relationships and onto her parental community. While Meena abused the use of her mother's credit card in a manipulative way, she was unconsciously making her mother mad and paying her mother back for the wrongs Meena perceived had been done to her.

Kohut's use of empathy is helpful in facilitating family health when empathic attunement is in order so that family members can relate to one another. Empathic relating results in the mutual understanding that needs must be communal in nature. According to Lee, people cannot understand themselves unless they understand others who are in them, he/she is included in them, as the reverse is true. . ... This unity presupposes difference in plurality. The unity of difference is possible through harmony and harmony is possible because of individual plurality.[7] The parable of the prodigal son (Luke 15:11–32) tells of the immense love of a father receiving back his younger son with celebration, a son who returns home after having squandered all of his inheritance. In that story, the father functions as the mediator and connector, though he is a part of the dominant, insider group. Yet the empathy in him brings him outside to receive his son and to bring him inside, restoring and continuing the relationship. Here, in Meena's story, each member has to see their ability to show empathy to one another and to restore the individual and family functionality.

ACTION/STRATEGIC INTERVENTION STAGE

The strategic goals in this case were primarily four: (1) to work with the family to enable them to find a way to resolve the problem relationally and foster empathy for one another, (2) to help the family to be aware of the cultural expectations and demands playing consciously or unconsciously in their interactions, (3) to educate them about the issues of those who live in-between cultures, and (4) to make them listen to each other in order to really "hear" what each one wants to tell the other.

The primary step for this family was to foster forgiveness and reconciliation. The family had a lot of disconnections and breakdowns in communication, especially between Meena, and Mathew. After several individual sessions with Meena, I invited Mercy to get a broader understanding of the picture and had a few sessions with her. Then, with her knowledge, I invited Mathew into the therapy. Initially Mathew, who was in his mid-fifties, was reluctant to come to therapy, though he knew me at a distant level. According to Mathew, "It is the problem of my daughter and my part is not needed in the therapy. Also, it is her mother who spoils her. She does everything without consulting with me." However, he came to me and we discussed various things related to their family issues. Mathew came to understand the family dynamic after four sessions and finally decided to join the family session as well. Mathew explained about Meena and her good manners and behaviors, her ability to learn in childhood, and concluded that it was her friendships that had spoiled her. I strongly sensed the emotional pain echoed in his voice. However, I was also aware about his role, disengagement, and frustration.

Both her parents worked hard to meet all Meena's needs and to provide everything for her so that their only child would not be put down by her peers. I worked with Mathew as a conversation partner, listening to him empathically. Then I invited Mathew and Mercy together to come to therapy and provided a safe space for them to discuss their present situation and their perspectives. Though there were different perspectives and misunderstandings those were resolved after a few sessions.

Finally, with everyone's knowledge and permission, a family meeting was arranged. As I provided them a safe space with non-anxious pastoral and healing presence and guided them with active and empathic listening, they began to pour out their feelings, views, expectations, and emotions that they had not shared in several years, though they were living in the same house. As their communication progressed, they began to see and understand their problem in an integrated manner. Using empathy and grace as the therapeutic tools, I also guided Meena, Mathew, and Mercy in talking about what it would look like to be in the others' shoes, at which point Meena and Mathew realized that they were focusing so hard on money they had neglected their only child. Mercy agreed that she was demanding and expected obedience, good grades, and good behavior from Meena in return for the material things she provided her. Meena, when hearing the intention and motivation of her parents, poured out all her anger and blocked emotional pain to her parents. Though it was embarrassing to the parents, they realized that Meena was verbalizing her pain as she apologized to both of her parents. Finally, they decided to let it go and begin a new life. They decided to spend family time and attend a church every Sunday after several years of ignoring their spiritual lives. In other words, they decided to reconnect among themselves, with others and with God. Meena recognized many of her behaviors as part of her sickness and decided to keep an accountability partner for herself. From this conversation, the entire family realized and agreed that the problem was a family problem that was affecting the functionality of all members in their family. They agreed that they were all dealing with the same feelings, just differently. They all agreed that they needed to move on toward the family functionality, for which they needed to encourage one another with more patience and grace, understanding each one's abilities and weaknesses.

NOTES

1. Though, three case studies were used in the research to test the applicability of this model, only two of those case studies are used in this book.
2. The names used in this case study are pseudonyms to maintain the confidentiality and protect the privacy of the participants.
3. Jung Young Lee, *Marginality: Key to Multicultural Theology* (Minneapolis, MN: Fortress Press, 1995), 121.
4. Ibid., 131.
5. The names used in this case study also are pseudonyms to maintain the confidentiality and protect the privacy of the participants.
6. This is the nickname given to people who speak the Malayalam language and behave in a traditional way.
7. Jung Young Lee, *Marginality: Key to Multicultural Theology*, 105.

APPENDIX

EMPIRICAL DATA, CODED, AND TABULATED

The charts and tables below indicate the findings of the data collected through a structured questionnaire. These findings were coded, analyzed and interpreted in order to find out how much the variables significantly determine these observations in the life of Indian immigrants who are living for many decades in the United States of America.

The following areas are the areas explored in this Questionnaire:

1. Intrafamily relationship between first- and second-generation immigrants
2. Communication, mutual acceptance and respect to cultural values
3. Emphasis/overemphasis on ethnic culture
4. Intergenerational conflict and individual/Family functionality
5. Role of religious and social institutions in educating acculturation and cultural struggles
6. Demographic details and multi ethnic identity.

© The Author(s) 2017
V. Jacob, *Counseling Asian Indian Immigrant Families*,
DOI 10.1007/978-3-319-64307-6

Section 1: Intrafamily Relationship Between
First- and Second-Generation Immigrants

The data in this section help us understand how the family relationship between husband and wife, parents and children operate within the family as different generations live together under the same roof.

Table 1   Family discussion on important family matters

My parents discuss all important family matters with me		Second-generation respondents	
		Number	Percentage
1	Disagree	61	61
2	Strongly disagree	03	03
3	Uncertain	15	15
4	Agree	21	21
5	Strongly agree	00	00
Total		100	100

I always discuss all family matters with my children		First-generation respondents	
		Number	Percentage
1	Disagree	05	05
2	Strongly disagree	00	00
3	Uncertain	45	45
4	Agree	50	50
5	Strongly agree	00	00
Total		100	100

The above tables explain that while 21 percent of second-generationrespondents agree that their parents discuss all family matters with them, 50 percent among the first-generation agree that they do so with their children.

Table 2   Parents who never restrict children to know family matters

My parents never restrict me to ask about anything what I need to know		**Second-generation** *respondents*	
		Number	*Percentage*
1	Disagree	89	89
2	Strongly disagree	05	05
3	Uncertain	00	00
4	Agree	06	06
5	Strongly agree	00	00
Total		100	100
I never restrict my children to ask about anything what they need to know		**First-generation** *respondents*	
		Number	*Percentage*
1	Disagree	07	07
2	Strongly disagree	00	00
3	Uncertain	45	45
4	Agree	48	48
5	Strongly agree	00	00
Total		100	100

The above data show that only a minority of respondents among second-generation immigrants (6 percent) agrees that their parents never restrict them to ask about anything what they need to know while 48 percent of respondents among first-generation immigrants agrees.

Table 3 Mutual respect in the family

My parents respect me like all other members in my family		Second-generation respondents	
		Number	Percentage
1	Disagree	15	15
2	Strongly disagree	01	01
3	Uncertain	06	06
4	Agree	78	78
5	Strongly agree	00	00
Total		100	100

I respect my children like all other members in my family		First-generation respondents	
		Number	Percentage
1	Disagree	00	00
2	Strongly disagree	00	00
3	Uncertain	14	14
4	Agree	86	86
5	Strongly agree	00	00
Total		100	100

The data in the above tables indicate that 78 percent of second-generation respondents and 86 percent of first-generation respondents agree that all members in their families are mutually respected.

Table 4 Perception about parents' traditionalism

I think my parents are too traditional		**Second-generation** *respondents*	
		Number	*Percentage*
1	Disagree	18	18
2	Strongly disagree	00	00
3	Uncertain	07	07
4	Agree	72	72
5	Strongly agree	03	03
Total		100	100
My children think that I am too traditional		**First-generation** *respondents*	
		Number	*Percentage*
1	Disagree	22	22
2	Strongly disagree	00	00
3	Uncertain	00	00
4	Agree	78	78
5	Strongly agree	00	00
Total		100	100

As per the above tables 75 percent of second-generation respondents agree or strongly agree that their parents are too traditional while 78 percent among first-generation also agrees that they are so.

Table 5   Children's ability to understand

My parents think their children don't understand as they do		Second-generation respondents	
		Number	Percentage
1	Disagree	04	04
2	Strongly disagree	00	00
3	Uncertain	00	00
4	Agree	68	68
5	Strongly agree	28	28
Total		100	100

I think my children don't understand everything as we their parents do		First-generation respondents	
		Number	Percentage
1	Disagree	16	16
2	Strongly disagree	00	00
3	Uncertain	00	00
4	Agree	84	84
5	Strongly agree	00	00
Total		100	100

According to the above tables, the large majority second-generation respondents (96 percent) agrees or strongly agrees that their parents think children don't understand as they do while 84 percent of first-generation respondents also agree with it.

Table 6   Children's right to express their opinion

I believe it is my right to say my opinion in the family or in the community		*Second-generation* respondents	
		Number	*Percentage*
1	Disagree	00	00
2	Strongly disagree	00	00
3	Uncertain	00	00
4	Agree	84	84
5	Strongly agree	16	16
Total		100	100

I believe my children have the right to share their opinion in the family or in the community		*First-generation* respondents	
		Number	*Percentage*
1	Disagree	09	09
2	Strongly disagree	00	00
3	Uncertain	16	16
4	Agree	75	75
5	Strongly agree	00	00
Total		100	100

As per the above table, all the second-generation respondents agree or strongly agree that it is their right to share their opinion in the family or in the community, while 75 percent of first-generation respondents also believe it is so.

Table 7 Children's knowledge to take care of themselves

I believe I have adequate knowledge to take care of myself		Second-generation respondents	
		Number	Percentage
1	Disagree	39	39
2	Strongly disagree	00	00
3	Uncertain	00	00
4	Agree	57	57
5	Strongly agree	04	04
Total		100	100

I believe that my children have adequate knowledge to take care of themselves		First-generation respondents	
		Number	Percentage
1	Disagree	85	85
2	Strongly Disagree	00	00
3	Uncertain	00	00
4	Agree	15	15
5	Strongly Agree	00	00
Total		100	100

Based on tables above, while 61 percent of second-generation respondents believe they have adequate knowledge to take care of themselves, only 15 percent of first-generation respondents believe so.

Table 8 Should children know everything in the family?

My parents believe that it is unnecessary for their children to know everything in the family		*Second-generation* respondents	
		Number	Percentage
1	Disagree	00	00
2	Strongly disagree	00	00
3	Uncertain	00	00
4	Agree	74	74
5	Strongly agree	26	26
Total		100	100

I don't think it is necessary for our children to know everything in the family		*First-generation* respondents	
		Number	Percentage
1	Disagree	06	06
2	Strongly disagree	00	00
3	Uncertain	00	00
4	Agree	04	04
5	Strongly agree	90	90
Total		100	100

Responding to the question regarding parents' attitude towards the need of children knowing *everything* that is going on in the family, all the 100 percent second-generation respondents agree that their parents believe it is unnecessary for their children to know everything in the family while 94 percent of first-generation respondents also agree that it is unnecessary for children to know everything in the family.

Table 9   Love languages/physical and verbal signs of affection

I think my parents don't show physical and verbal signs of affection		Second-generation respondents	
		Number	Percentage
1	Disagree	33	33
2	Strongly disagree	02	02
3	Uncertain	14	14
4	Agree	51	51
5	Strongly agree	00	00
Total		100	100

I show a lot of physical and verbal signs of affection (love languages)		First-generation respondents	
		Number	Percentage
1	Disagree	00	00
2	Strongly disagree	00	00
3	Uncertain	70	70
4	Agree	30	30
5	Strongly agree	00	00
Total		100	100

The data in the above tables reveal that while 51 percent of second-generation respondents agree that their parents don't show physical and verbal signs of affection, 30 percent of first-generation respondents agree and 70 percent are uncertain about it.

Table 10   Saving face in public

I believe my parents are too concerned with saving face in public		Second-generation respondents	
		Number	Percentage
1	Disagree	00	00
2	Strongly disagree	00	00
3	Uncertain	00	00
4	Agree	53	53
5	Strongly agree	47	47
Total		100	100

I am very concerned about saving my family's face in the community		First-generation respondents	
		Number	Percentage
1	Disagree	00	00
2	Strongly disagree	00	00
3	Uncertain	00	00
4	Agree	59	59
5	Strongly agree	41	41
Total		100	100

As per the above tables, while all the second-generation respondents agrees that their parents are too concerned about saving their face in public, all the first-generation respondents also agree that they are so.

Table 11 Parents' familiarity with American culture

I think my parents are not very familiar with the American culture		*Second-generation* respondents	
		Number	*Percentage*
1	Disagree	81	81
2	Strongly disagree	06	06
3	Uncertain	11	11
4	Agree	02	02
5	Strongly agree	00	00
Total		100	100
I think I am very familiar with the American Culture		*First-generation* respondents	
		Number	*Percentage*
1	Disagree	00	00
2	Strongly disagree	00	00
3	Uncertain	00	00
4	Agree	14	14
5	Strongly agree	86	86
Total		100	100

Data in the above tables show that a large majority second-generation respondent (87 percent) disagrees or strongly disagrees that their parents are familiar with the American culture while all the first-generation respondents agree or strongly agree with it.

Table 12   Parental expectation for children's behavior

My parents expect me to behave like a proper Indian male or female		**Second-generation** respondents	
		Number	Percentage
1	Disagree	00	00
2	Strongly disagree	00	00
3	Uncertain	00	00
4	Agree	81	81
5	Strongly agree	19	19
Total		100	100

I expect my children to behave like a proper Indian male or female		**First-generation** respondents	
		Number	Percentage
1	Disagree	00	00
2	Strongly disagree	00	00
3	Uncertain	08	08
4	Agree	92	92
5	Strongly agree	00	00
Total		100	100

The data in the above tables show that all the second-generation respondents agree or strongly agree that their parents expect them to behave like a proper or typical Indian male or female while 92 percent of first-generation respondents also agree with it.

Table 13   Parental demand for Children respecting elders

My parents demand that I should always show respect for elders		**Second-generation** *respondents*	
		Number	*Percentage*
1	Disagree	00	00
2	Strongly disagree	00	00
3	Uncertain	00	00
4	Agree	61	61
5	Strongly agree	39	39
Total		100	100

I expect my children to show respect for elders always		**First-generation** *Respondents*	
		Number	*Percentage*
1	Disagree	00	00
2	Strongly disagree	00	00
3	Uncertain	00	00
4	Agree	88	88
5	Strongly agree	12	12
Total		100	100

According to the above tables, while all the second-generation respondents agree that their parents demand them to show respect for elders, all the first-generation respondents also agree that their children should respect elders always.

Table 14 Perspective on respecting others

I believe those who deserve respect only should be respected		**Second-generation** *respondents*	
		Number	*Percentage*
1	Disagree	06	06
2	Strongly disagree	00	00
3	Uncertain	00	00
4	Agree	87	87
5	Strongly agree	07	07
Total		100	100
I believe that we should respect everyone older than us no matter who they are		**Second-generation** *respondents*	
		Number	*Percentage*
1	Disagree	00	00
2	Strongly disagree	00	00
3	Uncertain	13	13
4	Agree	68	68
5	Strongly agree	19	19
Total		100	100

As per the data in the above tables, while 94 percent of second-generation respondents agree or strongly agree that those who deserve respect only should be respected; 87 percent of first-generation respondents believe that everybody older than oneself should be respected no matter who they are. This is another sharp contradiction between the second and first-generation immigrants.

Table 15   Awareness of peer pressure in the school/workplace

My parents don't understand my peer pressure in the school/work place		Second-generation respondents	
		Number	Percentage
1	Disagree	43	43
2	Strongly disagree	00	00
3	Uncertain	51	51
4	Agree	06	06
5	Strongly agree	00	00
Total		100	100

I am aware of my children's peer pressure in the school/work place		First-generation respondents	
		Number	Percentage
1	Disagree	00	00
2	Strongly disagree	00	00
3	Uncertain	23	23
4	Agree	77	77
5	Strongly agree	00	00
Total		100	100

The above tables show that while 43 percent of second-generation respondents disagree that their parents don't understand their peer pressure in the school or at work, 77 percent among the first-generation immigrants agree that they are aware about their children's peer pressure in the school or at work.

Table 16 Parental control over phone conversation

My parents restrict me when I talk to my friends over the phone		*Second-generation* respondents	
		Number	Percentage
1	Disagree	65	65
2	Strongly disagree	00	00
3	Uncertain	00	00
4	Agree	35	35
5	Strongly agree	00	00
Total		100	100

I never restrict my children when they talk to their friends over the phone		*First-generation* respondents	
		Number	Percentage
1	Disagree	13	13
2	Strongly disagree	00	00
3	Uncertain	36	36
4	Agree	51	51
5	Strongly agree	00	00
Total		100	100

Based on the empirical data above, while 65 percent of second-generation respondents disagree that their parents restrict them when they talk to their friends over the phone, 51 percent of first-generation respondents agree that they never do so.

Table 17   Parental control over children choosing friends

My parents suggest who my friends should be		Second-generation respondents	
		Number	Percentage
1	Disagree	02	02
2	Strongly disagree	00	00
3	Uncertain	00	00
4	Agree	86	86
5	Strongly agree	12	12
Total		100	100

I never interfere in my children's decision of choosing friends		First-generation respondents	
		Number	Percentage
1	Disagree	92	92
2	Strongly disagree	08	08
3	Uncertain	00	00
4	Agree	00	00
5	Strongly agree	00	00
Total		100	100

The data in the above tables show that while 98 percent of second-generation respondents agree that their parents suggest who their friends should be, all the first-generation respondents disagree with the statement that they never interfere in their children's decision of choosing friends.

Table 18 Parental control over children choosing clothes

It is my parents who select my new clothes		*Second-generation respondents*	
		Number	*Percentage*
1	Disagree	32	32
2	Strongly disagree	01	01
3	Uncertain	00	00
4	Agree	67	67
5	Strongly agree	00	00
Total		100	100
I believe parents should have some control on selecting new clothes for children		*First-generation respondents*	
		Number	*Percentage*
1	Disagree	02	02
2	Strongly disagree	00	00
3	Uncertain	07	07
4	Agree	91	91
5	Strongly agree	00	00
Total		100	100

The above tables reveal that while 67 percent of second-generation respondents agree that their parents select clothes for them, 91 percent of first-generation respondents believes that parents should have some control when children selecting clothes for them.

Table 19   Parental expectation over children returning home everyday

My Parents insist me to return home every day on time		Second-generation respondents	
		Number	Percentage
1	Disagree	00	00
2	Strongly disagree	00	00
3	Uncertain	00	00
4	Agree	57	57
5	Strongly agree	43	43
Total		100	100

I expect my children to return home every day on time		First-generation respondents	
		Number	Percentage
1	Disagree	00	00
2	Strongly disagree	00	00
3	Uncertain	00	00
4	Agree	21	21
5	Strongly agree	79	79
Total		100	100

According to the above tables all the second-generation respondents agree that their parents insist that they return home every day on time, while all the parental respondents also agree that they do so.

Section 2: Communication, Mutual Acceptance and Respect to Cultural Values in the Family

The data in this section describe the communication pattern, mutual acceptance and respect for cultural values of two different generations living under the same roof.

Table 20   Quality conversational time between parents and children

My parents often spend quality conversational time with me		Second-generation respondents	
		Number	Percentage
1	Disagree	66	66
2	Strongly disagree	14	14
3	Uncertain	00	00
4	Agree	20	20
5	Strongly agree	00	00
Total		100	100

I often spend quality conversational time with my children		First-generation respondents	
		Number	Percentage
1	Disagree	07	07
2	Strongly disagree	00	00
3	Uncertain	54	54
4	Agree	39	39
5	Strongly agree	00	00
Total		100	100

Based on the above figures, while 20 percent of second-generation respondents agree that their parents spend quality conversational time with them 39 percent of first-generation respondents also agrees that they do so. However, the significant difference in the area of disagreement and uncertainty is noticeable. While 80 percent of second-generation respondents disagree or strongly disagree that their parents spend quality conversational time with them, 7 percent of first-generation respondents only disagree with this statement, though 54 percent of them are uncertain about it.

APPENDIX

Table 21 Active listening to communication

My parents actively listening to me when I talk to them		**Second-generation** *respondents*	
		Number	*Percentage*
1	Disagree	25	25
2	Strongly disagree	01	01
3	Uncertain	60	60
4	Agree	14	14
5	Strongly agree	00	00
Total		100	100

I actively listen to my children when they talk to me about something		**First-generation** *respondents*	
		Number	*Percentage*
1	Disagree	15	15
2	Strongly disagree	00	00
3	Uncertain	38	38
4	Agree	35	35
5	Strongly agree	12	12
Total		100	100

The above tables explain that while 14 percent of second-generation respondents agree that their parents actively listening to them, 47 percent of first-generation respondents agree or strongly agree with it.

Table 22 Dinner-time conversation

Mostly our dinner-time is a time for quality conversation		*Second-generation respondents*	
		Number	*Percentage*
1	Disagree	94	94
2	Strongly disagree	04	04
3	Uncertain	02	02
4	Agree	00	00
5	Strongly agree	00	00
Total		100	100

Mostly our dinner-time is a time for quality conversation		*First-generation respondents*	
		Number	*Percentage*
1	Disagree	82	82
2	Strongly disagree	07	07
3	Uncertain	11	11
4	Agree	00	00
5	Strongly agree	00	00
Total		100	100

According to the above data, 98 percent of second-generation respondents and 89 percent of first-generation respondents disagree or strongly disagree with the statement that their dinnertime is a time for quality conversation.

Table 23 Parents encouraging children to ask questions

My parents encourage me to ask questions to them		**Second-generation** *respondents*	
		Number	*Percentage*
1	Disagree	86	86
2	Strongly disagree	00	00
3	Uncertain	02	02
4	Agree	12	12
5	Strongly agree	00	00
Total		100	100

I encourage children to ask questions to their parents		**First-generation** *respondents*	
		Number	*Percentage*
1	Disagree	01	01
2	Strongly disagree	00	00
3	Uncertain	65	65
4	Agree	34	34
5	Strongly agree	00	00
Total		100	100

The above data show that while 12 percent of second-generation respondents agree that their parents encourage them to ask questions, 34 percent of first-generation respondents agree that they do so.

Table 24 Free and outgoing parents to associate with

My parents are very free and outgoing to associate with		Second-generation respondents	
		Number	Percentage
1	Disagree	63	63
2	Strongly disagree	04	04
3	Uncertain	00	00
4	Agree	33	33
5	Strongly agree	00	00
Total		100	100

I am very free and outgoing to associate with my children		First-generation respondents	
		Number	Percentage
1	Disagree	00	00
2	Strongly disagree	00	00
3	Uncertain	73	73
4	Agree	27	27
5	Strongly agree	00	00
Total		100	100

The data in the above tables indicate that while 33 percent of second-generation respondents agree that their parents are free and outgoing to associate with, only 27 percent among the first-generation respondents agrees with it.

Table 25   Perspective on inter-racial marriage

My parents are positive about inter-racial marriage		Second-generation respondents	
		Number	Percentage
1	Disagree	49	49
2	Strongly disagree	51	51
3	Uncertain	00	00
4	Agree	00	00
5	Strongly agree	00	00
Total		100	100

I am very positive about inter-racial marriage		First-generation respondents	
		Number	Percentage
1	Disagree	15	15
2	Strongly disagree	85	85
3	Uncertain	00	00
4	Agree	00	00
5	Strongly agree	00	00
Total		100	100

The data in the above tables reveal that while all the 100 percent second-generation respondents disagree or strongly disagree that the parental generation are positive towards the inter-racial marriages, all first-generation respondents also disagree with it.

Table 26   Talk about kissing, hugging, sex, marriage etc.

My parents talk about kissing, hugging, sex, marriage etc., with their children		*Second-generation respondents*	
		Number	Percentage
1	Disagree	78	78
2	Strongly disagree	22	22
3	Uncertain	00	00
4	Agree	00	00
5	Strongly agree	00	00
Total		100	100

I usually talk about kissing, hugging, sex, marriage etc., with our children		*Second-generation respondents*	
		Number	Percentage
1	Disagree	95	95
2	Strongly disagree	05	05
3	Uncertain	00	00
4	Agree	00	00
5	Strongly agree	00	00
Total		100	100

As per the above tables, all the respondents among both second-generation and first-generation immigrants disagree or strongly disagree that there is open communication about kissing, hugging, sex, marriage etc., between parents and children.

Table 27   Understanding on autonomy and interdependence

My parents consider that individual autonomy (independence) is bad		Second-generation respondents	
		Number	Percentage
1	Disagree	00	00
2	Strongly disagree	00	00
3	Uncertain	00	00
4	Agree	74	74
5	Strongly agree	26	26
Total		100	100

I consider interdependence is better than individual autonomy (independence)		Second-generation respondents	
		Number	Percentage
1	Disagree	00	00
2	Strongly disagree	00	00
3	Uncertain	00	00
4	Agree	35	35
5	Strongly agree	65	65
Total		100	100

According to the above tables, while all second-generation respondents agree or strongly agree that their parents consider individual autonomy as bad, all the first-generation respondents agree or strongly agree that interdependence is better than individual autonomy.

Table 28   Concept on talking back

My parents consider talking back is definitely disrespectful		*Second-generation* respondents	
		Number	*Percentage*
1	Disagree	00	00
2	Strongly disagree	00	00
3	Uncertain	00	00
4	Agree	53	53
5	Strongly agree	47	47
Total		100	100

Talking back to parents or older people is definitely disrespectful		*First-generation* respondents	
		Number	*Percentage*
1	Disagree	00	00
2	Strongly disagree	00	00
3	Uncertain	00	00
4	Agree	80	80
5	Strongly agree	20	20
Total		100	100

The above tables explain that while all the second-generation respondents agree/strongly agree that their parents consider back talking to parents or elders is definitely disrespectful, all the first-generation respondents also agree or strongly agree with it.

Table 29   Expectation of being obedient

My parents believe that their children should obey them in all things		Second-generation respondents	
		Number	Percentage
1	Disagree	00	00
2	Strongly disagree	00	00
3	Uncertain	00	00
4	Agree	77	77
5	Strongly agree	23	23
Total		100	100

Children are supposed to obey their parents in all things		First-generation respondents	
		Number	Percentage
1	Disagree	00	00
2	Strongly disagree	00	00
3	Uncertain	00	00
4	Agree	100	100
5	Strongly agree	00	00
Total		100	100

The above tables indicate that all the second-generation and first-generationrespondents agree or strongly agree that the parental generation expect their children to obey them in all things.

Table 30   Expectation to avoid shame on the family

My parents expect me not to bring shame on my family		*Second-generation* respondents	
		Number	*Percentage*
1	Disagree	00	00
2	Strongly disagree	00	00
3	Uncertain	00	00
4	Agree	45	45
5	Strongly agree	55	55
Total		100	100

I always expect my children not to bring shame on my family		*First-generation* respondents	
		Number	*Percentage*
1	Disagree	00	00
2	Strongly disagree	00	00
3	Uncertain	00	00
4	Agree	25	25
5	Strongly agree	75	75
Total		100	100

As per the above tables, while all the second-generation respondents agree or strongly agree that their parents expect them not to bring shame on their family, all the first-generation respondents also agree or strongly agree with it.

Table 31   Parental control in decision-making

My parents tell me what to do with my life while I want to make my own decisions		*Second-generation* respondents	
		Number	Percentage
1	Disagree	05	05
2	Strongly disagree	00	00
3	Uncertain	05	05
4	Agree	90	90
5	Strongly agree	00	00
Total		100	100

I often advise my children what to do with their life		*First-generation* respondents	
		Number	Percentage
1	Disagree	00	00
2	Strongly disagree	00	00
3	Uncertain	00	00
4	Agree	95	95
5	Strongly agree	05	05
Total		100	100

Regarding parental control in decision-making, while 90 percent of second-generation respondents agree that their parents advise them what to do with their life when they want to make their own decisions, all the first-generation respondents also agree or strongly agree that they often advise their children what to do with their life.

Table 32   Parental control on social life

My parents tell me that a social life is not very important at this age, though I think it is		**Second-generation** *respondents*	
		Number	*Percentage*
1	Disagree	31	31
2	Strongly disagree	00	00
3	Uncertain	65	65
4	Agree	04	04
5	Strongly agree	00	00
Total		100	100

I think a social life is not very important at the age of 18, 19, 20		**First-generation** *respondents*	
		Number	*Percentage*
1	Disagree	37	37
2	Strongly disagree	00	00
3	Uncertain	00	00
4	Agree	63	63
5	Strongly agree	00	00
Total		100	100

The data in the above tables describe that while a minority of 4 percent of second-generation respondents agree that their parents tell them a social life is not very important at their present age, 63 percent of first-generation respondents think a social life is not very important at the age of 18, 19, 20 for their children.

Table 33   Academic expectation

My parents' academic expectations always exceed my performance		Second-generation respondents	
		Number	Percentage
1	Disagree	34	34
2	Strongly disagree	00	00
3	Uncertain	00	00
4	Agree	63	63
5	Strongly agree	03	03
Total		100	100

My academic expectation about my children is always high		First-generation respondents	
		Number	Percentage
1	Disagree	00	00
2	Strongly disagree	00	00
3	Uncertain	00	00
4	Agree	69	69
5	Strongly agree	31	31
Total		100	100

While a significant majority of second-generation respondents (66 percent) believe that their parents' academic expectation always exceeds their performance, all the first-generation respondents also agree or strongly agree that they have a high academic expectation about their children.

Table 34   Fairness of sacrificing personal interest for family

I believe it is unfair to sacrifice personal interest for the sake of family interest		**Second-generation** respondents	
		Number	*Percentage*
1	Disagree	08	08
2	Strongly disagree	00	00
3	Uncertain	00	00
4	Agree	88	88
5	Strongly agree	04	04
Total		100	100
Sacrificing personal interest for the sake of family interest is not unfair		**First-generation** respondents	
		Number	*Percentage*
1	Disagree	00	00
2	Strongly disagree	00	00
3	Uncertain	00	00
4	Agree	80	80
5	Strongly agree	20	20
Total		100	100

As per the above tables, while 92 percent of second-generation respondents agree or strongly agree that it is unfair to sacrifice personal interest for the sake of family interest, all the first-generation respondents agree or strongly agree that is not unfair.

Table 35 Need for unconditional acceptance

I need my parents to accept me for being myself		**Second-generation** *respondents*	
		Number	*Percentage*
1	Disagree	00	00
2	Strongly disagree	00	00
3	Uncertain	00	00
4	Agree	87	87
5	Strongly agree	13	13
Total		100	100

I accept my children for being whatever they are		**First-generation** *respondents*	
		Number	*Percentage*
1	Disagree	00	00
2	Strongly disagree	00	00
3	Uncertain	30	30
4	Agree	70	70
5	Strongly agree	00	00
Total		100	100

Responding to question regarding unconditional acceptance from parents, while all the second-generation respondents agree or strongly agree that their parents need to accept them as whatever they are, only 70 percent of first-generation respondents accept their children for whatever they are.

Table 36 Preference of the kind of love

I prefer love with more physical and verbal signs of affection to mere housing, feeding, educating and meeting material needs		Second-generation respondents	
		Number	Percentage
1	Disagree	00	00
2	Strongly disagree	00	00
3	Uncertain	00	00
4	Agree	89	89
5	Strongly agree	11	11
Total		100	100

Meeting educational and material needs of my children are more important than showing mere love language		First-generation respondents	
		Number	Percentage
1	Disagree	73 (39* both)	73
2	Strongly disagree	00	00
3	Uncertain	00	00
4	Agree	27	27
5	Strongly agree	00	00
Total		100	100

Based on the above tables while all the second-generation respondents prefer love with more physical and verbal signs to mere housing, feeding, educating, and meeting material needs, 73 percent of first-generation respondents disagree with this. However, 39 respondents out of this 73 percent scribbled in a little space found at the end of the question that both are equally important.

Table 37 Entering into bed-/study-rooms without permission

I am OK with my parents entering into my room without my permission		Second-generation respondents	
		Number	Percentage
1	Disagree	78	78
2	Strongly disagree	19	19
3	Uncertain	00	00
4	Agree	03	03
5	Strongly agree	00	00
Total		100	100

I don't wait for the permission of my children to enter into their rooms		First-generation respondents	
		Number	Percentage
1	Disagree	21	21
2	Strongly disagree	00	00
3	Uncertain	22	22
4	Agree	57	57
5	Strongly agree	00	00
Total		100	100

As per the above data while 3 percent of second-generation respondents agree that they are OK with their parents entering into their room without their permission, 57 percent of first-generation respondents agree that they don't wait for their children's permission to enter into their rooms.

Table 38   Parents' complaining about children talking to opposite genders

My parents complain when I talk to my male/female friends		Second-generation respondents	
		Number	Percentage
1	Disagree	13	13
2	Strongly disagree	00	00
3	Uncertain	00	00
4	Agree	77	77
5	Strongly agree	10	10
Total		100	100

It's OK for children talking long time on the phone with their male/female friends		First-generation respondents	
		Number	Percentage
1	Disagree	88	88
2	Strongly disagree	00	00
3	Uncertain	00	00
4	Agree	12	12
5	Strongly agree	00	00
Total		100	100

Regarding children talking to opposite-gender friends; while 87 percent of second-generation respondents disagree that their parents are OK about children talking long time on the phone with their male/female friends, 88 percent of first-generation respondents also agree that they are not OK with it.

Table 39 Issue of dating Indians or non-Indians

My parents never encourage dating either Indians or non-Indians		**Second-generation** *respondents*	
		Number	*Percentage*
1	Disagree	00	00
2	Strongly disagree	00	00
3	Uncertain	00	00
4	Agree	54	54
5	Strongly agree	46	46
Total		100	100
I don't encourage my children dating either Indians or non-Indians		**First-generation** *respondents*	
		Number	*Percentage*
1	Disagree	00	00
2	Strongly disagree	00	00
3	Uncertain	00	00
4	Agree	73	73
5	Strongly agree	27	27
Total		100	100

According to the above data, all the second-generation respondents agree or strongly agree that they are not encouraged to date either Indians or non-Indians while all the first-generation respondents also agree or strongly agree that they don't encourage it.

Table 40   Encouragement to speak Indian vernacular at home

My parents encourage me to speak Indian vernacular at home		Second-generation respondents	
		Number	Percentage
1	Disagree	06	06
2	Strongly disagree	01	01
3	Uncertain	14	14
4	Agree	79	79
5	Strongly agree	00	00
Total		100	100

I encourage children speaking Indian vernacular at home		First-generation respondents	
		Number	Percentage
1	Disagree	00	00
2	Strongly disagree	00	00
3	Uncertain	17	17
4	Agree	83	83
5	Strongly agree	00	00
Total		100	100

As per the empirical data above, 79 percent of second-generation respondents and 83 percent of first-generation respondents agree that parents encourage children to speak Indian vernacular at home.

Table 41   Parents who make decision for their children

My parents decide major things (e.g., education, career, spouse etc.) for me		**Second-generation** *respondents*	
		Number	*Percentage*
1	Disagree	00	00
2	Strongly disagree	00	00
3	Uncertain	00	00
4	Agree	98	98
5	Strongly agree	02	02
Total		100	100

I usually decide major things like education, career, spouse etc., for my children		**First-generation** *respondents*	
		Number	*Percentage*
1	Disagree	00	00
2	Strongly disagree	12	12
3	Uncertain	33	33
4	Agree	55	55
5	Strongly agree	00	00
Total		100	100

According to the above tables, while all the second-generation respondents agree that it is their parents who make decisions on major things such as education, career, and spouse, only 55 percent of first-generation respondents agree with this. However, 48 out of these 55 percent are the fathers based on the gender indicated in the questionnaire.

Table 42 Feeling of children being parents' property

I often think that I am my parents' property		*Second-generation respondents*	
		Number	*Percentage*
1	Disagree	00	00
2	Strongly disagree	94	94
3	Uncertain	06	06
4	Agree	00	00
5	Strongly agree	00	00
Total		100	100
I don't think children are parents' property		*First-generation respondents*	
		Number	*Percentage*
1	Disagree	00	00
2	Strongly disagree	00	00
3	Uncertain	00	00
4	Agree	100	100
5	Strongly agree	00	00
Total		100	100

Responding to the question regarding feeling of children being parents' property, all the respondents among both second and first-generation immigrants agree that they don't believe children are parents' property.

Table 43   Language difference and communication difficulty at home

Communication with my parents is often difficult due to language differences		Second-generation respondents	
		Number	Percentage
1	Disagree	98	98
2	Strongly disagree	01	01
3	Uncertain	01	01
4	Agree	00	00
5	Strongly agree	00	00
Total		100	100

Communication with my children is not difficult because there is language differences		First-generation respondents	
		Number	Percentage
1	Disagree	00	00
2	Strongly disagree	00	00
3	Uncertain	00	00
4	Agree	100	100
5	Strongly agree	00	00
Total		100	100

Based on the above data, 99 percent of second-generation respondents and all the first-generation respondents agree that there is no communication difficulty between parents and children due to language difference.

Table 44   Gender discrimination in everyday life

My parents treat me differently because of my gender		**Second-generation** *respondents*	
		Number	*Percentage*
1	Disagree	68	68
2	Strongly disagree	00	00
3	Uncertain	31	31
4	Agree	01	01
5	Strongly agree	00	00
Total		100	100

I don't treat my children differently because of their gender difference		**First-generation** *respondents*	
		Number	*Percentage*
1	Disagree	00	00
2	Strongly disagree	00	00
3	Uncertain	08	08
4	Agree	92	92
5	Strongly agree	00	00
Total		100	100

According to the above figures, while 68 percent of second-generation respondents disagree that they are discriminated at home due to gender difference, 92 percent of first-generation respondents agree that they do not treat their children differently based on gender.

Table 45   Linking education success with life success

My parents link education successes with my life success		Second-generation respondents	
		Number	Percentage
1	Disagree	00	00
2	Strongly disagree	00	00
3	Uncertain	00	00
4	Agree	62	62
5	Strongly agree	38	38
Total		100	100

I think education success is a major part of life success		First-generation respondents	
		Number	Percentage
1	Disagree	00	00
2	Strongly disagree	00	00
3	Uncertain	00	00
4	Agree	12	12
5	Strongly agree	88	88
Total		100	100

The above tables describe that all the second-generation respondents agree or strongly agree that their parents link education success with life's success, while all the first-generation respondents also agree or strongly agree that education success is a major part of life success.

Table 46 Judging/disciplining based on Indian standards

My parents judge me based on their Indian standards		Second-generation respondents	
		Number	Percentage
1	Disagree	00	00
2	Strongly disagree	00	00
3	Uncertain	00	00
4	Agree	96	96
5	Strongly agree	04	04
Total		100	100

I discipline my children based on my understanding of child rearing		First-generation respondents	
		Number	Percentage
1	Disagree	00	00
2	Strongly disagree	00	00
3	Uncertain	04	04
4	Agree	96	96
5	Strongly agree	00	00
Total		100	100

According to the above data, while all the second-generation respondents agree or strongly agree that their parents judge them based on Indian standards, 96 percent of first-generation respondents agree that they discipline their children based on their Indian understanding of child rearing.

Table 47   Parental approval for kissing or making love in public

My parents do not approve kissing or making love in public with my boy/girl friend		**Second-generation** respondents	
		Number	*Percentage*
1	Disagree	00	00
2	Strongly disagree	00	00
3	Uncertain	00	00
4	Agree	77	77
5	Strongly agree	23	23
Total		100	100

I don't encourage children kissing and making love with their boy/girlfriend in public		**First-generation** respondents	
		Number	*Percentage*
1	Disagree	00	00
2	Strongly disagree	00	00
3	Uncertain	00	00
4	Agree	80	80
5	Strongly agree	20	20
Total		100	100

The data in the above tables indicate that all the second-generation respondents agree or strongly agree that parents do not approve children kissing or making love with their boy/girlfriend in public, while all the first-generation respondents also agree with it.

Table 48   Restrictions on hanging out with friends

My parents hardly allow me to hang out with my friends		*Second-generation respondents*	
		Number	*Percentage*
1	Disagree	52	52
2	Strongly disagree	00	00
3	Uncertain	00	00
4	Agree	47	47
5	Strongly agree	01	01
Total		100	100

I don't restrict my children hanging out with their friends		*First-generation respondents*	
		Number	*Percentage*
1	Disagree	23	23
2	Strongly disagree	00	00
3	Uncertain	30	30
4	Agree	47	47
5	Strongly agree	00	00
Total		100	100

The above data indicate that 48 percent of second-generation respondents agree or strongly agree that their parents hardly allow them to hang out with their friends, while 47 percent of first-generation respondents agree that they don't restrict children to hang out with their friends.

Table 49   Parents re-living their childhood through children

I think my parents seem to live their childhood life through their children		Second-generation respondents	
		Number	Percentage
1	Disagree	05	05
2	Strongly disagree	00	00
3	Uncertain	00	00
4	Agree	90	90
5	Strongly agree	05	05
Total		100	100

It makes me happy when I provide things that I could not enjoy in my childhood to my children		First-generation respondents	
		Number	Percentage
1	Disagree	00	00
2	Strongly disagree	00	00
3	Uncertain	00	00
4	Agree	74	74
5	Strongly agree	26	26
Total		100	100

According to the above data while all the second-generation respondents agree or strongly agree that their parents live their childhood through their children, the response received from all the first-generation respondents also support this idea.

Section 3: (Over)Emphasis on the Ethnic Culture

The data in this section helps us to understand how ethnic culture is emphasized or overemphasized in the family where different generations are living together.

Table 50   Emphasis on Indian culture/lifestyle

I am told that the Indian culture/lifestyle is the best		Second-generation respondents	
		Number	Percentage
1	Never	00	00
2	Rarely	02	02
3	Occasionally	41	41
4	Always	57	57
Total		100	100

I think Indian culture and lifestyle is the best		First-generation respondents	
		Number	Percentage
1	Never	00	00
2	Rarely	00	00
3	Occasionally	39	39
4	Always	61	61
Total		100	100

Based on the above data, while 57 percent of second-generation respondents have been always told that Indian culture and lifestyle is the best, 61 percent of first-generation respondents always believe it is so.

Table 51   Advise to maintain Indian culture at home and in community

I am always advised to maintain the Indian culture at home and in the community		**Second-generation** *respondents*	
		Number	Percentage
1	Never	00	00
2	Rarely	00	00
3	Occasionally	50	50
4	Always	50	50
Total		100	100
I advise my children to maintain the Indian culture at home and in the community		**First-generation** *respondents*	
		Number	Percentage
1	Never	00	00
2	Rarely	00	00
3	Occasionally	29	29
4	Always	71	71
Total		100	100

As per the above tables 50 percent of second-generation respondents always, and the other 50 percent occasionally, are advised to maintain Indian culture at home and in the community, while 71 percent of first-generation respondents always and 29 percent occasionally advise their children to do so.

Table 52 Spiritual belief and dating

I am taught that dating is against my spiritual belief and faith tradition		**Second-generation** *respondents*	
		Number	Percentage
1	Never	02	02
2	Rarely	33	33
3	Occasionally	24	24
4	Always	41	41
Total		100	100

I believe dating is against my spiritual belief and faith tradition		**First-generation** *respondents*	
		Number	Percentage
1	Never	00	00
2	Rarely	33	33
3	Occasionally	36	36
4	Always	41	41
Total		100	100

The data in the above tables reveal that 41 percent of second-generation respondents always and 24 percent occasionally are taught dating is against their spiritual belief and faith tradition while 41 percent of first-generation respondents always, and 36 percent occasionally, believe that dating is against their spiritual belief and faith tradition.

Table 53 Parents' belief about American culture

My parents believe that American culture is very loose and lack parental control		Second-generation respondents	
		Number	Percentage
1	Never	00	00
2	Rarely	02	02
3	Occasionally	42	42
4	Always	56	56
Total		100	100

I think American culture is very loose and lack parental control		First-generation respondents	
		Number	Percentage
1	Never	00	00
2	Rarely	04	04
3	Occasionally	69	69
4	Always	27	27
Total		100	100

According to second-generation immigrants, 56 percent of their parents always and 42 percent occasionally think American culture is very loose and lack parental control while 27 percent of first generation parents always and 69 percent occasionally believe that it is so.

Table 54   Ideas about Indian dress code

My parents believe that the Indian dress code is the modest way of dressing		**Second-generation** *respondents*	
		Number	*Percentage*
1	Never	02	02
2	Rarely	35	35
3	Occasionally	47	47
4	Always	16	16
Total		100	100

I believe that the Indian dress code is the modest way of dressing		**First-generation** *respondents*	
		Number	*Percentage*
1	Never	00	00
2	Rarely	48	48
3	Occasionally	43	43
4	Always	09	09
Total		100	100

Based on the response of second-generation immigrants, 16 percent of their parents always, and 47 percent occasionally, believe that Indian dress code is the modest way of dressing, while 9 percent first-generation respondents always and 43 percent occasionally believe it is so.

Table 55 Concept of individual autonomy and independence

My parents believe Individual autonomy and independence is Western and unhealthy		Second-generation respondents	
		Number	Percentage
1	Never	00	00
2	Rarely	02	02
3	Occasionally	27	27
4	Always	71	71
Total		100	100
In my understanding, Individual autonomy and independence is western and not very healthy		First-generation respondents	
		Number	Percentage
1	Never	00	00
2	Rarely	00	00
3	Occasionally	03	03
4	Always	97	97
Total		100	100

As per the above data while 71 percent of second-generation respondents always, and 27 percent occasionally, agree that their parents believe individual autonomy & independence is Western and unhealthy, 97 percent of first-generation respondents always and 3 percent occasionally believe that it is so.

Table 56   Understanding about American culture

My parents think American culture is very good to practice for their children		Second-generation respondents	
		Number	Percentage
1	Never	55	55
2	Rarely	45	45
3	Occasionally	00	00
4	Always	00	00
Total		100	100

I think American culture is very healthy and good to practice for my family		First-generation respondents	
		Number	Percentage
1	Never	36	36
2	Rarely	64	64
3	Occasionally	00	00
4	Always	00	00
Total		100	100

The above tables showe that 55 percent of second-generation respondents never, and 45 percent rarely, think their parents believe that American culture is very good to practice for their children while 36 percent first-generation respondents and 64 percent rarely think it is so.

Table 57   Response to sex-education curriculum used in US public schools

My parents are happy about the sex-education curriculum used in the US Public Schools		Second-generation respondents	
		Number	Percentage
1	Never	61	61
2	Rarely	39	39
3	Occasionally	00	00
4	Always	00	00
Total		100	100

I am happy about the sex-education curriculum used in the US Public Schools		First-generation respondents	
		Number	Percentage
1	Never	69	69
2	Rarely	31	31
3	Occasionally	00	00
4	Always	00	00
Total		100	100

According to the observation of the second-generation respondents 61 percent of their parents never, and 39 percent rarely, are happy about the sex-education curriculum used in the United States Public Schools, while 69 percent of first-generation respondents never, and 31 percent rarely, are happy about it.

Table 58   Parents comparing their children with other Indian kids

My parents compare me with the other Indian kids around us		**Second-generation** *respondents*	
		Number	Percentage
1	Never	11	11
2	Rarely	67	67
3	Occasionally	18	18
4	Always	04	04
Total		100	100

I often compare my children with other Indian kids around us		**First-generation** *respondents*	
		Number	Percentage
1	Never	03	03
2	Rarely	83	83
3	Occasionally	14	14
4	Always	00	00
Total		100	100

The data in the above tables reveal that 4 percent of second-generation respondents always, and 18 percent occasionally, are compared with other Indian kids around them, while 14 percent of first-generation respondents occasionally do so.

Table 59   Response to children marrying non-Indians

My parents have no problem if I marry a non-Indian male or female		**Second-generation** *respondents*	
		Number	Percentage
1	Never	96	96
2	Rarely	04	04
3	Occasionally	00	00
4	Always	00	00
Total		100	100

I am Okay if my children marry a non-Indian male or female		**First-generation** *respondents*	
		Number	Percentage
1	Never	91	91
2	Rarely	09	09
3	Occasionally	00	00
4	Always	00	00
Total		100	100

According to the above table 96 percent of second-generation respondents think their parents will never have no problem (meaning always will have a problem) if they marry a non-Indian male or female, while 91 percent of first-generation respondents agree that they are never okay if their children marry a non-Indian male or female.

Table 60 Low divorce rate and Indian culture

My parents believe that the low divorce rate among Indians is because of the Indian culture		**Second-generation** respondents	
		Number	*Percentage*
1	Never	00	00
2	Rarely	00	00
3	Occasionally	10	10
4	Always	90	90
Total		100	100

I believe that the low divorce rate among Indians is because of the Indian culture		**Second-generation** respondents	
		Number	*Percentage*
1	Never	00	00
2	Rarely	00	00
3	Occasionally	00	00
4	Always	100	100
Total		100	100

As per the observation of the second-generation respondents 90 percent of them always, and 10 percent occasionally, think their parents believe that the low divorce rate among Indians is because of Indian culture, while all the first-generation respondents believe that it is so.

Table 61   Parental desire to send children back to India during their teenage years

If there were some opportunities my parents would have sent me back to India during my teen age		Second-generation respondents	
		Number	Percentage
1	Never	00	00
2	Rarely	06	06
3	Occasionally	50	50
4	Always	44	44
Total		100	100

I Prefer/preferred to send my children back to India during their teen age		First-generation respondents	
		Number	Percentage
1	Never	00	00
2	Rarely	07	07
3	Occasionally	39	39
4	Always	54	54
Total		100	100

Responding to the question regarding cultural conflicts and teen age issues, 44 percent of second-generation respondents always, and 50 percent occasionally, think their parents would have sent them back to India during their teen age if there were some opportunities to do so, while 54 percent of first-generation respondents always, and 39 percent occasionally, preferred to send their children back to India during their teen age.

Table 62 Encouragement for dating

My parents encourage me for dating		*Second-generation* respondents	
		Number	Percentage
1	Never	93	93
2	Rarely	07	07
3	Occasionally	00	00
4	Always	00	00
Total		100	100
I encourage my children for dating		*First-generation* respondents	
		Number	Percentage
1	Never	96	96
2	Rarely	04	04
3	Occasionally	00	00
4	Always	00	00
Total		100	100

The above tables indicate that 93 percent of second-generation respondents never, and 7 percent rarely, are encouraged by their parents to date, while 96 percent of first-generation respondents never and 4 percent rarely encourage their children for dating.

Table 63   Preference of American food to Indian food

I prefer American food to Indian food		Second-generation respondents	
		Number	Percentage
1	Never	00	00
2	Rarely	00	00
3	Occasionally	12	12
4	Always	88	88
Total		100	100
I prefer American food to Indian food		First-generation respondents	
		Number	Percentage
1	Never	00	00
2	Rarely	23	23
3	Occasionally	77	77
4	Always	00	00
Total		100	100

Based on the above response, 88 percent of second-generation respondents always, and the remaining 12 percent occasionally, prefer American food to Indian, while none of the first-generation respondents always prefer American food, though 77 percent occasionally prefer it.

Table 64   Better country to live with sufficient money

My parents believe that if there is sufficient money, India is the better place to live		Second-generation respondents	
		Number	Percentage
1	Never	00	00
2	Rarely	00	00
3	Occasionally	09	09
4	Always	91	91
Total		100	100

I think India is better than US to live in if there is sufficient money		First-generation respondents	
		Number	Percentage
1	Never	00	00
2	Rarely	00	00
3	Occasionally	06	06
4	Always	94	94
Total		100	100

The data in the above tables indicate that a vast majority of second-generation respondents (91 percent) observes that their parents always think India is better than the United States to live if there is sufficient money, while 94 percent of first-generation respondents also always think it is so.

Table 65   Parental community's attitude towards American culture

My parental community is too judgmental about American Culture		Second-generation respondents	
		Number	Percentage
1	Never	00	00
2	Rarely	04	04
3	Occasionally	87	87
4	Always	09	09
Total		100	100

Indian Community is not very judgmental about American Culture		First-generation respondents	
		Number	Percentage
1	Never	00	00
2	Rarely	18	18
3	Occasionally	80	80
4	Always	02	02
Total		100	100

According to the above data, 87 percent of second-generation respondents observe that their parental community is occasionally too judgmental about American Culture, while 80 percent of first-generation respondents also agree that they are occasionally doing so.

Table 66   Parents and second-generationimmigrants

I believe that the second-generation Indian immigrants different from their parents		Second-generation respondents	
		Number	Percentage
1	Never	00	00
2	Rarely	00	00
3	Occasionally	21	21
4	Always	79	79
Total		100	100
I believe that the second generation Indian immigrants different from their parents		First-generation respondents	
		Number	Percentage
1	Never	00	00
2	Rarely	02	02
3	Occasionally	55	55
4	Always	43	43
Total		100	100

While 79 percent of second-generation respondents always believe that they are different from their parents, only 43 percent of the parental generation always believe so.

Table 67   Emphasis on Indian cultural values and traditions

My parents put too much emphasis on Indian cultural values and traditions		Second-generation respondents	
		Number	Percentage
1	Never	00	00
2	Rarely	18	18
3	Occasionally	21	21
4	Always	61	61
Total		100	100

I don't put too much emphasis on Indian cultural values and traditions		First-generation respondents	
		Number	Percentage
1	Never	00	00
2	Rarely	73	73
3	Occasionally	16	16
4	Always	11	11
Total		100	100

According to the data in the above tables, while 61 percent of second-generation respondents observe that their parents put too much emphasis on Indian cultural values and traditions, 73 percent of first-generation respondents agree that they rarely don't put (means always do) put too much emphasis on Indian cultural values and traditions, which agrees with the meaning of the second-generation's response.

Section 4: Intergenerational Conflict and Family/Individual Functionality

The data in this section help us to understand the intergenerational conflict and individual and/or family functionality among the Indian immigrant community living in the multiple cultural spaces of the United States.

Table 68   Family clash and back answering

Whenever there is a clash with my parents/grandparents, I talk back to them		*Second-generation* respondents	
		Number	*Percentage*
1	Disagree	28	28
2	Strongly disagree	00	00
3	Uncertain	00	00
4	Agree	66	66
5	Strongly agree	06	06
Total		100	100
My children back-answer to me whenever I confront them		*First-generation* respondents	
		Number	*Percentage*
1	Disagree	26	26
2	Strongly disagree	00	00
3	Uncertain	15	15
4	Agree	59	59
5	Strongly agree	00	00
Total		100	100

As per the above empirical data, while 72 percent of second-generation respondents agree that they talk back to their parents/grandparents, only 59 percent of first-generation respondents agree.

Table 69   Response when imposing something onto children

I quietly ignore my parents/grandparents when they try to impose something on me		Second-generation respondents	
		Number	Percentage
1	Disagree	48	48
2	Strongly disagree	00	00
3	Uncertain	06	06
4	Agree	42	42
5	Strongly agree	04	04
Total		100	100

My children quietly ignore me when I try to discipline them		First-generation respondents	
		Number	Percentage
1	Disagree	00	00
2	Strongly disagree	00	00
3	Uncertain	16	16
4	Agree	84	84
5	Strongly agree	00	00
Total		100	100

From the above tables, it is evident that while 46 percent of second-generation respondents ignore their parents/grandparents when imposing their cultural values on them, 84 percent of first-generation respondents agree that children do so when they try to discipline them. (This is an effort by parents to impress outsiders that their children are submissive and good.)

Table 70   Parental expectation to obey them

My parents/grant parents expect me to obey them whenever there is a clash with them		**Second-generation** *respondents*	
		Number	Percentage
1	Disagree	00	00
2	Strongly disagree	00	00
3	Uncertain	00	00
4	Agree	58	58
5	Strongly agree	42	42
Total		100	100

I expect my children to obey me whenever there is a clash with them		**First-generation** *respondents*	
		Number	Percentage
1	Disagree	00	00
2	Strongly disagree	00	00
3	Uncertain	00	00
4	Agree	66	66
5	Strongly agree	34	34
Total		100	100

According to the above figures, while all the second-generation respondents agree (58 percent) or strongly agree (42 percent) that their parents/grandparents expect them to obey them when there is a clash at home, all the first-generation respondents also agree that they expect the same from their children.

Table 71 Yelling and shouting ar second-generation

| *My parents yell and shout at me* | | *Second-generation* respondents | |
		Number	*Percentage*
1	Disagree	20	20
2	Strongly disagree	00	00
3	Uncertain	45	45
4	Agree	32	32
5	Strongly agree	03	03
Total		100	100

| *Occasionally I am forced to yell and shout at my children* | | *First-generation* respondents | |
		Number	*Percentage*
1	Disagree	10	10
2	Strongly disagree	00	00
3	Uncertain	52	52
4	Agree	38	38
5	Strongly agree	00	00
Total		100	100

The above tables explain that while 35 percent of second-generation respondents agree that their parents yell and shout at them, 38 percent of first-generation respondents also agree that they are occasionally forced to do so.

Table 72   Isolating oneself after every family fight

I lock myself in my room after a fight with my parents/grand parents		**Second-generation** *respondents*	
		Number	*Percentage*
1	Disagree	12	12
2	Strongly disagree	00	00
3	Uncertain	02	02
4	Agree	84	84
5	Strongly agree	02	02
Total		100	100

My children lock themselves in their rooms after a fight with me		**First-generation** *respondents*	
		Number	*Percentage*
1	Disagree	00	00
2	Strongly disagree	00	00
3	Uncertain	20	20
4	Agree	80	80
5	Strongly agree	00	00
Total		100	100

According to the above data, 86 percent of second-generation respondents and 80 percent of first-generation respondents agree that the second-generation immigrants lock themselves in their rooms after a fight with their parents/grandparents.

Table 73   Staying overnight after family fight

When my parents yell and shout at me I stay overnight with my friends		Second-generation respondents	
		Number	Percentage
1	Disagree	25	25
2	Strongly disagree	04	04
3	Uncertain	06	06
4	Agree	65	65
5	Strongly agree	00	00
Total		100	100

My children stay overnight with their friends when there is a clash at home		First-generation respondents	
		Number	Percentage
1	Disagree	27	27
2	Strongly disagree	00	00
3	Uncertain	09	09
4	Agree	64	64
5	Strongly agree	00	00
Total		100	100

According to the above data 65 percent of second-generation respondents and 64 percent of first-generation respondents agree that second-generation immigrants stay overnight with their friends following a clash at home.

Table 74   Not eating at home after family fight

I don't eat from home for days after a fight with my parents/grandparents		**Second-generation** respondents	
		Number	*Percentage*
1	Disagree	06	06
2	Strongly disagree	02	02
3	Uncertain	00	00
4	Agree	92	92
5	Strongly agree	00	00
Total		100	100

My children don't eat from home for days after a quarrel at home		**First-generation** respondents	
		Number	*Percentage*
1	Disagree	00	00
2	Strongly disagree	00	00
3	Uncertain	06	06
4	Agree	94	94
5	Strongly agree	00	00
Total		100	100

The data in the above tables indicate that 92 percent of second-generation respondents and 94 percent of first-generation respondents agree that the second-generation immigrants do not eat at home for days following a quarrel at home.

Table 75   Communication after family fights

I don't talk to my parents/grandparents for days after a fight with them		**Second-generation** respondents	
		Number	*Percentage*
1	Disagree	00	00
2	Strongly disagree	00	00
3	Uncertain	00	00
4	Agree	82	82
5	Strongly agree	18	18
Total		100	100

My children don't talk to me for days after a clash/fight at home		**First-generation** respondents	
		Number	*Percentage*
1	Disagree	00	00
2	Strongly disagree	00	00
3	Uncertain	06	06
4	Agree	94	94
5	Strongly agree	00	00
Total		100	100

All the second-generation respondents agree (82 percent) or strongly agree (18 percent) that they don't talk to their parents for days after a clash/fight at home, while 94 percent first-generation respondents also agree.

Table 76 Moving out after family fight

I move out from my parental home when my parents yell and shout at me		**Second-generation** respondents	
		Number	Percentage
1	Disagree	88	88
2	Strongly disagree	03	03
3	Uncertain	09	09
4	Agree	00	00
5	Strongly agree	00	00
Total		100	100

My children move out from my home after a family fight		**Second-generation** respondents	
		Number	Percentage
1	Disagree	94	94
2	Strongly disagree	00	00
3	Uncertain	5	5
4	Agree	01	01
5	Strongly agree	00	00
Total		100	100

As per the above tables 91 percent of second-generation respondents and 94 percent of second-generation respondents disagree that the second-generation immigrants move out from their parental home after family fights.

Table 77   Getting angry and arguing when imposing parental views and values

I get angry and argue with my parents/grandparents when they impose their views and values on me		**Second-generation** respondents	
		Number	*Percentage*
1	Disagree	07	07
2	Strongly disagree	02	02
3	Uncertain	00	00
4	Agree	81	81
5	Strongly agree	10	10
Total		100	100
My children get angry and argue with me when I try to teach them my views and values		**First-generation** respondents	
		Number	*Percentage*
1	Disagree	09	09
2	Strongly disagree	00	00
3	Uncertain	13	13
4	Agree	78	78
5	Strongly agree	00	00
Total		100	100

According to the above tables, while a large majority of second-generation respondents agree (91 percent) that they get angry and argue with their parents/grandparents when imposing parental views and values on them, only 78 percent among first-generation respondents agrees with it.

Table 78 Getting angry and destroying things when judged by Indian standards

I get angry and destroy things at home when I am judged by the Indian standards		Second-generation respondents	
		Number	Percentage
1	Disagree	29	29
2	Strongly disagree	04	04
3	Uncertain	08	08
4	Agree	53	53
5	Strongly agree	06	06
Total		100	100

My children get angry and destroy things at home when I discipline them based on Indian standards		First-generation respondents	
		Number	Percentage
1	Disagree	05	05
2	Strongly disagree	00	00
3	Uncertain	29	29
4	Agree	66	66
5	Strongly agree	00	00
Total		100	100

The above tables explain that 59 percent of second-generation respondents agree or strongly agree that second-generation immigrants get angry and destroy things at home when they are judged by Indian standards, while 66 percent among first-generation respondents also agrees with it.

Table 79   Using drugs, tobacco and liquor to handle stress

I use drugs, tobacco and/or liquor when there is constant fighting at home		**Second-generation** respondents	
		Number	Percentage
1	Disagree	61	61
2	Strongly disagree	36	36
3	Uncertain	03	03
4	Agree	00	00
5	Strongly agree	00	00
Total		100	100

My children use drugs, tobacco and/or liquor when there is constant fighting at home		**First-generation** respondents	
		Number	Percentage
1	Disagree	72	72
2	Strongly disagree	16	16
3	Uncertain	12	12
4	Agree	00	00
5	Strongly agree	00	00
Total		100	100

According to the above data, 97 percent of second-generation respondents disagree (61 percent) or strongly disagree (36 percent) that that they use drugs, tobacco and/or liquor when there is constant fighting at home while 88 percent among the first-generations also disagree (72 percent) or strongly disagree (16 percent) with this statement.

Table 80 Doing something to get in trouble with the police

After every fight at home I do something that I can get in trouble with the police		Second-generation respondents	
		Number	Percentage
1	Disagree	63	63
2	Strongly disagree	36	36
3	Uncertain	00	00
4	Agree	01	01
5	Strongly agree	00	00
Total		100	100

After every fight at home my children do something that they can get in trouble with the police		First-generation respondents	
		Number	Percentage
1	Disagree	54	54
2	Strongly disagree	23	23
3	Uncertain	22	22
4	Agree	01	01
5	Strongly agree	00	00
Total		100	100

The data in the above tables reveal that only 1 percent of respondents each from both first and second-generation immigrants agree that second-generation immigrants do something to get in trouble with the police after a fight at home.

Table 81   Poor appetite and reluctance to eat due to constant family fighting

Whenever there is a fight at home my appetite is poor and I don't like to eat		*Second-generation* respondents	
		Number	*Percentage*
1	Disagree	13	13
2	Strongly disagree	00	00
3	Uncertain	00	00
4	Agree	87	87
5	Strongly agree	00	00
Total		100	100

After every fight at home it seems my children do not eat and their appetite is poor		*First-generation* respondents	
		Number	*Percentage*
1	Disagree	04	04
2	Strongly disagree	00	00
3	Uncertain	26	26
4	Agree	70	70
5	Strongly agree	00	00
Total		100	100

As per the above tables, 87 percent of second-generation respondents and 70 percent of first-generation respondents agree that the appetite of the second-generation immigrants is poor and they don't like to eat following family fights.

Table 82 Depression due to irrational judgment

I feel depressed when I am judged based on the Indian standards		*Second-generation respondents*	
		Number	Percentage
1	Disagree	09	09
2	Strongly disagree	00	00
3	Uncertain	15	15
4	Agree	73	73
5	Strongly agree	03	03
Total		100	100
My children feel depressed when they are judged based on their parental principles		*First-generation respondents*	
		Number	Percentage
1	Disagree	00	00
2	Strongly disagree	00	00
3	Uncertain	32	32
4	Agree	68	68
5	Strongly agree	00	00
Total		100	100

As per the above tables, while 76 percent of second-generation respondents agree that they feel depressed when they are judged based on Indian standards, 68 percent of first-generation respondents also agree they observe the same in their children.

Table 83 Feeling of vain effort

When I am judged on Indian standards I feel that everything I do is an effort		*Second-generation respondents*	
		Number	*Percentage*
1	Disagree	00	00
2	Strongly disagree	00	00
3	Uncertain	02	02
4	Agree	97	97
5	Strongly agree	01	01
Total		100	100

My children often say that they are taking a lot of effort		*First-generation respondents*	
		Number	*Percentage*
1	Disagree	00	00
2	Strongly disagree	00	00
3	Uncertain	22	22
4	Agree	53	53
5	Strongly agree	25	25
Total		100	100

The data in the above tables demonstrate that while 98 percent of second-generation respondents feel that everything they do is an effort as they are constantly judged by Indian values and principles, 78 percent of second-generation respondents often hear their children saying the same.

Table 84   Irrational judgment that leads to Feeling worthlessness

I feel I am worthless when I am judged on the Indian standards		**Second-generation** respondents	
		Number	Percentage
1	Disagree	35	35
2	Strongly disagree	00	00
3	Uncertain	18	18
4	Agree	47	47
5	Strongly agree	00	00
Total		100	100

It seems my children occasionally think they are worthless		**First-generation** respondents	
		Number	Percentage
1	Disagree	58	58
2	Strongly disagree	00	00
3	Uncertain	13	13
4	Agree	29	29
5	Strongly agree	00	00
Total		100	100

While 47 percent of second-generation respondents agree that they feel worthless when they are constantly judged by Indian values and principles, 29 percent of second-generation respondents also agree that they sense it among their children.

Table 85 Irrational judgment that leads to feeling sadness

I feel sad when I am judged on Indian standards		**Second-generation** *respondents*	
		Number	*Percentage*
1	Strongly disagree	00	00
2	Disagree	00	00
3	Uncertain	00	00
4	Agree	94	94
5	Strongly agree	06	06
Total		100	100

My children feel sad when they are disciplined by their parental principles		**First-generation** *respondents*	
		Number	*Percentage*
1	Strongly disagree	00	00
2	Disagree	00	00
3	Uncertain	00	00
4	Agree	100	100
5	Strongly agree	00	00
Total		100	100

Responding to the question with regard to feeling sad when being judged by Indian cultural values and beliefs, all the second- and first-generation respondents agree that second-generation immigrants feel sad when they are disciplined and judged by Indian values and principles.

Table 86   Saving face over helping family

My parents are more concerned about saving their face in public rather than helping their family		**Second-generation** respondents	
		Number	Percentage
1	Disagree	00	00
2	Strongly disagree	00	00
3	Uncertain	00	00
4	Agree	28	28
5	Strongly agree	72	72
Total		100	100

Saving the image of my family in public is my first priority		**First-generation** respondents	
		Number	Percentage
1	Disagree	00	00
2	Strongly disagree	00	00
3	Uncertain	00	00
4	Agree	59	59
5	Strongly agree	41	41
Total		100	100

Based on the above tables, while all second-generation respondents agree (28 percent) or strongly agree (72 percent) that their parents are more concerned about saving their face in public rather than helping their family, all the second-generation respondents agree (59 percent) or strongly agree (41 percent) that saving the image of their family is their first priority.

Table 87   Fights that lead family life out of order

Everything goes out of order for days/weeks when there is a fight at home		*Second-generation respondents*	
		Number	*Percentage*
1	Disagree	01	01
2	Strongly disagree	00	00
3	Uncertain	01	01
4	Agree	97	97
5	Strongly agree	01	01
Total		100	100

Everything goes out of order for days/weeks when there is a fight at home		*First-generation respondents*	
		Number	*Percentage*
1	Disagree	00	00
2	Strongly disagree	00	00
3	Uncertain	00	00
4	Agree	78	78
5	Strongly agree	22	22
Total		100	100

As per the above tables, 98 percent of second-generation respondents and all the first-generation respondents agree (78 percent) or strongly agree (22 percent) with the statement that everything goes out of order for days/weeks when there is a fight at home.

Table 88   Family fight and family's pretension

When there is a family fight at home, my parents pretend that there is nothing special in it		*Second-generation* respondents	
		Number	Percentage
1	Disagree	01	01
2	Strongly disagree	00	00
3	Uncertain	02	02
4	Agree	89	89
5	Strongly agree	08	08
Total		100	100

Family fights are common and there is nothing great in it		*First-generation* respondents	
		Number	Percentage
1	Disagree	00	00
2	Strongly disagree	00	00
3	Uncertain	00	00
4	Agree	91	91
5	Strongly agree	09	09
Total		100	100

According to the above data, 97 percent of second-generation respondents and all the second-generation respondents agree that first-generation parents believe that family fights are common and there is nothing great in it.

Table 89   Family fights and professional help

We don't seek professional help even when there are constant fights and arguments at home		Second-generation respondents	
		Number	Percentage
1	Disagree	00	00
2	Strongly disagree	00	00
3	Uncertain	00	00
4	Agree	80	80
5	Strongly agree	20	20
Total		100	100

We don't go for counseling because there are fights and arguments at home		First-generation respondents	
		Number	Percentage
1	Disagree	00	00
2	Strongly disagree	00	00
3	Uncertain	00	00
4	Agree	86	86
5	Strongly agree	14	14
Total		100	100

The above table delineates that all the first and second-generation respondents agree or strongly agree that their families don't seek professional help though there are constant fights and arguments at home.

Table 90   Parental expectation of being good children

My parents always expect me to be a good man/woman, means to behave like a proper Indian		Second-generation respondents	
		Number	Percentage
1	Disagree	00	00
2	Strongly disagree	00	00
3	Uncertain	00	00
4	Agree	82	82
5	Strongly agree	18	18
Total		100	100

I expect my children to be a good man/woman; behaving like a proper Indian		First-generation respondents	
		Number	Percentage
1	Disagree	00	00
2	Strongly disagree	00	00
3	Uncertain	13	13
4	Agree	87	87
5	Strongly agree	00	00
Total		100	100

As per the above data, while all the second-generation respondents agree that their parents expect them to be good man/woman means to behave like a proper Indian, 87 percent of first-generation respondents also believe that being good means behaving like a proper Indian.

Table 91   Judgment that leads to rebellion

When I am judged by the Indian standards, I rebel with my parents and parental community	**Second-generation** respondents	
	Number	Percentage
1 Disagree	00	00
2 Strongly disagree	00	00
3 Uncertain	05	05
4 Agree	88	88
5 Strongly agree	07	07
Total	100	100

It seems that my children have always some reservation with the Indian community	**First-generation** respondents	
	Number	Percentage
1 Disagree	00	00
2 Strongly disagree	00	00
3 Uncertain	19	19
4 Agree	81	81
5 Strongly agree	00	00
Total	100	100

The above data explain that 95 percent of second-generation respondents agree that they rebel with their parents and parental community when they are constantly judged by Indian standards, while 81 percent of first-generation respondents also agree that their children always have some reservations with the Indian community.

Table 92   Parents' response towards premarital boy/girlfriend

My parents think that I don't need a boy/girlfriend prior to my marriage		**Second-generation** *respondents*	
		Number	*Percentage*
1	Disagree	00	00
2	Strongly disagree	00	00
3	Uncertain	00	00
4	Agree	83	83
5	Strongly agree	17	17
Total		100	100

I don't think my children need a boy/girlfriend prior to their marriage		**First-generation** *respondents*	
		Number	*Percentage*
1	Disagree	00	00
2	Strongly disagree	00	00
3	Uncertain	00	00
4	Agree	94	94
5	Strongly agree	06	06
Total		100	100

From the above tables, it is evident that all the second-generation respondents agree or strongly agree that their parents believe their children don't need a boy/girlfriend prior to their marriage, while all the first-generation respondents also agree or strongly agree with this statement.

Table 93   Discussion about girl/boyfriends with parents

I don't share anything about my girl/boyfriend with my parents		**Second-generation** respondents	
		Number	Percentage
1	Disagree	00	00
2	Strongly disagree	00	00
3	Uncertain	00	00
4	Agree	63	63
5	Strongly agree	37	37
Total		100	100

My children do not share anything about their girl/boyfriend with me		**First-generation** respondents	
		Number	Percentage
1	Disagree	00	00
2	Strongly disagree	00	00
3	Uncertain	18	18
4	Agree	82	82
5	Strongly agree	00	00
Total		100	100

According to the above figures while all the second-generation respondents agree or strongly agree that they don't share anything about their girl/boyfriend with their parents, 82 percent of first-generation respondents agree with them.

Table 94   Sharing peer pressure with parents

I talk about my peer pressure with my parents		**Second-generation** respondents	
		Number	*Percentage*
1	Disagree	21	21
2	Strongly disagree	41	41
3	Uncertain	13	13
4	Agree	25	25
5	Strongly agree	00	00
Total		100	100

My children always discuss their peer pressure with me		**First-generation** respondents	
		Number	*Percentage*
1	Strongly disagree	10	10
2	Disagree	00	00
3	Uncertain	61	61
4	Agree	29	29
5	Strongly agree	00	00
Total		100	100

The above tables explain that 25 percent of respondents among the second-generations and 29 percent among the first-generations agree that the peer pressure of the children is discussed with their parents.

Table 95   Hiding emotional needs from parents

I hide most of my emotional needs from my parents		**Second-generation** *respondents*	
		Number	*Percentage*
1	Disagree	01	01
2	Strongly disagree	00	00
3	Uncertain	02	02
4	Agree	82	82
5	Strongly agree	15	15
Total		100	100
My children never hide their emotional needs from me		**First-generation** *respondents*	
		Number	*Percentage*
1	Disagree	33	33
2	Strongly disagree	00	00
3	Uncertain	51	51
4	Agree	16	16
5	Strongly agree	00	00
Total		100	100

According to the data, 97 percent of second-generation respondents agree or strongly agree that they hide most of their emotional needs from their parents, only 16 percent of first-generation respondents agree that their children never hide their emotional needs from parents.

Table 96   Parents who fight each other

My parents get along well and never fight each other		*Second-generation respondents*	
		Number	*Percentage*
1	Disagree	22	22
2	Strongly disagree	00	00
3	Uncertain	36	36
4	Agree	42	42
5	Strongly agree	00	00
Total		100	100

I get along well with my spouse and never fight with him/her		*First-generation respondents*	
		Number	*Percentage*
1	Disagree	00	00
2	Strongly disagree	00	00
3	Uncertain	23	23
4	Agree	77	77
5	Strongly agree	00	00
Total		100	100

The above data show that while 22 percent of second-generation respondents disagree that their parents get along well and never fight each other, none of the first-generation respondents disagree with it, though 23 percent respond that they are uncertain about it.

Table 97   Parental control on family affairs

My parents control most of our family affairs		Second-generation respondents	
		Number	Percentage
1	Disagree	00	00
2	Strongly disagree	00	00
3	Uncertain	24	24
4	Agree	76	76
5	Strongly agree	00	00
Total		100	100

I control most of my family affairs		First-generation respondents	
		Number	Percentage
1	Disagree	19	19
2	Strongly disagree	00	00
3	Uncertain	23	23
4	Agree	58	58
5	Strongly agree	00	00
Total		100	100

As per the above table, while 76 percent of second-generation respondents agree that it is their parents who control most of their family affairs, only 58 percent of first-generation respondents agree with this.

Table 98   Authoritarian fathers

My Father is very authoritarian		*Second-generation respondents*	
		Number	*Percentage*
1	Disagree	46	46
2	Strongly disagree	01	01
3	Uncertain	25	25
4	Agree	26	26
5	Strongly agree	02	02
Total		100	100
I am not authoritarian Father		*First-generation respondents*	
		Number	*Percentage*
1	Disagree (Not Applicable/Mothers)	50	50
2	Strongly disagree	00	00
3	Uncertain	17	17
4	Agree	33	33
5	Strongly agree	00	00
Total		100	100

According to the above table, while 28 percent of second-generation respondents agree or strongly agree that their fathers are authoritarians, 33 percent of first-generation respondents also agree that they are so.

Table 99　Controlling mothers

My mother is controlling		Second-generation respondents	
		Number	Percentage
1	Disagree	41	41
2	Strongly disagree	00	00
3	Uncertain	22	22
4	Agree	35	35
5	Strongly agree	02	02
Total		100	100
I am not a controlling Mother		First-generation respondents	
		Number	Percentage
1	Disagree (Not Applicable/Fathers)	50	50
2	Strongly disagree	00	00
3	Uncertain	36	36
4	Agree	14	14
5	Strongly agree	00	00
Total		100	100

Based on the data in the above table while 37 percent of second-generation respondents agree that their mothers are controlling, only 14 percent of first-generation respondents agrees that they are so.

Table 100   Happy relationship with parents and children

I am happy in my relationship with my parents		**Second-generation** *respondents*	
		Number	*Percentage*
1	Disagree	24	24
2	Strongly disagree	00	00
3	Uncertain	39	39
4	Agree	37	37
5	Strongly agree	00	00
Total		100	100
My children have a cordial relationship with me		**First-generation** *respondents*	
		Number	*Percentage*
1	Disagree	18	18
2	Strongly disagree	00	00
3	Uncertain	32	32
4	Agree	50	50
5	Strongly agree	00	00
Total		100	100

The data in the above tables show that 37 percent of second-generation respondents and 50 percent of first-generation respondents agree that they have a happy relationship.

Table 101   Implicit obedience to parental principles and values

I cannot implicitly obey my parents' principles and values		Second-generation respondents	
		Number	Percentage
1	Disagree	00	00
2	Strongly disagree	00	00
3	Uncertain	00	00
4	Agree	87	87
5	Strongly agree	13	13
Total		100	100

My children obey all principles I implement at home		First-generation respondents	
		Number	Percentage
1	Disagree	91	91
2	Strongly disagree	00	00
3	Uncertain	09	09
4	Agree	00	00
5	Strongly agree	00	00
Total		100	100

While all the second-generation respondents agree or strongly agree that they cannot implicitly obey their parents' principles and values, none of the first-generation respondents agree that their children obey all principles they implement at home.

Table 102   Children behaving like Indians

I try to behave like an Indian at home and in the community		*Second-generation* respondents	
		Number	*Percentage*
1	Disagree	62	62
2	Strongly disagree	00	00
3	Uncertain	29	29
4	Agree	09	09
5	Strongly agree	00	00
Total		100	100

My children try to behave like an Indian at home and in the community		*First-generation* respondents	
		Number	*Percentage*
1	Disagree	39	39
2	Strongly disagree	00	00
3	Uncertain	47	47
4	Agree	14	14
5	Strongly agree	00	00
Total		100	100

According to the above data, a minority of second-generation respondent (9 percent) and a slightly more (14 percent) first-generation respondents agree that second-generation immigrants try to behave like an Indian at home and in the community.

Table 103   Parents who judge with Indian principles and values

My parents judge me with their Indian principles and values		Second-generation respondents	
		Number	Percentage
1	Disagree	00	00
2	Strongly disagree	00	00
3	Uncertain	02	02
4	Agree	98	98
5	Strongly agree	00	00
Total		100	100

I think I discipline my children based on my Indian understanding		First-generation respondents	
		Number	Percentage
1	Disagree	09	09
2	Strongly disagree	00	00
3	Uncertain	19	19
4	Agree	72	72
5	Strongly agree	00	00
Total		100	100

As per the above tables, while a significant majority of second-generation respondents (98 percent) agree that their parents judge them by Indian cultural values and principles, only 72 percent of first-generation respondents agree that they do so. However, for the first generation it is not judging but rather disciplining. Again, these are two different levels of understanding.

Section 5: Role of Religious and Social Institutions in Educating Cultural Struggles and Acculturation

The data in this section help us to understand the role that religious and social institutions play in making immigrant communities aware of their cultural struggles, stress related to acculturation, and the need for acculturation.

Table 104   Respondents attending Indian English Church/ Temple/ Mosque

I attend an Indian English Church/ Temple/ Mosque		Second-generation respondents	
		Number	Percentage
1	Disagree	63	63
2	Strongly disagree	04	04
3	Uncertain	00	00
4	Agree	29	29
5	Strongly agree	04	04
Total		100	100

I attend an Indian English Church/ Temple/ Mosque		First-generation respondents	
		Number	Percentage
1	Disagree	67	67
2	Strongly disagree	00	00
3	Uncertain	00	00
4	Agree	33	33
5	Strongly agree	00	00
Total		100	100

As per the above tables 33 percent of respondents each from both first and second-generation immigrants attend churches/ temples/ mosques conducting services in the English language.

Table 105   Respondents attending Indian vernacular Church/ Temple/ Mosque

I attend an Indian vernacular Church/ Temple/ Mosque		Second-generation respondents	
		Number	Percentage
1	Disagree	33	33
2	Strongly disagree	00	00
3	Uncertain	00	00
4	Agree	67	67
5	Strongly agree	00	00
Total		100	100
I attend an Indian vernacular Church/ Temple/ Mosque		First-generation respondents	
		Number	Percentage
1	Disagree	33	33
2	Strongly disagree	00	00
3	Uncertain	00	00
4	Agree	67	67
5	Strongly agree	00	00
Total		100	100

According to the above table, while 67 percent of respondents each from both first and second-generation immigrants attend Churches/ Temples/ Mosques that conduct service in an Indian vernacular.

Table 106   Respondents attending American English Church/ Temple/ Mosque

I attend an American English Church/ Temple/ Mosque		Second-generation respondents	
		Number	Percentage
1	Disagree	96	96
2	Strongly disagree	04	04
3	Uncertain	00	00
4	Agree	00	00
5	Strongly agree	00	00
Total		100	100

I attend an American English Church/Temple/Mosque		First-generation respondents	
		Number	Percentage
1	Disagree	100	100
2	Strongly disagree	00	00
3	Uncertain	00	00
4	Agree	00	00
5	Strongly agree	00	00
Total		100	100

The above tables explain that none of the respondents either among first or second-generation immigrants attend American English church/ temple/ mosque.

Table 107   Church/ Temple/ Mosque that speaks about immigrants' cultural struggles

My Church/ Temple/ Mosque often speaks about the cultural struggles of immigrants		*Second-generation* respondents	
		Number	Percentage
1	Disagree	40	40
2	Strongly disagree	04	04
3	Uncertain	29	29
4	Agree	25	25
5	Strongly agree	02	02
Total		100	100

My Church/ Temple/ Mosque often speaks about the cultural struggles of immigrants		*First-generation* respondents	
		Number	Percentage
1	Disagree	06	06
2	Strongly disagree	00	00
3	Uncertain	61	61
4	Agree	33	33
5	Strongly agree	00	00
Total		100	100

The data in these tables reveal that 27 percent of second-generation respondents and 33 percent of first-generation respondents agree that their Church/ Temple/ Mosque often speaks about cultural struggles of immigrants.

Table 108   Church/ Temple/ Mosque that often exalts the Indian culture

My Church/ Temple/ Mosque often teaches that Indian culture is the best		Second-generation respondents	
		Number	Percentage
1	Disagree	00	00
2	Strongly disagree	00	00
3	Uncertain	11	11
4	Agree	53	53
5	Strongly agree	36	36
Total		100	100

My Church/ Temple/ Mosque often teaches that Indian culture is the best		First-generation respondents	
		Number	Percentage
1	Disagree	00	00
2	Strongly disagree	00	00
3	Uncertain	29	29
4	Agree	71	71
5	Strongly agree	00	00
Total		100	100

According to the above tables, 89 percent of second-generation respondents and 71 percent of first-generation respondents agree that their church /temple/ mosque often teaches that Indian culture is the best.

Table 109   Church/ Temple/ Mosque that helps immigrants to live in both cultures

My Church/Temple/Mosque helps immigrant families to live simultaneously in both American and Indian cultures		Second-generation respondents	
		Number	Percentage
1	Disagree	54	54
2	Strongly disagree	12	12
3	Uncertain	19	19
4	Agree	15	15
5	Strongly agree	00	00
Total		100	100

My Church/Temple/Mosque helps immigrant families to live simultaneously in both American and Indian cultures		First-generation respondents	
		Number	Percentage
1	Disagree	32	32
2	Strongly disagree	00	00
3	Uncertain	64	64
4	Agree	04	04
5	Strongly agree	00	00
Total		100	100

As per the table, 66 percent of second-generation respondents and 32 percent of first-generation respondents disagree that their church/temple/ mosque helps immigrant families to live simultaneously in both American and Indian cultures. The percentage of second-generation respondents is double the size of first-generation respondents.

Table 110   Seminars, workshops and conferences on immigrants' issues

My Church/ Temple/ Mosque conducts seminars, workshops and conferences on the sociocultural struggles of the Indian immigrants in US		Second-generation respondents	
		Number	Percentage
1	Disagree	54	54
2	Strongly disagree	08	08
3	Uncertain	12	12
4	Agree	26	26
5	Strongly agree	00	00
Total		100	100

My Church/ Temple/ Mosque conducts seminars, workshops, and conferences, on the sociocultural struggles of the Indian immigrants in US		First-generation respondents	
		Number	Percentage
1	Disagree	35	35
2	Strongly disagree	00	00
3	Uncertain	33	33
4	Agree	32	32
5	Strongly agree	00	00
Total		100	100

According to the above data, 62 percent of second-generation respondents and 35 percent of first-generation respondents disagree that their church/temple/mosque conducts seminars, workshops and conferences on the sociocultural struggles of immigrants in their church/ temple/ mosque.

Table 111 Debates and discussions on immigrants' issues

My Church/ Temple/ Mosque encourages debates and discussions on the immigrants' issues		Second-generation respondents	
		Number	Percentage
1	Disagree	51	51
2	Strongly disagree	04	04
3	Uncertain	20	20
4	Agree	25	25
5	Strongly agree	00	00
Total		100	100

My Church/ Temple/ Mosque encourages debates and discussions on the immigrants' issues		First-generation respondents	
		Number	Percentage
1	Disagree	41	41
2	Strongly disagree	00	00
3	Uncertain	25	25
4	Agree	34	34
5	Strongly agree	00	00
Total		100	100

The data in the above tables reveal that 55 percent of second-generation respondents and 41 percent of first-generation respondents disagree or strongly disagree that their church/ temple/ mosque encourages debates and discussions on the immigrants' issues.

Table 112 Teaching on interracial marriages

My Church/ Temple/ Mosque teaches about interracial marriage		Second-generation respondents	
		Number	Percentage
1	Disagree	31	31
2	Strongly disagree	54	54
3	Uncertain	15	15
4	Agree	00	00
5	Strongly agree	00	00
Total		100	100

My Church/ Temple/ Mosque teaches about interracial marriage		First-generation respondents	
		Number	Percentage
1	Disagree	74	74
2	Strongly disagree	00	00
3	Uncertain	26	26
4	Agree	00	00
5	Strongly agree	00	00
Total		100	100

Based on the above data, 85 percent of second-generation respondents and 74 percent of first-generation respondents disagree that their church/ temple/ mosque teaches about interracial marriages.

Table 113   Teaching about the need of acculturation

My Church/ Temple/ Mosque often teaches about the need of acculturation		Second-generation respondents	
		Number	Percentage
1	Disagree	81	81
2	Strongly disagree	03	03
3	Uncertain	13	13
4	Agree	03	03
5	Strongly agree	00	00
Total		100	100

My Church/ Temple/ Mosque often teaches about the need of acculturation		First-generation respondents	
		Number	Percentage
1	Disagree	74	74
2	Strongly disagree	00	00
3	Uncertain	25	25
4	Agree	01	01
5	Strongly agree	00	00
Total		100	100

As per the above table, 84 percent of second-generation respondents and 74 percent of first-generation respondents disagree or strongly disagree that their church/ temple /mosque often teaches about the need of acculturation.

Table 114   Listening to the concerns of second-generationIndian immigrants

My Church/ Temple/ Mosque always listens to the concerns of the second-generation Indian immigrants		**Second-generation** respondents	
		Number	Percentage
1	Disagree	16	16
2	Strongly disagree	51	51
3	Uncertain	02	02
4	Agree	31	31
5	Strongly agree	00	00
Total		100	100

My Church/ Temple/ Mosque always listens to the concerns of the second generation Indian immigrants		**First-generation** respondents	
		Number	Percentage
1	Disagree	64	64
2	Strongly disagree	00	00
3	Uncertain	19	19
4	Agree	17	17
5	Strongly agree	00	00
Total		100	100

Based on the above data, 67 percent of second-generation respondents and 64 percent of first-generation respondents disagree or strongly disagree that their churches/temples/mosques always listen to the concerns of the second generation Indian immigrants.

Table 115 Different views about first-generation and second-generation immigrants

My Church/ Temple/ Mosque has two different views about first- and second-generation Indian immigrants		Second-generation respondents	
		Number	Percentage
1	Disagree	48	48
2	Strongly disagree	04	04
3	Uncertain	04	04
4	Agree	36	36
5	Strongly agree	08	08
Total		100	100

My Church/ Temple/ Mosque has two different views about the first- and second-generation Indian immigrants		First-generation respondents	
		Number	Percentage
1	Disagree	13	13
2	Strongly disagree	00	00
3	Uncertain	13	13
4	Agree	74	74
5	Strongly agree	00	00
Total		100	100

According to the above tables, while 44 percent of second-generation respondents agree that their church/ temple/ mosque has two different views about first- and second-generation immigrants, 74 percent of first-generation respondents agree with the same statement.

Table 116 Use of Indian vernacular in teaching and preaching

My Church/ Temple/ Mosque always uses an Indian vernacular to teach and preach		*Second-generation* respondents	
		Number	*Percentage*
1	Disagree	35	35
2	Strongly disagree	00	00
3	Uncertain	00	00
4	Agree	43	43
5	Strongly agree	22	22
Total		100	100
My Church/ Temple/ Mosque always uses an Indian vernacular to teach and preach		*First-generation* respondents	
		Number	*Percentage*
1	Disagree	32	32
2	Strongly disagree	00	00
3	Uncertain	05	05
4	Agree	00	00
5	Strongly agree	63	63
Total		100	100

The above tables delineate that 65 percent of second-generation respondents and 63 percent of first-generation respondents agree that their church/ temple/ mosque always uses Indian vernacular to teach and preach.

Table 117   Ability to understand the Indian English accent

I fully understand the English accent used by Indian teachers/ preachers in my Church/ Temple/ Mosque		Second-generation respondents	
		Number	Percentage
1	Disagree	35	35
2	Strongly disagree	00	00
3	Uncertain	10	10
4	Agree	55	55
5	Strongly agree	00	00
Total		100	100

My children fully understand the English accent used by Indian teachers/preachers in my Church/ Temple/ Mosque		First-generation respondents	
		Number	Percentage
1	Disagree	06	06
2	Strongly disagree	00	00
3	Uncertain	37	47
4	Agree	57	57
5	Strongly agree	00	00
Total		100	100

The data in the above tables explain that 55 percent of second-generation respondents and 57 percent of first-generation respondents agree that second-generation immigrants understand the English accent used by Indian teachers/preachers in their church/temple/mosque.

Table 118 Concerns about emotional, spiritual, and cultural needs of second generationimmigrants

My Church/ Temple/ Mosque considers the emotional, spiritual, cultural needs of second-generationimmigrants very seriously		Second-generation respondents	
		Number	Percentage
1	Disagree	25	25
2	Strongly disagree	56	56
3	Uncertain	00	00
4	Agree	19	19
5	Strongly agree	00	00
Total		100	100
My Church/ Temple/ Mosque considers the emotional, spiritual, cultural needs of second-generation immigrants very seriously		First-generation respondents	
		Number	Percentage
1	Disagree	20	20
2	Strongly disagree	00	00
3	Uncertain	71	71
4	Agree	09	09
5	Strongly agree	00	00
Total		100	100

As per the above empirical data, while 81 percent of second-generation respondents disagree or strongly disagree that their church/ temple/ mosque considers the emotional, spiritual, cultural needs of second-generation immigrants very seriously, only 1/5th (20 percent) of first-generation respondents disagree with this statement.

Table 119 Church/Temple/Mosque that tries to make second generations proper Indians

Indian Church/ Temple/ Mosque in my area tries to make me a proper Indian		*Second-generation* respondents	
		Number	*Percentage*
1	Disagree	16	16
2	Strongly disagree	00	00
3	Uncertain	28	28
4	Agree	56	56
5	Strongly agree	00	00
Total		100	100

Indian Church/ Temple/ Mosque in my area tries to make our children proper Indians		*First-generation* respondents	
		Number	*Percentage*
1	Disagree	10	10
2	Strongly disagree	00	00
3	Uncertain	28	28
4	Agree	62	62
5	Strongly agree	00	00
Total		100	100

Data in the above tables show that majority of respondents among both second- (56 percent) and first-generations (62 percent) agree that the church/ temple/ mosque in their area tries to make second-generation immigrants proper Indians.

Table 120   Major concerns of Church/ Temple/ Mosque

My Church/ Temple/ Mosque is more concerned about spiritual issues than sociocultural and emotional issues		*Second-generation* respondents	
		Number	*Percentage*
1	Disagree	14	14
2	Strongly disagree	02	02
3	Uncertain	00	00
4	Agree	48	48
5	Strongly agree	36	36
Total		100	100
My Church/ Temple/ Mosque is more concerned about spiritual issues than socio-cultural and emotional issues		*First-generation* respondents	
		Number	*Percentage*
1	Disagree	00	00
2	Strongly disagree	00	00
3	Uncertain	10	10
4	Agree	90	90
5	Strongly agree	00	00
Total		100	100

According to the above figures, 74 percent of second-generation respondents and 90 percent of first-generation respondents agree or strongly agree that their church/ temple/ mosque is more concerned about the spiritual issues of its members than sociocultural and emotional issues.

Table 121   Consideration for second-generation immigrants

My Church/ Temple/ Mosque considers second-generation immigrants as fully Indians		Second-generation respondents	
		Number	Percentage
1	Disagree	34	34
2	Strongly disagree	03	03
3	Uncertain	05	05
4	Agree	56	56
5	Strongly agree	02	02
Total		100	100
My Church/ Temple/ Mosque considers second-generation immigrants as fully Indians		First-generation respondents	
		Number	Percentage
1	Disagree	34	34
2	Strongly disagree	00	00
3	Uncertain	18	18
4	Agree	48	48
5	Strongly agree	00	00
Total		100	100

According to the above tables, 58 percent of second-generation respondents and 48 percent of first-generation respondents agree that their church/ temple/ mosque considers second generation immigrants as fully Indians, the same as Indians born and raised in India.

Table 122   Sense of religious/social belonging

My Church/ Temple/ Mosque is primarily not for me but for my parents		*Second-generation respondents*	
		Number	*Percentage*
1	Disagree	27	27
2	Strongly disagree	06	06
3	Uncertain	00	00
4	Agree	19	19
5	Strongly agree	48	48
Total		100	100
My Church/ Temple/ Mosque is for me and for my children		*First-generation respondents*	
		Number	*Percentage*
1	Disagree	01	01
2	Strongly disagree	00	00
3	Uncertain	18	18
4	Agree	81	81
5	Strongly agree	00	00
Total		100	100

According to the above data, 67 percent of second-generation respondents agree or strongly agree their current church/ temple/ mosque is primarily not for them but for their parents, while 81 percent of second-generation respondents agree that it is for them and also for their children.

Table 123   Separate services/programs in different languages

My Church/ Temple/ Mosque conducts separate services in an Indian vernacular for our parents and in English for us		*Second-generation* respondents	
		Number	Percentage
1	Disagree	86	86
2	Strongly disagree	00	00
3	Uncertain	00	00
4	Agree	14	14
5	Strongly agree	00	00
Total		100	100

My Church/ Temple/ Mosque conducts separate services in an Indian vernacular for us and in English for our children		*First-generation* respondents	
		Number	Percentage
1	Disagree	74	74
2	Strongly disagree	00	00
3	Uncertain	00	00
4	Agree	26	26
5	Strongly agree	00	00
Total		100	100

The above data shows that only 14 percent of second-generation respondents agree that they have separate English service in their church/temple/mosque, while 26 percent of first-generation respondents agree that they have separate services in different languages for first and second-generation immigrants.

Section 6: Demographic Details and Multi Ethnic Identity

This section deals with general information with regard to the gender, age, education, marital status and other personal and familial details of the sample population.

Table 124 Gender

Your gender		Second-generation respondents	
		Number	Percentage
1	Male	50	50
2	Female	50	50
Total		100	100
Your gender		*First-generation respondents*	
		Number	Percentage
1	Male	50	50
2	Female	50	50
Total		100	100

The above tables reveal that the percentage of male and female respondents among both second and first-generation respondents is 50 percent.

Table 125   Age group

Your age group is between:		Second-generation respondents	
		Number	Percentage
1	17–19	42	42
2	20–22	48	48
3	23–24	10	10
Total		100	100
Your age group is between:		First generation-respondents	
		Number	Percentage
1	35–45	00	00
2	46–55	61	61
3	56–65	39	39
Total		100	100

Based on the above data, while the majority of second-generation respondents (48 percent) are within the age group of 20–22, 42 percent are in the age group 17–19. So also, the largest majority among first-generation respondents (61 percent) falls in the age group of 46–55 and the next majority (39 percent) is in age group 56–65.

Table 126   Present educational status

Are you student, employee or both?		*Second-generation respondents*	
		Number	*Percentage*
1	Student	55	55
2	Employee	10	10
3	Both	35	35
Total		100	100
Are you employed or retired		*First-generation respondents*	
		Number	*Percentage*
1	Employed	94	94
2	Retired	06	06
Total		100	100

According to the above data, 55 percent of second-generation respondents are students, 10 percent are employees and 35 percent are employees–cum-students, 94 percent of first-generation respondents are employees and 6 percent are retired or unemployed.

Table 127   Parents' marital status during majority of children's life

What has been the marital status of your parents for the majority of your life		*Second-generation* respondents	
		Number	Percentage
1	Married	99	99
2	Divorced	00	00
3	Widowed	01	01
4	Remarried	00	00
5	Separated	00	00
Total		100	100
What is your marital status for the majority of your life?		*First-generation* respondents	
		Number	Percentage
1	Married	100	100
2	Divorced	00	00
3	Widowed	00	00
4	Remarried	00	00
5	Separated	00	00
Total		100	100

Based on the data in the above tables, while 99 percent of second-generation respondents responded that their parents were married for the majority of their life, all the first-generation respondents agreed that their marital status for the majority of their life was married.

Table 128   Parents' current marital status

What is your parents' marital status at present?		*Second-generation respondents*	
		Number	*Percentage*
1	Married	95	95
2	Divorced	00	00
3	Widowed	00	00
4	Remarried	05	05
5	Separated	00	00
Total		100	100

What is your current marital status?		*First-generation respondents*	
		Number	*Percentage*
1	Married	95	95
2	Divorced	00	00
3	Widowed	00	00
4	Remarried	05	05
5	Separated	00	00
Total		100	100

As per the above data, the current marital status of 95 percent of second-generation respondents is "married" and 5 percent are remarried.

Table 129   Primary language of communication with parents

What is the primary language that you use to speak to your parents?		*Second-generation* respondents			
		Mother	Father	Number	Percentage
1	Mostly Indian dialect and some English	03	03	06	06
2	Indian dialect and English about equally	08	08	16	16
3	Mostly English and some Indian dialect	39	39	78	78
4	English only	00	00	00	00
Total		50	50	100	100

What is the primary language that you use to speak to your children?		*First-generation* respondents	
		Number	Percentage
1	Mostly Indian dialect and some English	27	27
2	Indian dialect and English about equally	61	61
3	Mostly English and some Indian dialect	12	12
4	English only	00	00
Total		100	100

The data in the above tables delineate that 78 percent of second-generation respondents use mostly English and some Indian dialect to communicate with their parents, while 61 percent of first-generation respondents use Indian dialect and English about equally to communicate with their children.

Table 130   Parents' highest level of education

What is your parents' highest level of education?		**Second-generation** *respondents*			
		Mother	*Father*	*Number*	*Percentage*
1	Don't know	00	00	00	00
2	Some high school	00	00	00	00
3	High school graduate	03	04	07	07
4	Some college	06	08	14	14
5	Undergraduate	04	02	06	06
6	Graduate	07	06	13	13
7	Postgraduate	09	13	22	22
8	Professional	21	17	38	38
Total		50	50	100	100

What is your highest level of education?		**First-generation** *respondents*			
		Mother	*Father*	*Number*	*Percentage*
1	Don't know	00	00	00	00
2	Some high school	00	00	00	00
3	High school graduate	03	02	05	05
4	Some college	04	06	10	10
5	Undergraduate	07	03	10	10
6	Graduate	06	12	18	18
7	Postgraduate	05	05	10	10
8	Professional	25	22	47	47
Total		50	50	100	100

According to second-generation respondents, 38 percent of their parents hold professional degrees and 22 percent hold postgraduate degrees. However, according to first-generation respondents, 47 percent of them hold professional degrees, 10 percent postgraduate degrees and 18 percent hold graduate degrees.

Table 131   Place where highest education is completed

Did your parents complete this education in the USA?		*Second-generation* respondents			
		Mother	*Father*	*Number*	*Percentage*
1	Yes	06	09	15	15
2	No	44	41	85	85
Total		50	50	100	100

Did you complete this education in the USA?		*First-generation* respondents			
		Mother	*Father*	*Number*	*Percentage*
1	Yes	06	09	15	15
2	No	44	41	85	85
Total		50	50	100	100

According to the above tables both second and first-generation respondents agree that 85 percent of parental immigrants completed their highest education in India itself.

Table 132   Parents' profession

What is your parents' profession?		*Second-generation respondents*			
		Mother	*Father*	*Number*	*Percentage*
1	Physician, RNs, LVNs	31	09	40	40
2	Software/ITs, research, attorneys	12	21	33	33
3	Business	00	11	11	11
4	Technicians, CNAs	07	00	07	07
5	Insurance, Teachers	00	00	00	00
6	Accountants, CPAs and bankers	00	06	06	06
7	Retired/unemployed	00	03	03	03
8	Security/factory job	00	00	00	00
Total		50	50	100	100

What is your current profession?		*First-generation respondents*			
		Mother	*Father*	*Number*	*Percentage*
1	Physician, RNs, LVNs	31	09	40	40
2	Software/ITs, research, attorneys	12	21	33	33
3	Business	00	11	11	11
4	Technicians, CNAs	07	00	07	07
5	Insurance, Teachers	00	00	00	00
6	Accountants, CPAs and bankers	00	06	06	06
7	Retired/unemployed	00	03	03	03
8	Security/factory job	00	00	00	00
Total		50	50	100	100

According to both second- and first-generation respondents 40 percent of first-generation immigrants are health care professionals such as physicians and nurses, and 33 percent are IT Professionals and attorneys. Another 11 percent are business people.

Table 133   Family's annual income

What is your family's annual income? (Give your best guess if you are not sure)		**Second-generation** respondents	
		Number	Percentage
1	Less than $ 10,000	00	00
2	$ 10,001–20,000	00	00
3	$ 20,001–40,000	00	00
4	$ 40,001–60,000	05	05
5	$ 60,001–80,000	23	23
6	$ 80,001–100,000	44	44
7	$ 100,000 and above	28	28
Total		100	100

What is your family's annual income? (Give your best guess if you are not sure)		**First-generation** respondents	
		Number	Percentage
1	Less than $ 10,000	00	00
2	$ 10,001–20,000	00	00
3	$ 20,001–40,000	00	00
4	$ 40,001–60,000	06	06
5	$ 60,001–80,000	25	25
6	$ 80,001–100,000	48	48
7	$ 100,000 and above	21	21
Total		100	100

According to the above table, 44 percent of families of second-generation respondents live with an annual income between $ 80,001–100,000 and 21 percent with $ 100,000 and above. However, according to the first-generation respondents 48 percent of them live with an annual income between $ 80,001–100,000 and 21 percent of families live with an annual income of $ 100,000 and above.

Table 134 Different ways in which respondents think of themselves

There are many different ways in which people think of themselves. Which ONE of the following most closely describes how you view yourself	Second-generation respondents	
	Number	Percentage
1 I consider myself as an Asian Indian, though I live and study/work in US	00	00
2 I consider myself as an American though I have Asian Indian background and characteristics	73	73
3 I consider myself as an Indian-American, though deep down I always know I am an Indian	01	01
4 I consider myself as an Indian-American, though deep down I view myself as an American first	14	14
5 I consider myself as an Indian-American, I have both Indian and American characteristics and a blend of both	12	12
Total	100	100

There are many different ways in which people think of themselves. Which ONE of the following most closely describes how you view yourself	First-generation respondents	
	Number	Percentage
1 I consider myself as an Asian Indian, though I live and study/work in US	42	42
2 I consider myself as an American though I have Asian Indian background and characteristics	00	00
3 I consider myself as an Indian-American, though deep down I always know I am an Indian	52	52
4 I consider myself as an Indian-American, though deep down I view myself as an American first	00	00
5 I consider myself as an Indian-American, I have both Indian and American characteristics and I view myself as a blend of both	06	06
Total	100	100

As per the above data, 73 percent of second-generation respondents consider themselves as Americans though they have Asian Indian Background and characteristics while 14 percent consider themselves as Indian-American, though deep down they view themselves as American first. At the same time, while 52 percent first-generation respondents consider themselves as Indian-Americans, though deep down they always know they are Indians, 42 percent consider themselves as Asian Indians, though they live and study/work in the United States.

Table 135   Being comfortable with ethnic identity

How comfortable are you with your ethnic identity as an Indian-American		Second-generation respondents	
		Number	Percentage
1	Extremely uncomfortable	00	00
2	Very uncomfortable	73	73
3	Somewhat uncomfortable	14	14
4	Comfortable	13	13
5	Very comfortable	00	00
6	Extremely comfortable	00	00
Total		100	100

How comfortable are you with your ethnic identity as an Indian-American		First-generation respondents	
		Number	Percentage
1	Extremely uncomfortable	00	00
2	Very uncomfortable	00	00
3	Somewhat uncomfortable	00	00
4	Comfortable	00	00
5	Very comfortable	47	47
6	Extremely comfortable	53	53
Total		100	100

As per the above data, 73 percent of second-generation respondents are very uncomfortable and 14 percent are somewhat uncomfortable with their ethnic identity as Indian-American, while 43 percent of first-generation respondents are very comfortable and 53 percent are extremely comfortable with their ethnic identity as Indian American.

REFERENCES

Abbott, Douglas A., Julie Johnson, John Defrain, and Rochelle L. Dalla, eds. 2009. *Strengths and Challenges of New Immigrant Families: Implications for Research, Education Policy and Service*. New York: Lexington Books.

Abraham, Margaret. 1991. Sexual Abuse in South Asian Immigrant Marriages. *Violence Against Women* 5 (6): 591–618.

Abrams, Phillip. 1982. The Historical Sociology of Individuals: Identity and the Problem of Generations. In *Historical Sociology*, ed. Phillip Abrams, 191–227. Ithaca: Cornell University Press.

Ahmed, K. 1999. Adolescent Development for South Asian American Girls. In *Emerging Voices: South Asian American Women Redefine Self, Family and Community*, ed. S.R. Gupta, 37–49. Walnut Creek: Alta Mira Press.

Alexander, George P. 1997. *New Americans: The Progress of Asian Indians in America*. Cypress: P&P Enterprises.

American Psychiatric Association. 2000. *Diagnostic and Statistical Manual of Mental Disorders*. 4th ed. Arlington: American Psychiatric Association.

———. 2013. *Diagnostic and Statistical Manual of Mental Disorders*. 5th ed. Arlington: American Psychiatric Association.

Aravamudan, M.K. 2003. *Conflict Continuity and Change: Indian Americans Negotiate Ethnic Identity and Gender Through Decisions About Dating and Marriage*. PhD dissertation, Northwestern University.

Arendell, Terry. 1997. *Contemporary Parenting: Challenges and Issues*. Thousand Oaks: Sage.

Arles, Nalini. 1998. Spirituality and Culture in the Practice of Pastoral Care and Counseling. In *Spirituality and Culture in the Practice of Pastoral Care and Counseling: Voices from Different Contexts*, ed. John Foskett and Emmanuel Larety, 89–96. Fairwater: Cardiff Academic Press.

© The Author(s) 2017

V. Jacob, *Counseling Asian Indian Immigrant Families*,

DOI 10.1007/978-3-319-64307-6

Arora, P. 1995. Imperiling the Prestige of the White Woman: Colonial Anxiety and Film Censorship in India. *Visual Anthropology Review* 11 (2): 36–49.

Atkinson, Donald, and Ruth H. Gim. 1989. Asian American Cultural Identity and Attitudes Towards Mental Health Services. *Journal of Counseling Psychology* 36 (2): 209–212.

Augsburger, David W. 1986. *Pastoral Counseling Across Cultures*. Philadelphia: The Westminster Press.

Bacon, J. 1999. Constructing Collective Ethnic Identities: The Case of Second Generation Asian Indians. *Qualitative Sociology* 22 (2): 141–160.

Balasubramaniam, V. 2005. *The Relationship Between Ethnic Identity, Self Concept, and Acculturation in Asian Indian Adolescents*. PhD dissertation, University of Houston.

Baptiste, D.A. 2005. Family Therapy with East Indian Immigrant Parents Rearing Children in the United States: Parental Concerns, Therapeutic Issues, and Recommendations. *Contemporary Family Therapy, An International Journal* 27 (3): 345–366.

Bentley, William. 1962. *The Diary of William Bentley*. Salem: The Essex Institute.

Berry, John W., Jean S. Phinney, David L. Sam, and Paul Vedder, eds. 2006. *Immigrant Youth in Cultural Transition: Acculturation, Identity and Adaptation Across National Contexts*. Hillsdale: Lawrence Erlbaum Associates, Publishers.

Bhatacharya, Gauri. 1998. Drug Use Among Asian Indian Adolescents: Identifying Protective/Risk Factors. *Adolescence* 33 (129): 169–184.

Bhattacharjee, A. 1992. The Habit of Ex-Nomination: Nation, Women, and the Indian Immigrant Bourgeoisies. *Public Culture* 5 (1): 19–44.

Bhatti, Ghazala. 1999. *Asian Children at Home and School*. London: Routledge.

Blake, John. 2002. South Asian Atlantans Feel Burden of Model Minority Myth. *Atlanta Journal Constitution*. http://modelminority.com/printout177.html. Accessed 19 Nov 2012.

Browning, Don S. 1991. *A Fundamental Practical Theology*. Minneapolis: Fortress Press.

Carter, Robert T. 1995. *The Influence of Race and Racial Identity in Psychotherapy: Toward a Racially Inclusive Model*. New York: Wiley.

Chandrasekar, S., ed. 1984. *From India to America: A Brief History of Immigration: Problems of Discrimination: Adaptation and Assimilation*. La Jolla: Population Review Publication.

Chen, A. 1997. Shaping a Philippine-Chinese American Identity. *Filipino Reporter*, July 24.

Cherian, Leela. 2010. Hitting Out: Violent Behaviors in Asian Indian American Homes. In *Caring for the South Asian Soul: Counseling South Asians in the Western World*, ed. Thomas Kulanjiyil and T.V. Thomas, 43–52. Bangalore: Primalogue.

Clandinin, Jean, and Michael Connelly. 2000. *Narrative Inquiry: Experience and Story in Qualitative Research*. San Francisco: Jossey-Bass.

Corey, Gerald. 1996. *Theory and Practice of Counseling and Psychotherapy*. 5th ed. Pacific Grove: Brooks/Cole Publishing Company.

Das, A.K., and S.F. Kemp. 1997. Between Two Worlds: Counseling South Asian Immigrants. *Journal of Multicultural Counseling and Development* 25 (1): 23–33.

Dasgupta, S. 1998. Gender Roles and Cultural Continuity in the Asian Indian Immigrant Community in the United States. *Sex Roles: A Journal of Research* 38 (11/12): 953–975.

Dugsin, Raban G. 2001. Conflict and Healing in Family Experience of Second-Generation Immigrants from India Living in North America. *Family Process* 40 (2): 233–241.

Durvasula, R.S., and G.A. Mylvaganam. 1994. Mental Health of Asian Indians: Relevant Issues and Community Implications. *Journal of Community Psychology* 22 (2): 97–108.

Espiritu, Y.L. 1997. *Asian American Men and Women: Love, Labor, Laws*. Thousand Oaks: Sage.

Espiritu, Y.L., and F.N. Wolf. 2001. The Paradox of Assimilation: Children of Filipino Immigrants in San Diego. In *Ethnicities: Children of Immigrants in America*, ed. Rubén G. Rumbaut and Alejandro Portes, 157–186. Berkeley: University of California Press.

Ewen, Robert B. 1988. *An Introduction to Theories of Personality*. Hillsdale: Lawrence Erlbaum Associate Publishers.

Fan, Xiaoyan. 2012. *Positive Factors Against Intergenerational Conflict in Chinese Immigrant Families: A Pilot Study*. PhD dissertation, Loyola University, Chicago.

Feagin, Joe R. 1978. *Racial and Ethnic Relations*. New York: Prentice Hall.

Foner, Nancy, ed. 2009. *Across Generations: Immigrant Families in America*. New York: New York University Press.

Fong, Timothy. 2002. *The Contemporary Asian American Experience: Beyond the Model Minority*. Englewood Cliff: Prentice Hall.

Foskett, John, and Emmanuel Larety, eds. 1998. *Spirituality and Culture in the Practice of Pastoral Care and Counseling: Voices from Different Contexts*. Fairwater: Cardiff Academic Press.

Foster, Charles R. 1987. *Ethnicity in the Education of the Church*. New York: Scarit Press.

Gaikwad, V.R. 1965. *The Anglo Indians: A study in the Problems and Process Involved in Emotional and Cultural Integration*. Bombay: Asia Publishing House.

Gardner, R.W., B. Robey, and P.C. Smith. 1989. Asian Americans: Growth, Change, and Diversity. *Population Bulletin* 40 (4): 1–43.

Chopra, Mallika. 2005. *100 Promises to My Baby*. Emmaus: Rodale Inc.

Garner, Murphy. 1953. *In the Minds of Men*. New York: Basic Books.

Gawle, Rupa. 2002. Desi Chameleon: Gen X Indian Americans Need the Right Blend of East and West. *India Abroad*, An Asian News Paper, November 22.

Geertz, Clifford. 1972. Myth, Symbol and Culture. *Journal of the American Academy of Arts and Sciences* 101 (1): 169–187.

George, Sam. 2006. *Coconut Generation: Ministry to the Americanized Asian Indians*. Niles: Mall Publishing Co.

Gidoomal, Ram. 2010. Displacement: Effect of Immigration on Families. In *Caring for the South Asian Souls*, ed. Thomas Kulanjiyil and T.V. Thomas, 9–20. Bangalore, IN: Primalogue Publishing & Media.

Goldberg, Arnold, and Paul E. Stepansky, eds. 1984. *How Does Analysis Cure?* Chicago: The University of Chicago Press.

Gonzalez, Gabriella C. 2005. *Educational Attainment in Immigrant Families: Community, Context and Family Background (The New Americans)*. Ramsey, FL: LFB Scholarly Publishing LLC.

Graham, Elaine, Heather Walton, and Frankie Ward. 2005. *Theological Reflection: Methods*. London: SCM Press.

Gupta, S. 1999. Forged by Fire: Indian-Americans Reflect on Their Marriages, Divorces, and on Rebuilding Lives. In *Emerging Voices: South Asian American Women Redefine Self, Family, and Community*, ed. S.R. Gupta, 193–221. Walnut Creek: Alta Mira Press.

Gutierrez, Elizabeth. 1996. The Dotbuster Attacks: Hate Crime Against Asian Indians in Jersey City, New Jersey. *Middle States Geographer*, pp. 30–38. http://geographyplanning.buffalostate.edu/MSG%201996/5_Gutierrez.pdf. Accessed 29 Aug 2012.

Hall, Gordon, C. Nagayama, and Sumie Okazaki, eds. 2002. *Asian American Psychology: The Science of Lives in Context*. Washington, DC: American Psychological Association.

Hanson, M., E. Lynch, and K. Wayman. 1990. Honoring the Cultural Diversity of Families When Gathering Data. *Topics in Early Childhood Special Education*. 10 (1): 112–131.

Hartman, Heniz. 1958. *Ego Psychology and the Problem of Adaptation*. New York: International Universities Press.

Hedge, Radha. 1998. Translated Enactments: The Relational Configurations of the Asian Indian Immigrant Experience. In *Reading in Cultural Contexts*, ed. J. Martin, T. Nakayama, and L. Flores, 315–321. Mountain View: Mayfield.

Helweg, Arthur H. 2004. *Strangers in a Not-So-Strange Land: Indian American Immigrants in the Global Age*. Ontario: Thompson Wadsworth.

Herbert, Paul G. 1985. *Anthropological Insight for Missionaries*. Grand Rapids: Baker Book House.

Hong, George K., and MaryAnna Domokos-Cheng Ham. 2001. *Psychotherapy and Counseling with Asian American Clients: A Practical Guide.* Thousand Oaks: Sage.

Inman, A.G., M.G. Constantine, and N. Ladany. 1999. Cultural Value Conflict: An Examination of Asian Indian Women's Bicultural Experience. In *Asian and Pacific Islander Americans: Issues and Concerns for Counseling and Psychotherapy,* ed. D.S. Sandhu, 31–41. New York: Nova Science Publishers.

Jambunathan, S., and D.C. Burts. 2003. Comparison of Perception of Self-Competence Among Five Ethnic Groups of Preschoolers in the United States. *Early Child Development and Care* 173 (6): 651–660.

Jambunathan, S., and K.P. Counselman. 2002. Parenting Attitudes of Asian Indian Mothers Living in the United States and in India. *Early Child Development and Care* 172 (6): 657–662.

Jambunathan, Saigeetha, Diane C. Burts, and Sarah Pierce. 2000. Comparisons of Parenting Attitudes Among Five Ethnic Groups in the United States. *Journal of Comparative Family Studies* 31 (4): 395–406.

Jeremias, Jehoachim. 1981. *Jersalem in the Time of Jesus.* Philadelphia: Fortress Press.

Johal R.S. 2002. *The World Is Ours: Second Generation South Asians Reconcile Conflicting Expectations.* M.Ed. thesis, York University.

Kakar, Sudhir, ed. 1978. *The Inner World: A Psychoanalytic Study of Childhood and Society in India.* Delhi: Oxford University Press.

———, ed. 1992. *Identity and Adulthood.* Delhi: Oxford University Press.

———, ed. 1996. *The Indian Psyche.* Delhi: Oxford University Press.

———. 2007. *Culture and Psyche: Selected Essays.* 2nd ed. Delhi: Oxford University Press.

Kerr, M.E., and M. Bowen. 1988. *Family Evaluation.* New York: Norton.

Kluckholn, C., and H. Murray. 1948. *Personality in Nature, Society, and Culture.* New York: Alfred Knopf.

Kohut, Heinz. 1971. *Analysis of Self.* New York: International Universities Press.

———. 1977. *The Restoration of the Self.* New York: International Universities Press.

Kulanjiyil, Thomas, and T.V. Thomas, eds. 2003. *Culture and Psychology: Understanding Indian Culture and Its Implications for Counseling Asian Indian Immigrants in the United States.* PhD dissertation, Wheaton College Graduate School IL.

———, eds. 2010. *Caring for the South Asian Souls: Counseling South Asians in the Western World.* Bangalore: Primalogue Publishing & Media.

Kurien, Prema A. 2005. Being Young, Brown, and Hindu: The Identity Struggles of the Second Generation Indian Americans. *Journal of Contemporary Ethnography* 34 (4): 434–469.

Lartey, Emmanuel Y. 2003. *In Living Color: An Intercultural Approach to Pastoral Care and Counseling*. Philadelphia: Thompson-Shore, Inc.

———. 2006. *Pastoral Theology in an Intercultural World*. Cleveland: Pilgrim Press.

Lee, Jung Yung. 1995. *Marginality: The Key to Multicultural Theology*. Minneapolis: Fortress Press.

Lee, E. 1997. *Working with Asian Americans: A Guide for Clinicians*. New York: Gilford Press.

Lee, Jee-Sook. 2004. *International Conflict, Ethnic Identity and Their Influence on Problem Behaviors Among Korean American Adolescents*. PhD dissertation, University of Pittsburgh.

Leonard, Karen Isaksen. 1992. *Making Ethnic Choices: California's Punjabi Mexican Americans*. Philadelphia: Temple University Press.

———. 1997. *The South Asian Americans*. Westport: Greenwood Press.

Lyman, Stanford M. 1977. *The Asian in North America*. Santa Barbara: ABC Clio Inc.

Mahalingam, Ramaswami, ed. 2006. *The Cultural Psychology of Immigrants*. Hillsdale: Lawrence Earlbaum Associates, Publishers.

Marable, Manning. 1990. The Rhetoric of Racial Harmony: Finding Substance in Culture and Ethnicity. *Sojourners* 19 (7): 14–18.

Matthew, Jamie. 2002. *Trials: Children of Post-1965 Indian Immigrants*. http://thekkattil.net/documents/1093377989_content.pdf. Accessed 12 Dec 2012.

McGolderick, Monica, ed. 1998. *Revisioning Family Therapy: Race, Culture and Gender in Clinical Practice*. New York: The Guildford Press.

Melwani, Lavina. 1995. Forging an Indian American Identity: How Authentic an Indian Are You? *Little India*, October 31.

Mio, J., and G. Iwamasa, eds. 2003. *Culturally Diverse Mental Health: The Challenges of Research and Resistance*. New York: Brunner-Routledge.

Moltmann, Jürgen. 2006. *The Crucified God*. New York: Harper & Raw.

Nagel, Joane. 1994. Constructing Ethnicity: Creating & Recreating Ethnic Identity and Culture. *Social Problems* 41 (1): 152–176.

Newman, Sally, and Steven W. Brummel, eds. 1989. *Intergenerational Programs: Imperatives, Strategies, Impacts, Trends*. New York: Haworth Press, Inc.

Ng, David. 1987. Sojourners Bearing Gifts: Pacific Asian American Christian Education. In *Ethnicity in the Education of the Church*, ed. Charles R. Foster, 12–26. Nashville: Scarit Press.

Nichols, Michael P., ed. 2006. *Family Therapy: Concepts and Methods*. Boston: Pearson Education, Inc.

Nouwen, Henry J.M. 1968. Anton Boison and Theology Through Living Human Documents. *Pastoral Psychology* 19 (7): 49–63.

Noy, Pinchas. 1969. A Revision of Psychoanalytic Theory of the Primary Purpose. *International Journal of Psychoanalysis* 50 (2): 155–178.

O'Sullivan, Tony. 1999. *Asian-American Affairs: A Face Saved Is a Face Earned*. New York: Russell Sage.

Ong, Paul M., Lucie Cheng, and Leslie Evans. 1992. Migration of Highly Educated Asians and Global Dynamics. *Asian and Pacific Migration Journal*. 1 (3–4): 543–567.

Ornestein, Paul H., ed. 1978. *The Search for the Self: Selected Writings of Heinz Kohut, 1950–1978*. New York: International University Press.

Park, Robert E. 1926. Our Racial Frontier on the Pacific. *Survey Graphic* 56 (3): 192–196.

———. 1961. *Introduction to Everett V*. In *Stonequist's the Marginal Man: A Study in Personality and Cultural Conflict*. New York: Russell and Russell.

Phinney, Jean S., and Linda Line Alipuria. 1987. *Ethnic Identity in Older Adolescents from Four Ethnic Groups*. Paper Presented at the Biennial Meeting of the Society for Research in Child Development, Baltimore, April 30.

Portes, A., and R. Rambaut. 2001. *Legacies: The Story of the Immigrant Second Generation*. Berkley: University of California Press.

Prathikanti, Sudha. 1997. East Indian Families. In *Working with Asian Americans: A Guide for Clinicians*, ed. Evelyn Lee, 113–125. New York: Guilford Press.

Ranganath, V.M., and V.K. Ranganath. 1997. Asian Indian Children. In *Transcultural Child Development: Psychological Assessment and Treatment*, ed. William Arroyo, Gloria Johnson-Powell, Joe Yamamoto, and Gail Wyatt, 103–125. New York: Wiley.

Rao, V., S. Channabassavanna, and R. Parthasarathy. 1994. Transitory Status Image of Working Women in Modern India. *India Journal of Social Work* 45 (2): 198–202.

Rosmarin, David H., Joseph S. Bigda-Peyton, Sarah J. Kertz, Nasya Smith, Scott L. Rauch, and Throstur Bjorgvinsson. 2012. A Test of Faith in God and Treatment: The Relationship of Belief in God to Psychiatric Treatment Outcomes. *Journal of Affective Disorders* 146 (3): 41–46.

Rumbaut, Ruben G., and Alejandro Portes, eds. 2001. *Ethnicities: Children of Immigrants in America*. Berkley: University of California Press.

Sala, M.J. 2002. *The Conflict Between Collectivism and Individualism in Adolescent Development: Asian Indian Female Decision-Making in Regard to Cultural Normative Behavior*. PhD dissertation, Loyola University, Chicago.

Sandhu, D.S., P.R. Portes, and S.A. McPhee. 1996. Assessing Cultural Adaptation: Psychometric Properties of the Cultural Adaptation Pain Scale. *Journal of Multicultural Counseling and Development* 24 (1): 15–25.

Saran, Parmatma. 1985. *The Asian Indian Experience in the United States*. Cambridge, MA: Schenkman Press.

Saran, Parmatma, and E. Eames. 1991. *The New Ethnics: Asian Indians in the United States*. New York: Praeger.

Scupin, Raymond. 2003. *Ethnicity in Race and Ethnicity*. Englewood Cliff: Prentiece Hall.

Segal, U. 1991. Cultural Variables in Asian Indian Families. *Families in Society* 72 (4): 233–241.

———. 1998. Asian Indian Families. In *Ethnic Families in America: Patterns and Variations*, ed. Mindel Charles, R. Habenstein, and Wright Rooswelt Jr., 331–360. Upper Saddle River: Prentice Hall.

Sethi, Brij B., V.R. Thakore, and S.C. Gupta. 1965. Changing Patterns of Culture and Psychiatry in India. *American Journal of Psychotherapy* 19 (1): 50–64.

Shams, R., and R. Williams. 1995. Differences in Perceived Parental Care and Protection and Related Psychological Distress between British Asian and Non-Asian Adolescents. *Journal of Adolescence* 18 (3): 329–348.

Sharma, Meena. 2008. *Walking a Cultural Divide: The Lived Experiences of Second Generation Asian Indian Females in Canada and the United States*. Detroit: Wayne State University.

Siegel, Allen M. 1996. *Heinz Kohut and the Psychology of the Self*. New York: Rutledge.

Singh, Narinder. 1994. *Canadian Sikhs: History, Religion and Culture of Sikhs in North America*. Ottawa: Canadian Sikh's Studies Institute.

Sodowsky, Gargi Roysircar, and John C. Carey. 1988. Relationships Between Acculturation Related Demographics and Cultural Attitudes of an Asian Indian Immigrant Group. *Journal of Multicultural Counseling and Development* 16 (3): 117–136.

Sohrabji, Sunita. 2012a. Indian Americans Most Educated, Richest Says Pew Report. *India-West*, June 29. A10. http://www.pewsocialtrends.org/2012/06/19/the-rise-of-asian-americans/2/#indian. Accessed 29 June 2012.

———. 2012b. Breaking: At Least Seven Killed, Many Injured at Wisconsin Sikh Temple. *India-West*, August 5. A10. www.indiawest.com/news/5879/breaking-at-least-seven-killed-many -injured-at-wisconsin-sikh-temple.html. Accessed 8 Oct 2012.

———. 2013. Suicide Amongst Indian Americans: We're Stressed, Depressed, But Who's Listening? *India West Newspaper*, July 12. http://www.indiawest.com/news/12062-suicide-amongst-indian-americans-we-re-stressed-depressed-but-who-s-listening.html?utm_source=Newsletter+-+2013+-+July+12&utm_campaign=DNL+-+July+12%2C+2013&utm_medium=email. Accessed 16 July 2013.

Sotomayor, Mao. 1997. Language, Culture, Ethnicity in Developing Self-Concept. *Social Case Work* 111 (4): 195–203.

Srinivas, M.N. 1966. *Social Change in Modern India*. Berkley: University of California Press.

St. Clair, Michael, and Jody Wigren. 2004. *Object Relations and Self- Psychology*. Belmont: Thomson Learning.

Stonequist, Everett V. 1961. *The Marginal Man: A Study in Personality and Cultural Conflicts.* New York: Russell and Russell.

Sunaina, Maira. 1969. *Desis in the House: Indian American Youth Culture in NYC.* Philadelphia: Temple University Press.

Takaki, Ronald. 1998. *Strangers from a Different Shore: A History of Asian Americans.* Toronto: Little Brown & Co.

Taylor, J.H. 1976. *The Halfway Generation: A Study of Asian Youth in Newcastle-Upon-Tyne.* Atlantic Highlands: Humanities Press.

Tiwari, N., A.G. Inman, and D.S. Sandhu. 2003. South Asian Americans: Culture, Concerns and Therapeutic Concerns. In *Culturally Diverse Mental Health: The Challenges of Research and Resisitance,* ed. J. Mio and G. Iwamasa, 191–209. New York: Brunner-Routledge.

Uba, Laura. 1994. *Asian Americans: Personality Patterns, Identity and Mental Health.* New York: Guildford Press.

United States Census Bureau. 2000. *Figures 9 and 12.*http://www.census.gov/prod/2002pubs/c2kbr01-16.pdf. Accessed 10 Mar 2012.

Vanaja, Dhruvarajan. 1993. Ethnic Cultural Retention and Transmission Among First Generation Hindu Asian Indians in Canadian Prairie City. *Journal of Comparative Family Studies* 24 (1): 63–79.

Wagon, Frank Milstead. 1994. *The Will to Be Known: The Development of a Pastoral-Theological Model of the Self Based upon Deitrich Bonhoeffer and Heinz Kohut.* PhD dissertation, The Southern Baptist Theological Seminary.

Wakil, S.P., C.M. Siddique, and F.A. Wakil. 1981. Between Two Cultures: A Study in Socialization of Children of Immigrants. *Journal of Marriage and the Family* 43 (3): 929–940.

Wei, William. 1993. *The Asian American Movement.* Philadelphia: Temple University Press.

Whitehead, Alfred North. 1978. *Process and Reality.* New York: Free Press.

Whitehead, James D., and Evelyn Eaton Whitehead. 1981. *Method in Ministry: Theological Reflection and Christian Ministry.* New York: The Seabury Press.

Winnicott, Donald W. 2005. *Playing and Reality.* New York: Routledge.

Yao, E.L. 1988. Working Effectively with Asian Immigrant Parents. *Phi Delta Kappa* 70 (3): 223–225.

Zacharias, Oscar Ravi. 2006. *Walking from East to West: God in the Shadows.* Grand Rapids: Zondervan.

Zhou, M. 1997. Growing Up American: The Challenges Confronting Immigrant Children and Children of Immigrants. *Annual Review of Sociology* 23 (1): 63–95.

———. 2004. Are Asian Americans Becoming 'White'? *Contexts* 3 (1): 29–35.

INDEX

Note: Page numbers followed by "n" refer to notes.

© The Author(s) 2017
V. Jacob, *Counseling Asian Indian Immigrant Families*,
DOI 10.1007/978-3-319-64307-6

Multigenerational transmission, 197
Multi-level assessments, 207
Multi-perspectival approach, 207
Multiple cultural generations, 202
Multiple generations, 55, 76, 77, 88, 89, 105
Multiple identities, 150, 188
Murray, H., 102, 104n11
Mute, 157
Mutual acceptance, 12, 245, 265–294
Mutuality, 109
Mutual misunderstanding, 39
Mutual respect, 73, 74, 201
Mylvaganam, G. A., 33, 34, 49n44
Myths, 14, 69n4
"Myth, Symbol and Culture", 49n37

N
Nagayama Hall, Gordon C., 48n21
Nagel, Joanne, 15, 19n19
Nanny, 216, 232, 233
Narcissism, 106, 121, 122, 124, 197, 237
  healthy narcissism, 221
  normal narcissism, 221
Narcissistic child, 126
Narcissistic disturbances, 126
Narcissistic libido, 128
Narcissistic personality disorders, 125
Narcissistic rage, 128
Narcissistic transference, 124, 126
Narcissus, 125
Narrative counseling approach, 206
Narrative inquiry space, 205
Narrative perspective, 205
Narrative therapy approach, 194, 205
National cultures, 46
National identity, 14
Nationality, 150
National origin, 67
National origins system, 23
Native-born peers, 39

Native country, 57
Native villages, 58
Nature, 28
Nature of a child, 118
Nature of healing, 185
Nazareth, 157
Nazareth Manifesto, 163
Nazi movement, 122
Need for acceptance, 132
Need for acculturation, 99
Need for healing, 185
Need of acculturation, 349, 358
Negation, 151, 155, 157–159
Negative experience, 153
Negative influences, 2
Neglected, 236
Neither/nor, 151, 154, 155, 157, 158, 162, 180
Neither/nor way of thinking, 151
Neonatal sex discrimination tests, 88
Network of relationships, 195
Neurologist, 122
New age, 159
New Americans, 47n3, 49n38, 49n39
New arrivals, 11
Newborn infant, 118
New center, 159
New church, 166
New cultural forms, 14
New culture, 11, 41
New environment, 44
New ethnics, 50n61, 50n66
New identity, 120
New immigrants, 101
New marginal community, 159, 184
New marginal in-beyond, 155
New marginality, 158, 160, 163, 171, 180, 182, 183
New marginalized community, 165
New marginalized person, 157, 163
New marginal people, 163, 166, 171, 184, 226